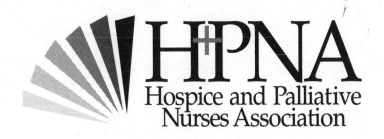

Hospice and Palliative
Nurses Association

CORE CURRICULUM FOR THE GENERALIST HOSPICE AND PALLIATIVE NURSE

Second Edition

Coordinating Editor:

Patricia H. Berry, PhD, APRN, BC-PCM
Assistant Professor
University of Utah College of Nursing
Salt Lake City, Utah

KENDALL/HUNT PUBLISHING COMPANY
4050 Westmark Drive   Dubuque, Iowa 52002

TABLE OF CONTENTS

CHAPTER   I: AN OVERVIEW OF HOSPICE AND PALLIATIVE CARE

CHAPTER   II: INTERDISCIPLINARY COLLABORATIVE PRACTICE IN THE HOSPICE AND PALLIATIVE CARE SETTINGS

CHAPTER VI: **CARE OF THE PATIENT AND FAMILY**

CHAPTER VII: **THE DYING PERSON IN VARIOUS CARE SETTINGS**

CHAPTER VIII: END-OF-LIFE CARE FOR THE CHILD AND FAMILY

CHAPTER IX: INDICATORS OF IMMINENT DYING

CHAPTER X: ECONOMIC AND POLICY ISSUES IN HOSPICE AND PALLIATIVE CARE

CHAPTER XI: TRENDS FOR THE FUTURE

CHAPTER XII: **ADVANCE CARE PLANNING: THE ROLE OF THE NURSE**

CHAPTER XIII: **ETHICAL ISSUES IN END-OF-LIFE CARE**

CONTRIBUTORS

Terry Altilio, RN, MSN, CHPN®, LMSW
Social Work Coordinator
Department of Pain Medicine and Palliative Care
Beth Israel Medical Center
New York, NY

Patricia H. Berry, PhD, APRN, BC-PCM (Editor)
Assistant Professor
University of Utah College of Nursing
Salt Lake City, UT

Linda Briggs, MA, MSN, RN
Assistant Director
Respecting Choices® and Ethics Consultant
Gundersen Lutheran Medical Foundation
La Crosse, WI

Cathleen A. Collins, RN, MSN, CHPN®
Assistant Professor
Texas Tech University Health Sciences Center
School of Nursing
Lubbock, TX

Constance Dahlin, RN, APRN, BC-PCM
Palliative Care Nurse Practitioner
Massachusetts General Hospital
Palliative Care Service
Boston, MA

Deanna Dockter, BSN, CHPN®
RN Case Manager for Cancer Pain
University of Washington Cancer Center
    Pain Clinic
University of Washington
Seattle, WA

Judith B. Eighmy, RN, BSN, CHPN®
Partner, Pacific Healthcare Consultants
Rolling Hills Estates, CA

Mary Ersek, PhD, RN
Research Scientist
Pain Research Department
Swedish Medical Center
Seattle, WA

Betty R. Ferrell, PhD, FAAN
Research Scientist
City of Hope National Medical Center
Duarte, CA

Marlene A.S. Foreman, BSN, MN, APRN-BC,
    CHPN®
Clinical Nurse Specialist
Hospice of Acadiana
LaFayette, LA

Rose Anne Indelicato, MSN, APRN, BC-PCM,
    OCN
Program Manager: Pain Management and
    Palliative Care
Visiting Nurse Services in West Chester
White Plains, NY

Kathy Kalina, RN, BSN, CHPN®
Director of Inpatient Services
Community Hospice of Ft. Worth, TX

Jeanne M. Martinez, RN, MPN, CHPN®
Quality and Education Specialist
Northwest Memorial Home Health Care
Chicago, IL

Marianne L. Matzo, PhD, APRN, FAAN
Professor and Frances E. & A. Earl Zigler Chair in
    Palliative Care Nursing
University of Oklahoma
Oklahoma City, OK

Sandra L. Muchka, RN, MS, CS, CHPN®
CNS Palliative Care
Medical College of Wisconsin
Milwaukee, WI

Patricia Murphy, RN, MA
Chief Executive Officer
Hospice of Martin & St. Lucie
Stuart, FL

Elayne J. Nahman, MSW, LCSW
Partner, Pacific Healthcare Consultants
Rolling Hills Estates, CA

Judith A. Paice, PhD, RN, FAAN
Director Cancer Pain
Northwestern University
School of Medicine
Division of Hematology-Oncology
Chicago, IL

Darrell Owens, PhD, CHPN®
Palliative Care Specialist
University of Washington at
    Harborview Med Center
Seattle, WA

Joanne E. Sheldon, RN, MEd, CHPN®, CIC
Education Coordinator of the Hospice Institute
Hospice of the Western Reserve
Euclid, Ohio

Lizabeth H. Sumner, RN, BSN
Consultant and Educator
Palliative Care for Infants, Children and
    Across the Life Span
Vista, CA

Barbara G. Volker, RN, MSN, CHPN®
Consultant/Educator—Hospice and Palliative Care
Volker Consulting Service
Fresno, CA

Ashby C. Watson, RN, MS, CS, OCN
Psychosocial Oncology Clinical Nurse Specialist
MCV Hospitals & Physicians of the Virginia
    Commonwealth University Health System
Richmond, VA

Margery A. Wilson, MSN, FNP, CHPN®, APRN,
    BC-PCM
Palliative Care Nurse Practitioner
Wellmont Health System
Bristol, TN

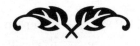

EXPERT REVIEWERS

Lynn Borstelmann, RN, MN, CHPN®, AOCN
Director, Oncology Services
The Nebraska Medical Center
Omaha, NE

Harriett Driss-McTighe, BSN, RN
Staff Nurse/Case Manager
Shepherd Home
Rochester, NY

Sharmon Figenshaw, RN, MN, CHPN®, ARNP
Hospice/Palliative Nurse Practitioner
Providence Hospice and Home Care of
    Snohomish County
Everett, WA

Kenneth Conrad Jackson, II, PharmD,
    BS Pharmacy
Clinical Pharmacy/Clinical Associate Professor
University of Utah Health Sciences Center
Pain Management Center
Salt Lake City, UT

Karen A. Kehl, RN, MS, CHPN®
Research Assistant/On-call Nurse
University of Wisconsin-Madison
School of Nursing/HospiceCare, Inc.
Madison, WI

Candace A. Kinser, RN, CHPN®
Public Relations Director and Staff Nurse
Inspiration Hospice
Salt Lake City, UT

Fran Koubek, RN, MSN, CHPN®
Nurse Specialist
Hospice of Dayton
Dayton, OH

Judy Lentz, RN, MSN, NHA
CEO
Hospice and Palliative Nurses Association
Pittsburgh, PA

David J. Maxwell, RN, BSN, CHPN®
Staff Nurse
Marian Franciscan Center
Milwaukee, WI

Mary Lynn McPherson, PharmD, BCPS
Associate Professor
University of Maryland
School of Pharmacy
Hospice Consultant Pharmacist
Baltimore, MD

Marie T. Nolan, DNSc, RN
Associate Professor
Johns Hopkins University
School of Nursing
Baltimore, MD

Annice O'Doherty, RN, CHPN®
Hospice Case Manager
Hospice of the Chesapeake
Annapolis, MD

Patricia Pollina, RN, BSN, CHPN®
Staff RN
Nathan Adelson Hospice
Las Vegas, NV

Sue Robertson, RN, PhD(c), MSEd
Part-time Faculty
California State University, Fullerton
Per Diem Staff Nurse
San Diego Hospice and Palliative Care
Fullerton, CA

M. Colleen Scanlon, RN, JD
Senior Vice President, Advocacy
Catholic Health Initiatives
Denver, CO

Pam Stephenson, BN, MSN, CS, AOCN, CHPN®
Clinical Nurse Specialist
Forum Health-Cancer Care Centers
Youngstown, OH

Dena Jean Sutermaster, RN, MSN, CHPN®
Director of Education/Research
Hospice and Palliative Nurses Association
Pittsburgh, PA

Glenn Townsend, RN, BSN
Registered Nurse
St. Josephs Hospital
Phoenix, AZ

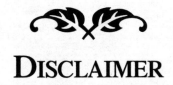

DISCLAIMER

The Hospice and Palliative Nurses Association,
its officers and directors and the authors and reviewers of this Core Curriculum
make no claims that buying or studying it will guarantee a passing score
on the CHPN® Certification examination.

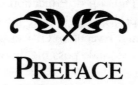

PREFACE

There is a popular saying, *"We all stand on the shoulders of those who came before us,"* that comes to mind when I think of the Hospice and Palliative Nurses Association, and in particular, this most recent edition of the *Core Curriculum for the Generalist Hospice and Palliative Nurse.* We are fortunate to have such a strong foundation of talented, knowledgeable, and committed hospice and palliative nurses and the wisdom and insight of literally millions of patients and family members to teach and encourage us. I gratefully acknowledge all of those authors who contributed to the study guides, practice review, and the first edition of the Core Curriculum that preceded this work. They laid the strong foundation upon which the Core Curriculum is built.

The groundwork for this publication, the *Core Curriculum for the Generalist Hospice and Palliative Nurse, 2nd edition,* began in 1994 when nurses prepared to take the first hospice nurse certification examination. In many cases these early hospice nurses had not taken an exam since state boards and were just as apprehensive about this one. Review courses were developed to help in the preparation process which resulted in the first publication, the *Hospice Nurses Certification Exam Review: A Self-Study Guide* authored by Ken Zeri, Kathleen Egan and Virginia Shubert (1994). That first effort was followed in 1997 by the second edition, *The Hospice Nurse's Study Guide: A Preparation for the CRNH Candidate* authored by myself, Ken Zeri and Kathleen Egan.

In 1997 The Hospice Nurses Association became the Hospice and Palliative Nurses Association (HPNA). Subsequently, the certification designation changed from Certified Registered Nurse in Hospice (CRNH) to Certified Hospice and Palliative Nurse (CHPN®). In 1999 the Study Guide was transformed into the *Hospice and Palliative Nursing Practice Review,* edited by Barbara Volker, with eleven contributors. With an emphasis beyond preparation for the certification exam, it became the standard for the basic level of nursing knowledge in hospice and palliative care.

The first edition of the *Core Curriculum for the Generalist Hospice and Palliative Nurse,* was published in 2002. This 2nd edition is an update of that publication, and as with the first edition, is intended for hospice and palliative nurses as well as those in other practice settings. In addition to serving as a departure point to prepare for the CHPN certification exam, the *Core Curriculum* can also be of benefit to any nurse caring for persons with life-limiting progressive illness. It includes, in addition to the basics of hospice and palliative care, content on pediatric palliative care, the challenges of providing palliative care in hospitals, intensive care units, long-term care, and assisted living settings, and the economic and policy trends in the palliative care and hospice fields. This second edition revision also includes separate chapters on ethics and advance care planning, both critical topics in the care of patients and their families facing life limited and progressive illness and death.

A project of this scope would be impossible without the help of many. Sincere thanks are due the writers and reviewers of this book from a wide range of hospice and palliative care disciplines including nursing, (including advanced practice, research, and academia), pharmacy, social work, and public relations. They all represent leaders in the field, and we are fortunate to have their contributions. Thanks to Amy Killmeyer, HPNA's Assistant Administrator/Office Manager who carefully formatted each chapter before it went to press. Her skills, especially organizing the text into outline form and formatting references are truly rare and admirable! Thanks also to the HPNA education committee, chaired by Beverly Paukstis, for their vision of the second edition. I owe a special debt of gratitude to Dena Jean Sutermaster, RN, MSN, CHPN®, HPNA's Director of Education/Research without whose help, sense of humor, organization, and persistence, this project would have never been completed. Finally, sincere thanks to Judy Lentz, RN, MSN, NHA, Chief Executive Officer of HPNA. Her vision, energy, and tireless advocacy for hospice and palliative care have made possible the vibrant HPNA of today.

Patricia Berry, PhD, APRN, BC-PCM

CHAPTER I

AN OVERVIEW OF HOSPICE AND PALLIATIVE CARE

Barbara G. Volker, RN, MSN, CHPN®
Patricia H. Berry, PhD, APRN, BC-PCM

First Edition Authors
Barbara G. Volker, RN, MSN, CHPN®, Ashby C. Watson, RN, MS, CS, OCN

I. History of Hospice and Palliative Care

A. Hospice

1. Concept antedates 475 AD

2. The term "hospes," from which the term hospice is derived, means to be both host and guest; implies an interaction and mutual caring between patient, family and hospice staff

3. Self-sustained communities evolved after 335 AD where ill, weary, homeless and dying persons received care

4. During the early middle ages, words *hospice, hospital* and *hostel* were used interchangeably

5. Also during the middle ages *hospitia* or traveler's rests provided food, shelter, as well as care for those sick or dying

6. The care and support of the whole person (the soul, mind, spirit) evolved in these early hospices

7. Evolved to care for the sick and incurables in 1800's

8. The word *hospice* became synonymous with care of the terminally ill late in the 1800's with the founding of Our Lady's Hospice in Dublin by Sister May Aikenhead of the Irish Sisters of Charity, who was a colleague of Florence Nightingale

9. St. Joseph's Hospice established in 1900 in London; Dame Cicely Saunders began refining the ideas and protocols that form the cornerstone of modern hospice care in the 1950's and 60's

10. Cicely Saunders, MD opened St. Christopher's Hospice in 1960's in suburban London, marking the beginning of the modern hospice movement

11. Cicely Saunders, MD visited the United States in 1963 and spoke to the medical and nursing students and interested others at Yale University

12. Florence Wald, Dean of Yale School of Nursing, resigned to plan and found the Connecticut Hospice

13. The Palliative Care service at the Royal Victoria Hospital, Montreal, Canada, started by Balfour Mount, MD opened in 1975; first use of the term "palliative care" to refer to a program of care for terminally ill persons and their families; this became the first hospice palliative care program in North America

14. The Connecticut Hospice incorporated in 1971, began seeing home care patients in 1974, 44 bed inpatient facility opened in 1979; the first hospice in the United States

15. 1983 Tax Equity Fiscal Responsibility Act created the Medicare Hospice Benefit; defines hospice care in the United States

B. Palliative Care

1. David Tasma, a Polish Jew who died of cancer in a London hospital in 1948—left Cicely Saunders a small legacy, saying, "I want to be a window in your home"

2. She acknowledges her interaction with him as the beginning of her work with thousands of dying patients, from which she established the science of palliative medicine

   a) Attends to the whole person

   b) Is limited to those who have progressive predictable disease

   c) Uses scientific rigor in developing treatment for pain and symptoms[1]

3. Contrasting views exist about the evolution of palliative care

   a) Hospice and palliative care are often seen as synonymous, e.g., in England and Canada, hospice is also called palliative care[2]

   b) Hospice is thought to be a subset of palliative care[3]

   c) Palliative care found its roots in hospice[4]

   d) Hospice includes the elements of palliative care, but not all palliative care includes all the elements of hospice care[5]

II. Development of Modern Hospice and Palliative Care Movements

A. Hospice Landmark Events

1. Development of current concepts of palliative care are, in large part, through the work of Dame Cicely Saunders at St. Christopher's Hospice in London, including the use of scheduled oral opioids for pain management

2. Elizabeth Kübler-Ross's work in the 1960's demystified death and dying and opened the debate on care of the dying for healthcare professionals and the lay public; *On Death and Dying* was published in 1969

3. Increased knowledge and research regarding grief, loss and bereavement

4. General dissatisfaction (among the public and some factions of the healthcare system) about how dying persons and their families are treated in the US healthcare system which generally emphasizes technological intervention and over treatment to prevent death

5. Development of the holistic nursing practice model

6. Issues related to cost of care versus quality of life

7. Physician assisted suicide movement and the 1995 results of the SUPPORT study, showing high incidence of uncontrolled pain (from 74% to 95%) in very ill and dying adults in spite of planned interventions from nurses to encourage physicians to attend to pain control[6]

8. The "natural death" consumer movement similar to the natural childbirth movement

9. Publication by the National Hospice Organization (NHO) of *A Pathway for Patients and Families Facing Terminal Illness* (1997)

10. Development by the National Hospice and Palliative Care Organization (NHPCO) of *Hospice Standards of Practice* (2001)

11. National Consensus Project Practice Guidelines (2004)

B. Palliative Care

1. Major factors have influenced the recent development of palliative care programs in the United States

   a) Consumer demand

      i. Aging of the population

      ii. Growing public interest in assisted suicide and euthanasia

      iii. Growing gap between what people with life-threatening illness desire and what they experience from healthcare systems and providers

      iv. Supreme Court's ruling on the right to die and its affirmation of right to care at the end of life

   b) Acknowledgment by medical community that care of dying is poor

      i. SUPPORT Study results[6]

      ii. Institute of Medicine's report on End of Life Care (1997)

      iii. Development of WHO Standards for Cancer Pain Relief (1996)

      iv. WHO Guidelines on Cancer Pain Relief and Palliative Care (1990)

      v. AHCPR Cancer Pain Guidelines (now Agency for Healthcare Research and Quality [AHRQ]); newly revised by the American Pain Society[7]

      vi. Grassroots development of State Cancer Pain Initiatives (now American Alliance of Cancer Pain Initiatives)

      vii. Efforts of Project on Death in America, LAST ACTS Initiative and Center to Improve the Care of the Dying[8]

      viii. Americans for Better Care of the Dying (ABCD)

      ix. Center for Palliative Care (CAPC)

      x. In 2001, JCAHO includes pain assessment and management as part of the accreditation process for hospitals, home health, long-term care, long-term care pharmacies, ambulatory care, behavioral health, managed behavioral health, healthcare networks

      xi. Clinical Practice Guidelines for Quality Palliative Care

III.   Hospice Philosophy

A.   Definitions of Hospice

1.   Medicare describes hospice as: an approach to caring for terminally ill individuals that stresses palliative care (relief of pain and uncomfortable symptoms), as opposed to curative care. In addition to meeting the patient's medical needs, hospice care addresses the physical, psychosocial and spiritual needs of the patient, as well as the psychosocial needs of the patient's family/caregiver. The emphasis of the hospice program is on keeping the hospice patient at home with family and friends as long as possible

2.   The National Hospice and Palliative Care Organization (NHPCO) describes hospice as a specialized form of multidisciplinary healthcare which is designed to provide palliative care, alleviate the physical, emotional, social and spiritual discomforts of an individual who is experiencing the last phase of life due to the existence of a life-limiting, progressive disease, to provide supportive care to the primary care giver and the family of the hospice patient

3.   Hospice and Palliative Nurses Association (HPNA) defines hospice nursing as the provision of palliative nursing care for the terminally ill and their families with the emphasis on their physical, psychosocial, emotional and spiritual needs. This care is accomplished in collaboration with an interdisciplinary team through a service that is available 24 hours a day, 7 days a week. The service comprises pain and symptom management, bereavement and volunteer components. Hospice nursing, then, is holistic practice conducted within an affiliative matrix. The hospice nurse, in developing and maintaining collaborative relationships with other members of the interdisciplinary team, must be flexible in dealing with the inevitable role blending that takes place. In functioning as a case manager, coordinating the implementation of the interdisciplinary team developed plan of care, the hospice nurse also shares an advocacy role for patients and their families with other members of the team

B.   Key Concepts in Hospice Philosophy

1.   The patient and family (as defined by the patient) are considered the single unit of care

2.   Hospice uses a core interdisciplinary team to address the physical, social, emotional and spiritual needs of the patient and family

3.   Hospice provides for the medical treatment of pain and other distressing symptoms associated with the life-limiting, progressive illness, but does not provide interventions to cure the disease or prolong life

4.   The interdisciplinary team develops the overall plan of care, in accordance with the wishes of the patient and family, in order to provide coordinated care that emphasizes supportive services such as home care, pain management and limited inpatient services

5.   Hospice care actively engages the community by utilizing volunteer support in delivering hospice services

6.   The patient's home or place of primary residence no matter where that may be (skilled nursing or residential care facilities, prisons, shelters, daycare centers for the elderly, etc.), is the primary site of hospice care

7.   The philosophy of hospice emphasizes comfort, dignity and quality of life, with the focus on spiritual and existential issues throughout dying, death and bereavement

8. Patients and families are empowered to achieve as much control over their lives as possible

C. Desired Goals for End-of-Life Care[9]

1. Self-determined life closure: terminally ill patients who are mentally competent should have freedom to decide how the rest of their life is spent within the options allowed by law

2. Safe and comfortable dying: patients are able to die free of distressing symptoms

3. Effective grieving: surviving family members/significant others are supported through the normal grieving process

D. Issues for Hospice

1. Six months life expectancy (should the disease run its usual course) or less may be seen as a death sentence by some physicians who thus may be reluctant to refer to hospice

2. Insurers may not pay for high-tech care and may limit access to specialists

3. Physicians may be reluctant to discuss Do Not Resuscitate (DNR) orders; patient and family may not be ready to accept them although DNR orders are not required for hospice admission

4. Referrals often occur when death is imminent, thus rushing hospice to quickly bond with family and initiate symptom management in crisis mode

5. Significant barriers to the management of pain continue to exist

IV. Philosophy of Palliative Care

A. Definitions of Palliative Care

1. The World Health Organization, in 2002, revised its definition of palliative care

  a) Palliative care is an approach to care which improves quality of life of patients and their families facing life-threatening illness, through the prevention and relief of suffering by means of early identification and impeccable assessment and treatment of pain and other problems, physical, psychosocial and spiritual[10]

2. The National Consensus Project for Quality Palliative Care in 2004 defined palliative care as

  a) The goal of palliative care is to prevent and relieve suffering and to support the best possible quality of life for patients and their families, regardless of the stage of the disease or the need for other therapies. Palliative care is both a philosophy of care and an organized, highly structured system for delivering care. Palliative care expands traditional disease-model medical treatments to include the goals of enhancing quality of life for patient and family, optimizing function, helping with decision-making and providing opportunities for personal growth. As such, it can be delivered concurrently with life-prolonging care or as the main focus of care[11]

3. The National Hospice and Palliative Care Organization (NHPCO) defines palliative care as treatment that enhances comfort and improves the quality of an individual's life during the last phase of life. No specific therapy is excluded from consideration. The test of palliative treatment lies in the agreement between the individual, physician(s), primary caregiver and

the hospice team that the expected outcome is relief from distressing symptoms, the easing of pain and/or enhancing the quality of life

B. **Core elements of palliative care, according to the National Consensus Project for Quality Palliative Care**[11]

1. Patient population: includes patients of all ages experiencing a debilitating chronic or life-threatening illness, condition or injury

2. Patient and family-centered care: the family is defined by the patient

3. Timing of palliative care: begins at the diagnosis of a life-threatening illness and continues through cure or until death and into the family's bereavement period

4. Comprehensive care: multidimensional assessments identify and relieve suffering through the prevention or alleviation of physical, psychological, social and spiritual distress

5. Interdisciplinary team: the core group of professionals include professionals from medicine, nursing and social work and may include some combination of volunteer coordinators, bereavement coordinators, chaplains, psychologists, pharmacists, nursing assistants and home attendants, physical-, occupational-, art-, play-, music- and child-life-therapists, case managers and trained volunteers

6. Attention to the relief of suffering: the primary goal of palliative care is to prevent or relieve the many and various burdens imposed by diseases and their treatments and consequent suffering

7. Communication skills: effective communication with all individuals involved in the care of patients and their families is essential in palliative care

8. Skill in the care of the dying and bereaved: knowledge regarding the full spectrum of patient and family needs is essential in palliative care

9. Continuity of care across settings: palliative care is integral to all healthcare delivery system settings; prevention of crises and unnecessary transfers are important outcomes

10. Equitable access: equitable access to palliative care across all ages and patient populations, all diagnostic categories, all healthcare settings including rural communities, regardless of race, ethnicity, sexual preference or ability to pay

11. Quality Improvement: a commitment to the pursuit of excellence and high quality of care is an essential core element of palliative care

C. **The eight domains of palliative care as defined by National Consensus Project for Quality Palliative Care. Excellence in specialist-level palliative care requires expertise in the following areas**[11]

1. Structure and processes of care

2. Physical aspects of care

3. Psychological and psychiatric aspects of care

4. Social aspects of care

5. Spiritual, religious and existential aspects of care

6. Cultural aspects of care

    7.   Care of the imminently dying patient

    8.   Ethical and legal aspects of care

D. Issues for Palliative Care

    1.   Patients, families and staff may have difficulty transitioning from curative to palliative care

    2.   Most programs are located in hospital-based, hierarchical medical institutions

    3.   Some programs may not provide continuity and communication with primary care physicians and community-based programs

    4.   Some programs may not provide supportive services, such as social work, spiritual, volunteer or bereavement follow-up

V. Hospice Care in the United States[12]

A. Programs

    1.   In 2003 there were approximately 3,300 operational hospice programs in all 50 states, Puerto Rico and Guam. This number includes both primary and multiple locations for individual hospices

        a)   67% were nonprofit

        b)   29% were for-profit

        c)   4% were government-run

        d)   94.7% were Medicare certified

        e)   64% were accredited; accreditation is not mandatory for hospices

    2.   Most states have hospice licensure laws that define specific requirements for operating as a hospice program

B. Patients

    1.   In 2003, an estimated 950,000 patients were served by hospice programs

        a)   54% were female; 46% male

        b)   63% were age 75 or older

        c)   81.2% were Caucasian

        d)   9% were Black or African American

        e)   4.3% were Hispanic or Latino

        f)   0.9% were Asian or Hawaiian/Pacific Islander

        g)   4.6% were classified as multiracial or "another race"

C. Reimbursement

1. Medicare: in 2002 Medicare spent about 2.7% of its total payments ($4.02 billion) on hospice[13]

2. Medicaid: hospice is covered under Medicaid in 43 states and the District of Columbia

3. Private insurance: most private insurance plans include a hospice benefit

D. Patient Information

1. Diagnosis

    a) 49% cancer

    b) 11% end-stage heart disease

    c) 9.6% dementia

    d) 6.8% lung disease

    e) 2.8% end-stage kidney disease

    f) 1.6% end-stage liver disease

2. Average length of service in 2003 was 55 days; median length of service was 22 days

3. Place of death for patients served by a hospice program

    a) 50% died at home

    b) 23% died in a nursing facility

    c) 7% died in a hospice unit

    d) 9% died in a hospital

    e) 7% died in a free-standing inpatient facility operated entirely by the hospice

    f) 4% died in a residential facility

VI. Palliative Care in the United States[14]

A. Programs

1. 1st U.S. formal program was St. Luke's in New York City started in 1970's, relied on philanthropic support

    a) Comprehensive interdisciplinary team saw patients in the ER and on nursing units

    b) Closed in mid 1980's for lack of support

2. A number of palliative care services have recently opened; similarities and differences include

    a) Payor sources

    b) Funding sources

    c) Diagnoses

    d) Research and grant funding sources

e) Organizational/administrative structure

f) Programs offered

g) Revenue/cost savings projected/reported; the Center to Advance Palliative Care (CAPC) has a formula to assist hospitals in projecting cost saving and increased revenue from instituting a palliative care program[15]

3. Nine pioneer palliative care programs have been developed

a) Balm of Gilead Center, Cooper Green Hospital, Birmingham, Alabama

b) Palliative Care Programs, Beth Israel Deaconess Medical Center/Care Group, Boston, Massachusetts

c) The Harry R. Horvitz Center for Palliative Medicine, The Cleveland Clinic Foundation, Cleveland, Ohio

d) Massachusetts General Hospital Palliative Care Hospital, Boston, Massachusetts

e) Palliative Care Program, Medical College of Virginia Hospitals and Physicians, Virginia Commonwealth University Health System, Richmond, Virginia

f) Pain and Palliative Care Service, Memorial Sloan-Kettering Cancer Center, New York, New York

g) The Lilian and Benjamin Hertzberg Palliative Care Institute, Mount Sinai School of Medicine, New York, New York

h) Palliative Care and Home Hospice Program, Northwestern Memorial Hospital, Chicago, Illinois

i) Comprehensive Palliative Care Service, University of Pittsburgh, Pittsburgh, Pennsylvania

B. Patient Preferences for Care at the End of Life

1. Two Gallop polls found that 9 out of 10 respondents preferred to be cared for at home if they were terminally ill with less than 6 months left to live[16]

2. In the 1996 Gallop survey 70% of respondents said they would seek hospice care, but 62% indicated that they would still seek curative care

C. Reimbursement

1. Medicare (36–74%)

2. Medicaid (0–20%)

3. Private insurance (10–34%)—includes HMO, Blue Shield, commercial insurances

4. Indigent Funds (17–20%)

5. Self-Pay (2–11%)

6. Medicaid SSI (0–6%)

D. Funding Sources for Research and Clinical Programs

1. Federal Grants

2. Private and public foundations

3. Industry grants

4. Endowments and other philanthropic efforts

5. In-kind support

E. Accreditation

1. There is currently no mandatory nationwide certification or accreditation for palliative care

2. JCAHO accreditation for hospitals covers inpatient palliative services, but no specialized accreditation is available as of yet

3. Some palliative care services with hospice components have sought Medicare certification

F. Patient Information

1. Diagnoses

    a) Cancer (53–100%)

    b) HIV (2–12%)

    c) Dementia (3–7%)

    d) Cardiovascular (6–19%)

    e) End-Stage Disease

        i. Lung (3–7%)

        ii. Liver (5–7%)

        iii. Renal (1–4%)

    f) Neurological (0–5%)

    g) Other (0–5%)

2. Length of Service (LOS)

    a) Average LOS range (5 days–71 days)

3. Location of death (regionally dependent on available beds)

    a) Hospital (6–51%)

    b) At home (22–68%)

    c) Nursing home (2–20%)

    d) Inpatient hospice (11–29%)

    e) Other (6–29%)

4.   Ethnicity

a)   Black (11–70%)

b)   White (27–75%)

c)   Hispanic (1–23%)

d)   Black Hispanic (1%)

e)   Asian Indian (2%)

f)   Asian (1%)

g)   American Indian (1%)

h)   Other (1%)

i)   Unknown (2–7%)

5.   Examples of patients who may be appropriate for palliative care rather than hospice care include

a)   Those on experimental protocols and/or who are receiving palliative chemotherapy and radiation therapy[17]

b)   Those individuals who are terminally ill but who are not ready to profess an acceptance of death as an inevitable event[18,19]

c)   Those patients who are still receiving active treatment for their incurable illness but who can also benefit from support services[20]

d)   Children with severe birth defects who will die quickly; often in the hospital[21]

e)   Those with a life-threatening illness but who are considered to be far from the terminal stage[22]

G.   Cost Savings and Revenue

1.   Goal of Palliative Care Units is to improve quality of care

2.   Fiscal argument is secondary to quality of care argument

3.   Potential savings for third party payors and for patients/families

a)   Palliative Care Unit (PCU) frees up beds for other patients

b)   Shortened hospital stays

c)   Reduced ancillary costs

d)   Reduces unnecessary tests and procedures

4.   Increasing data exists on palliative care outcomes and cost savings

a)   One study[23] found that PCU stay when compared to ICU and non-PCU unit stays, reduced "other" charges (medications, diagnostics) by 74%; charges were reduced overall 66%. (80% of patients had cancer, followed by vascular events, AIDS, organ failure)

i.   Costs were significantly reduced, especially variation in costs. In many cases, cost/day in the PCU was low enough to be covered by the Medicare hospice per diem

ii.   Both costs and charges were significantly reduced in a case control study

iii. Patient and family satisfaction was high

iv.   Results indicate that appropriate care given to terminally ill patients in a high volume medical center appears to significantly lower costs

b) Project Safe Conduct, a collaborative venture between Hospice of the Western Reserve and the Ireland Cancer Center at Case Western Reserve University and University Hospitals of Cleveland

   i.   The key goals of this project is to make palliative care accessible to persons suffering from advanced lung cancer even as they may be pursuing life-prolonging treatments

   ii. Outcomes include more referrals to hospice. Before Project Safe Conduct, 13% of patients with advanced lung cancer were referred to hospice; now, 80% of patients with that diagnosis access hospice, with length of stays, on average 10 days longer[24]

c) Research continues on the impact of palliative care teams and units on cost. One such program, at Virginia Commonwealth University Massey Cancer Center and the Medical College of Virginia, in Richmond, VA, found that with the implementation of appropriate standardized care of medically complex terminally ill patients can significantly lower costs by between 40 and 70%[25, 26]

CITED REFERENCES

1. Conner SR. New initiatives transforming hospice care. *The Hospice Journal*, 1999;14(3/4):193–203.

2. O'Connor P. Hospice vs. palliative care. *The Hospice Journal*. 1999;14(3/4):123–137.

3. Byock IR. Hospice and palliative care: a parting of the ways or a path to the future. *Journal of Palliative Medicine*. 1998;1:165–176.

4. Portenoy PR. *Defining Palliative Care*. Newsletter, Dept. of Pain and Palliative Care—Beth Israel Medical Center; 1998.

5. Brenner R. Hospice care and palliative care: a perspective from experience. *The Hospice Journal*. 1999;14(3/4):155–166.

6. The SUPPORT Principal Investigators. A controlled trial to improve care for seriously ill patients. *JAMA*. 1995;274:1591–1598.

7. Miaskowski C, Cleary J, Burney R, Coyne P, Finley R, Foster R, Grossman S, Janjan N, Ray J, Syrjala K, Weisman S, Zahrbock C. Guidelines for the management of cancer pain in adults and children. *APS Clinical Practice Guidelines Series*. No 3. Glenview, IL: American Pain Society; 2005.

8. Matzo ML, Sherman DW. *Palliative Care Nursing: Quality Care to the End of Life*. New York, NY: Springer Publishing; 2001.

9. National Hospice Organization. *A Pathway for Patients and Families Facing Terminal Illness*. Arlington, VA: National Hospice Organization; 1997:5–6.

10. World Health Organization. *National Cancer Control Programs: Policies and Managerial Guidelines*. 2nd ed. Author: 2002.

11. National Consensus Project for Quality Palliative Care. *Clinical Practice Guidelines for Quality Palliative Care*. Pittsburgh, PA: National Consensus Project for Quality Palliative Care; 2004. Can be accessed at www.nationalconsensusproject.org.

12. National Hospice and Palliative Care Organization, *Facts and Figures 2003*. Arlington, VA: National Hospice and Palliative Care Organization; 2004.

13. U.S. Department of Health and Human Services, *2003 CMS statistics*. Available at: http://www.cms.hhs.gov/researchers/pubs/03cmsstats.pdf.

14. *Pioneer Programs in Palliative Care: Nine Case Studies*. New York, NY: Milbank Memorial Fund; 2000. The Center to Advance Palliative Care, 2005.

15. Center to Advance Palliative Care (CAPC). Available at http://www.capc.org/. Accessed April 24, 2005.

16. Foreman J. 70% would pick hospice. *The Boston Globe*, 1996;250(96)(October 4):A3.

17. Beresford L. The questions of growth. *Hospice*. 1995;6(4):24–26.

18. Levetown M. Different—and needing to be more available. *Hospice*. 1995; 6(5): 15–16,36.

19. Ewald R. Orphaned by AIDS. *Hospice*. 1995;6(5):28–32.

20. Clark D, Neale B, Heather P. Contracting for palliative care. *Social Sciences and Medicine*. 1995;40(9):1193–1202.

21. Rogers B. When young life is lost. *Hospice*. 1995;6(5):24–27.

22. Lewis L. Many-party harmony. *Hospice*. 1995;6(5):8–9.

23. Payne SK. *A High Volume Specialist Palliative Care Unit (PCU) and Team Reduces End of Life (EOL) Costs*. 2001 ASCO Annual Meeting. American Society of Clinical Oncology.

24. Innovations in End of Life Care, Project Safe Conduct Integrates Palliative Goals into Comprehensive Cancer Care, An Interview with Pitorak EF, Armour M. Available at: http://www2.edc.org/lastacts/archives/archivesJuly02/featureinn.asp. Accessed April 24, 2005.

25.   Payne SK, Coyne P, Smith TJ. The health economics of palliative care. *Oncology.* 2002;16:808, 811–812.

26.   Smith TJ, Coyne P, Cassel B, Penberthy L, Hopson A, Hager MA. A high-volume specialist palliative care unit and team may reduce in-hospital end of life care costs. *Journal of Palliative Medicine.* 2003;6:699–705.

ADDITIONAL REFERENCES AND RESOURCES

Abu-Saad HH. Palliative care: An international view. *Patient Education and Counseling.* 2000;41:15–22.

Ferrell BR, Coyle N, eds. *Textbook of Palliative Nursing.* New York, NY: Oxford University Press; 2001.

Krisman-Scott MA. Origins of hospice in the United States: the care of the dying, 1945–1975. *Journal of Hospice and Palliative Nursing.* 2002:5(4):205–210.

Saunders C. The evolution of palliative care. *Patient Education and Counseling.* 2000;.41:7–13.

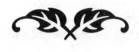

Chapter II

Interdisciplinary Collaborative Practice in the Hospice and Palliative Care Settings

Darrell Owens, Ph.D., CHPN®
Deanna Dockter, RN, BSN, CHPN®

I. **Introduction**

   A. **Interdisciplinary team (IDT) work is a key component in the successful provision of care and services to patients with a life-limiting illness and their families. Nurses, in addition to those from other disciplines such as medicine, counseling, spiritual care, dietary, social work, pharmacy, bereavement and allied therapies work collaboratively to assess, develop, implement and evaluate and monitor a patient and family centered palliative plan of care**

II. **Scope and Standards of Hospice and Palliative Care Practice**

   A. **In accordance with Standard VI, the hospice and palliative nurse collaborates with the patient and family, members of the interdisciplinary/healthcare team and other healthcare providers in providing patient and family care**

III. **Conceptual Models for End-of-Life Care**

   A. **Whole person suffering (Dame Cicely Saunders)**

      1. Four dimensions to suffering

         a) Physical, psychological, social, spiritual dimensions

         b) Each area of suffering is addressed to achieve comfort at end of life

   B. **Interdimensional Care Model[1]**

      1. As multidimensional beings, each change in health status initiates changes in the multiple dimensions of the person: the physical, the functional, the interpersonal, the wellbeing and the transcendent

      2. Care teams whose members possess expertise in these various dimensions and work in coordination with one another are well suited to aid the patient/family in adapting to these changes

C. **Tasks in Dying**[1]

1. Dying involves the completion of developmental tasks, to the extent chosen by the patient/family

2. Effective care teams provide a safe, encouraging, nurturing milieu to facilitate developmental task completion as the patient/family desires

D. **Patient Focused, Family Centered Model (serves as the basis for the NHPCO family evaluation of care)**[3]

1. Domains of care that define quality end-of-life care

a) Providing dying persons with desired physical comfort

b) Helping dying persons control decisions about medical care and daily routines

c) Relieving family members of the burden of being present at all times to advocate for their loved one

d) Educating family members so they felt confident to care for their loved ones at home

e) Providing family members with emotional support both before and after the patient's death

IV. **Healthcare Teams**

A. **The Multidisciplinary Team**

1. Most common team used in healthcare today

2. Individual professionals perform assessments, create goals and interventions based on their knowledge and expertise, in relative isolation from one another

3. Professional identity is clearly defined, team membership is secondary

4. Communication between team members occurs primarily through the legal record

5. Care goals may be uncoordinated or contradictory

6. Power distribution is usually hierarchical, with the physician at the center

a) Individuals lower on the hierarchy may not be asked for information that only they have

b) Individuals lower on the hierarchy may enjoy freedom from accountability, with lesser motivation to achieve desired outcomes

c) Hierarchy may thwart efforts by individuals to move from dependency to autonomy and interdependence

B. **The Interdisciplinary Team**

1. Typically used for care delivery by hospice and palliative care providers

2. Forms a caring community with the patient/family at its center

3. Is accountable as a unit for care outcomes

4. Team membership identity exceeds professional role

5.   Assigns leadership based on who has the most knowledge/expertise for the patient/family goals and needs

6.   Communicates through established channels toward the development, implementation, evaluation and revision of a common care plan

7.   Functions through the process of collaboration

   a)   Collaboration: from Latin roots, meaning "laboring together"

   b)   Defined in healthcare as sharing of decision-making, based on shared power and accountability. Nonhierarchical; assigns power based on knowledge or expertise as opposed to role or function

      i.   Collaborators interact both cooperatively and assertively

      ii.   Collaborators search for understanding; bargain; discuss issues face-to-face

8.   Members cover for each other in providing patient/family support

   a)   Some role blending, for example, all members carry responsibility to assess for the presence of pain

C.   **Advantages of the Interdisciplinary Team Model**

1.   Each team member has a unique patient/family relationship and therefore unique information, to bring to the care planning process

2.   Team members may easily consult with one another through formalized interactional team processes and informal processes

3.   Team members are able to cover for each others' weaknesses and compliment others' strengths

4.   Creative problem-solving is enhanced if each member's contribution is respected, resulting in new ways of viewing clinical and ethical dilemmas

5.   Members become multi-skilled practitioners who have gained knowledge through interactions with members of different professions

6.   Interacting team members provide each other an avenue for personal self-care: sharing of feelings

7.   Role blending speeds response to patient/family needs during a crisis

D.   **Additional Benefits for Interdisciplinary Team Members**

1.   Members share difficult decisions and burdens of care

2.   Members enjoy a sense of fun, camaraderie and belonging

V.   **Conflict within the Interdisciplinary Team**

A.   **Sources of Team Conflict**

1.   Role ambiguity, role overload, interpersonal conflict, inadequate communication, leadership dilemmas

B.   Manifestations of Team Conflict

1.   Underground communication (gossip), dominant member, isolated member, team factions, team secrets

C.   Effect on Creativity

1.   Presence of conflict may enhance creativity

a)   Diverse ideas yield deeper dialogue, patients and families benefit

b)   Uniformity may stifle creativity

D.   Management of Conflict

1.   If no risk to the patient, the program or the self, may ignore and view positively

a)   Monitor closely for effect; workplace dynamics can play a major role in a care providers sense of well-being

2.   If parties are willing to address the issue, are able to work together on the problem and if time allows and resources exist, attempt conflict resolution

a)   Facilitate trust development, communication and feelings expression

b)   When goals are not mutually exclusive, encourage collaboration or compromise; true consensus is generally considered to be the optimal outcome in conflict

c)   If goals are mutually exclusive, use persuasion, arbitration, hierarchy or vote

VI.   Promoting Collaboration[3]

A.   Individual Behaviors to Promote Collaboration

1.   Be assertive, ask directly, confront inappropriate behavior in a calm and assertive manner without using disclaimers or tag questions (for example, "I'm a good worker, aren't I?")

2.   Team members support one another, welcome new members to the team and orient them properly, avoid blaming and back-biting, mentor

3.   Be a life-long learner, keep skills up-to-date, read, research, learn, obtain certification, be an expert in your field

4.   Enhance your self-esteem: stop perfectionist thinking, strive for continuous improvement instead

5.   Recognize your strengths and make the most of them

6.   Take care of yourself, manage your stress, learn what nurtures you and then do it

7.   Ask for mutual commitment to establishing a trusting, respectful relationship in which there is mutual forgiveness of the past and commitment to problem solving

VII.   The Hospice and Palliative Care Interdisciplinary Team[1]

A.   Registered Nurse—the registered nurse assumes primary responsibility for the physical care of the patient providing expert pain and symptom management. In addition to their expertise in pain and symptom management, hospice and palliative care nurses must also

possess the skills necessary to recognize spiritual and psychosocial issues for patient and families. The RN generally serves at the coordinator of the IDT

B.   **Psychosocial Professionals**—psychosocial professionals are those members of the hospice and palliative care team primarily responsible for the provision of psychosocial assessment and treatment. Most often they are social workers and counselors with expertise in grief and bereavement counseling. In addition to the provision of psychosocial assessment and treatment, they may also provide assistance and/or counseling related to financial issues, legal issues, advance directives and funeral arrangements

C.   **Spiritual Care Professionals**—spiritual care professionals, also known as chaplains, spiritual care counselor or clergy are primarily responsible for the provision of spiritual care that focuses on healing, forgiveness and a sense of meaning

D.   **Patient's Physician**—as a member of the interdisciplinary team the patient's primary physician is responsible for oversight of care provided. He/she may continue to provide medical care for the patient should the patient so desire

E.   **Medical Director**—the hospice medical director often assumes overall responsibility for the medical management of all patients on the team or service. As a member of the interdisciplinary team the medical director assumes responsibility for medical care provided by the team or service and in some programs may also assume administrative duties. When the patient's physician remains involved, the Medical Director serves in an advisory/consultative role to him/her and to the interdisciplinary team

F.   **Home Health Aide or Nursing Assistant**—the home health aide or nursing assistant is responsible for provision of basic personal care. This personal care may include, but is not limited to: bathing, toileting, mouth care, skin care and transfers

G.   **Patient Care Volunteer**—patient care volunteers provide a variety of care and services to hospice and palliative care patients. Volunteers are members of the interdisciplinary team and may provide support including companionship, making deliveries and running errands

H.   **Consultative Members**—consultative members of the interdisciplinary team represent a variety of disciplines that are involved on an 'as needed' basis. These members include, but are not limited to: consulting physicians, pain specialists, pharmacists, nutritionists, psychiatrists, respiratory therapists, as well as physical, occupational and speech therapists

VIII. Hospice and Palliative Care Nursing Collaborative Practice Issues

A.   **Advance Directives and the Advance Care Planning Process**

1.   Understand the applicable laws regarding advance directives in the state of licensure

2.   Educate the general and healthcare communities regarding the implication and uses of: Durable Power of Attorney for Healthcare, Living Will, Informed Consent and the right to accept or refuse treatment in accordance with the Patient Self Determination Act of 1991

3. Based on the current literature regarding CPR, educate the general and healthcare communities on the appropriateness of do not resuscitate orders, allowing for patients and families to make informed decisions regarding resuscitation

4. Refer to Chapter 12 for a complete discussion of this topic

B. **Consumer Education**

1. Participate in the development and review of media materials (print, audio and video) related to hospice and palliative care, insuring information distributed is consistent with current standards of practice

2. Serve as a hospice and palliative care ambassador and resource to the general and healthcare communities via participation in community education classes and seminars

IX. **Professional Development**

A. **Participate in ongoing educational activities that increase knowledge, skill and competence in hospice and palliative care nursing**

B. **Serve as a role model, mentor, preceptor and educator for professional colleagues, students and other members of the healthcare community**

C. **Seek and obtain status as a certified hospice and palliative care nurse**

D. **Participate in the development and implementation of programs that increase knowledge of hospice and palliative nursing in the greater healthcare community**

E. **Seek membership in national organizations that support hospice and palliative nursing for example**

1. Hospice and Palliative Nurses Association

a) National

b) Chartered Chapters

2. American Nurses Association

3. Oncology Nursing Society

4. National Hospice and Palliative Care Organization

5. State hospice and palliative care organizations

X. **Research**

A. **Participate in, conducts and/or supports research related to hospice and palliative nursing**

B. **Participate in the writing and review of articles related to hospice and palliative nursing, submitting for publication when appropriate**

C. **Remain informed of current research and evidenced-based practice guidelines**

CITED REFERENCES

1.   Egan K, Labyak M. Hospice care: a model for quality end-of-life care. In: Ferrell BR, Coyle N, eds. *Textbook of Palliative Nursing*. New York, NY: Oxford University Press; 2001:7–26.

2.   Blickensdorf L. Nurses and physicians: creating a collaborative environment. *Journal of IV Nursing*, 1996;19(3):127–131.

3.   Teno JM, Casey VA, Welch LC, Edgman-Levitan S. Patient-focused, family-centered end-of-life medical care: views of the guidelines and bereaved family members. *Journal of Pain Symptom Management*. 2001;22:738–751.

ADDITIONAL REFERENCES AND RESOURCES

Abbott P, Derby S, Dahlin C, Ryan M, Sheehan D, Sherman D. *Scope and Standards of Hospice and Palliative Nursing Practice*. Washington, DC: American Nurses Publishing; 2002.

Cartwright J, Kayser-Jones J. End-of-life care in assisted living facilities: perceptions of residents, families and staffs. *Journal of Hospice and Palliative Nursing*. 2002:5(3):143–151.

Crawford G, Price S. Team working: palliative care as a model of interdisciplinary practice. *Medical Journal of Australia*. 2003;179(6 suppl):S32–34.

Egan KA, Abbott P. Interdisciplinary team training: preparing new employees for the specialty of hospice and palliative care. *Journal of Hospice and Palliative Nursing*. 2002:4(3):153–160.

Gilbert T. Nursing: empowerment and the problem of power. *Journal of Advanced Nursing*. 1995;21:865–871.

Krammer L, Ring A, Martinez J, Jacobs M, Williams M. The nurse's role in interdisciplinary and palliative care. In: Matzo M, Sherman D, eds. *Palliative Care Nursing*: *Quality Care to the End of Life*. New York, NY: Springer Publishing Company; 2001.

Larson E. The impact of physician-nurse interaction on patient care. *Holistic Nursing Practice*. 1999;13(2):38–46.

Lovelady B, Sword T. Hospice care planning: an interdisciplinary roadmap. *Journal of Hospice and Palliative Nursing*. 2002:6(4):223–231.

Mazanec P, Bartel J, Buras D, Fessler P, Hudson J, Jacoby M, Montana B, Phillips M. Transdisciplinary pain management: a holistic approach. *Journal of Hospice and Palliative Nursing*. 2002:4(4):228–234.

Pike A. Moral outrage and moral discourse in nurse-physician collaboration. *Journal of Professional Nursing*. 1991;7(6):351–363.

Stein L, Watts D, Howell T. The nurse-doctor game revisited. *New England Journal of Medicine*, 1990;322:546–549.

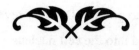

CHAPTER III

PATTERNS OF DISEASE PROGRESSION

Marlene Foreman, BSN, MN, APRN-BC, CHPN®

First Edition Authors
Constance Dahlin, RN, APRN, BC-PCM
Kathy Kalina, RN, BSN, CHPN®

I. **HIV/AIDS (Human Immunodeficiency Virus/Acquired Immunodeficiency Disease Syndrome)**

A. **Cumulative Number of AIDS Cases**

1. United States > 900,000 persons with the disease

2. Worldwide 36.1 million persons estimated with the disease

3. Total Deaths

a) United States—438,795 persons have died from AIDS

b) Worldwide—21.8 million deaths

c) Largest number is males from ages 30-45

B. **Definition: AIDS is characterized by infections and cancers that are the consequence of extreme immunodeficiency caused by infection with the human immunodeficiency virus (HIV). AIDS is the most advanced stage of HIV infection. HIV is a retrovirus that attaches to a cell and enters it**

C. **Transmission Occurs from**

1. Sexual Contact—rectal, vaginal and more rarely, oral contact with an infected person

2. Contaminated blood products

3. Contaminated needles shared by intravenous drug users

4. Organ transplant and insemination from infected donors

5. Prenatal and perinatal exposure for newborns (pregnancy, childbirth and breastfeeding)

6. Occupational injuries (e.g., needle sticks, sharps)

D. **Pathogenesis**

1. HIV infection with progression to AIDS

2. Virus attaches to T4 lymphocytes (CD4 cell) and macrophages facilitated by cytokine receptors

3. Uncoating of the virus

4. Conversion of viral RNA to proviral DNA by reverse transcriptase

5. Proviral DNA incorporated into the cell nucleus

6. Transcription of DNA into RNA

7. RNA expression and formation of infectious virion translates cell into proteins and enzymes

8. Replication of the virus within host cells

E. Disease Progression

1. Primary or Acute Infection

   a) Occurs when virus enters the body and replicates in the blood and lymphatics

   b) Initial decrease of T cells

   c) Viral load increases >100,000 copies/ml

   d) Within 5–30 days of exposure, flu-like symptoms characteristic of infection include fever, sore throat, skin rash and lymphadenopathy and myalgia

   e) Seroconversion usually within 6–12 weeks

2. Clinical Latency

   a) Chronic, asymptomatic state where clinically stable

   b) Resolution of flu-like symptoms

   c) Virus continues to replicate, most likely at some individually defined set point or rate

3. Early Symptomatic Stage

   a) Often occurs after years of infection

   b) CD4 counts drops below 500 cells/mm^3

   c) HIV viral load increases

4. Late Symptomatic Stage

   a) CD4 counts drop below 200 cells/mm^3

   b) HIV viral load increases above 100,000/ml

   c) Opportunistic infections occur including

      i. PCP

      ii. HIV encephalopathy/dementia

      iii. HIV wasting

      iv. Multiresistant TB, pulmonary and other organ involvement

      v. Bacterial infections

      vi. Oral/fungal candidiasis

        vii.   AIDS related malignancies

            (a)   Kaposi's sarcoma

            (b)   Non-Hodgkin's lymphoma

            (c)   Invasive cervical/anal cancer

       viii. Hepatitis C

        ix.   Sexually transmitted diseases

5.   Advanced HIV Disease

    a)   CD4 counts drop below 50 cells/mm^3

    b)   Immune system severely impaired

    c)   Further AIDS related infections/diagnoses

    d)   Pneumonia—Pneumocystis carinii, Mycobacterium tuberculosis

    e)   Skin Lesions—Kaposi's sarcoma, herpes simplex, molluscum contagiosum, scabies

    f)   Psychological—anxiety, depression, isolation

    g)   Neurological—dementia, meningitis, toxoplasmosis

    h)   CMV Retinitis

    i)   Fatigue

    j)   Poor functional status

    k)   Wasting syndrome

    l)   Pain

    m)   GI—diarrhea, anal and perirectal lesions, incontinence

6.   Comorbid illnesses predicting poor outcome

    a)   Liver decompensation

    b)   Lymphomas unresponsive to treatment

    c)   Progressive encephalopathy

    d)   Metastatic neoplasms

    e)   Substance abuse

    f)   Opportunistic infections unresponsive to treatment

F.   Issues in Progressive Illness

1.   The "roller coaster" unpredictable nature of the disease and its progression

2.   The treatable nature of the opportunistic infections

3.   Uncertainty of prognosis

4.   Availability of new conventional and non-traditional treatments

5.   AIDS is more a "chronic" and less a "terminal" disease

6. When/if to discontinue treatment: often it remains appropriate to continue ganciclovir (for CMV retinitis/blindness prevention) and some other antiretrovirals and opportunistic infection prophylaxis until the final stages of the illness

7. Death not from HIV/AIDS itself, but from complications caused by it

G. Potential Care Differences in the Person with HIV/AIDS

1. Non-traditional lifestyles and values

2. Alternative family structures

3. Large network for consumer advocacy and education about treatment and support

4. Youth of most patients

5. Multiple losses within their community

H. Hospice and Palliative Care Program Issues

1. Financial concerns regarding available treatments and medications

2. Need for staff education regarding unique care issues and fears arising from stigma of diseases and ignorance

3. Inflexibility of hospice admission criteria

4. When does a change from palliative care outside of a hospice framework to palliative care within a hospice framework become appropriate?

5. When to discontinue antiretroviral medications—the patient will usually want to decide this if they are able

I. Special Grief Issues in AIDS Bereavement

1. For family of origin, friends and professional caregivers—lack of recognition in care giving process. Result may be increased expressions of rage, fear, shame, guilt, helplessness, physical symptoms, self-destructiveness, insecurity, numbness and cynicism

2. Disenfranchised grief

3. Homophobia and heterosexism

4. Stigma of substance abuse

5. Stigma of AIDS and HIV leads to secrecy and isolation

6. Guilt of survivors

7. The feelings, fears related to the illness itself, complications and uncertainty regarding the course of the disease

8. Multiple and continuing losses

J. Treatment

1. Therapy recommended for all patients with primary HIV infections and symptomatic individuals

2. Antiviral therapy: antiretroviral drugs, protease inhibitors, nucleoside reverse-transcriptase inhibitors may be maintained until end of life unless difficulty swallowing prohibits, non-nucleoside reverse-transcriptase inhibitors

AIDS-RELATED CONDITIONS[a]

Condition	General Information Signs and Symptoms	Treatments[6]
Opportunistic Infections		
Fungal:		*(Note: meds ending in "zole" treat fungal infections)*
• Aspergillus	Rare; usually seen in end stage disease; cough, elevated LDH, fever, pleuritic chest pain	Amphotericin-B, itraconazole
• Candida	Often first opportunistic infection, can occur in (mouth, esophagus, vagina, rectum, skin), white, furry or cheesy patches on mucous membranes with burning pain and dysphagia, loss of appetite, vaginal or rectal burning, itching, & discharge	Nystatin, fluconazole, chlotrimazole, miconazole Amphotericin-B
• Coccidiodomycosis	Lung primary site of infection, may affect skin meninges, lymph nodes, liver; cough, fatigue, fever, malaise, pleuritic chest pain, weight loss	Amphotericin-B, fluconazole
• Cryptococcus Meningitis	Malaise, nausea, fatigue, behavior changes, headache, memory loss, mental status changes, photophobia, occasionally pneumonia	Amphotericin-B, fluconazole
• Histoplasmosis	Begins in lungs, may become systemic; lymphadenopathy, fever, cough, anemia, leukopenia, thrombocytopenia, hepatosplenomegaly, malaise, weight loss, skin lesions, dyspnea, anemia	Amphotericin-B, Itraconazole or fluconazole
Bacterial: • MAI/MAC (Mycobacterium Avium Complex)	Occurs late in HIV infection, approx. 50% incidence; fever, weight loss, fatigue, diarrhea, anorexia, thrombocytopenia, hepatospleno-megaly, night sweats, abdominal pain, weakness, dizziness, palpable abdominal lymphadenopathy	Macrolide, (clarithromycin or azithromycin), & rifabutin, & ethambutol for acute treatment. Prophylaxis with rifabutin or clarithromycin or ethambutol *(Combination treatment is most effective; rx & condition similar to TB)*
• Nocardiosis	Causes liquefaction, necrosis, abscesses, common in lung and CNS, may affect abdomen; *lung:* fever, malaise, night sweats, productive cough, weight loss; *CNS:* brain abscesses; *abdomen:* abdominal pain and tenderness, ascites, fever	TMP sulfa

(continued)

Condition	General Information Signs and Symptoms	Treatments[6]
• Salmonellosis	Incidence in patients with AIDS is 100 times greater than in the general population, usual cause is ingestion of contaminated food or direct fecal oral spread; anorexia, chills, diarrhea, fever, sweats, weight loss	Ampicillin or fluoroquinolone or ceftriaxone or Cipro® or TMP sulfa for acute treatment. TMP sulfa or amoxicillin for maintenance. Consider rifampin for synergistic effects
• Tuberculosis	May be first sign of immunocompromise, multi-drug resistance, approx. 75% have disease outside lung (pleura, lymph nodes, bone marrow, peripheral blood, GI and GU tract, brain, bone, skin, soft tissue, pericardium; cough, hemoptysis, night sweats, weight loss, fever	Isoniazid, rifampin, pyrazinamide & streptomycin or ethambutol. Prophylaxis with isoniazid or rifampin for those without current active TB
Protozoal *(parasitic infections):* • Cryptosporidium	Nausea, vomiting, fever, severe watery diarrhea, flatulence, malaise, myalgias, abdominal cramping, weakness, weight loss	Restore immune system with HAART. No currently approved specific agent. Try paromomycin or nitrazoxanide
• Isosporiasis	Biliary tract obstruction, intractable diarrhea, malabsorption, malnutrition, weakness, weight loss	TMP sulfa or pyrimethamine for acute treatment
• PCP (Pneumocystis carinii)	Most common opportunistic infection in persons with HIV, >65% develop PCP; cough, diarrhea, malaise, rales, wheezes, tachypnea, fever, dry cough, weight loss, night sweats, fatigue, dyspnea, weakness	TMP sulfa or dapsone as first line drugs. Pentamidine or clindamycin *as secondary drugs TMP sulfa (often taken as a prophylactic; reduces incidence by 90%)*
• Toxoplasmosis	Cats and birds often serve as reservoirs for the organism, most common cause of focal encephalitis in patients with AIDS; lethargy, confusion, delusions, paralysis, sensory deficits, focal neurologic deficits, seizures, headache, fever, coma (can cause symptoms in lung, heart and eyes)	Pyrimethamine & folinic acid to treat acute infection. Second line treatment with clindamycin or atovaquone or clarithromycin or azithromycin.TMP sulfa for prophylaxis in those with CD4 $< 100/mm^3$
Viral: • CMV (Cytomegalovirus) colitis	Can be sexually transmitted, latent virus in general population, CMV most common with CD4 counts < 50; weight loss, fatigue, diarrhea (often bloody), cramps, diffuse mucosal ulceration, erythema, esophagitis, gastritis, submucosal hemorrhage	High dose treatment with ganciclovir or foscarnet. Life-long daily maintenance with one of the two medications

(continued)

Condition	General Information Signs and Symptoms	Treatments[6]
• CMV (Cytomegalovirus) retinitis	Can be sexually transmitted, latent virus in general population, CMV most common with CD4 counts < 50; blurred vision, perivascular exudate, retinal hemorrhages, scotoma, loss of vision, unilateral visual field loss	Ganciclovir, foscarnet
• Herpes Simplex	Common sexually transmitted disease, disseminated HSV infection can be life-threatening; *general:* pain, painful vesicular eruption, ulcers; *genital lesions:* adenopathy, dysuria, lesions in genital area; *orolabial lesions:* adenopathy, vesicular eruptions on lips, tongue and oral mucosa; *rectal lesions:* painful, invasive lesions	Acyclovir
• Herpes Zoster	Caused by reactivation of the virus in dorsal root ganglia, may be first sign of immunocompromise; itching, deep, aching pain, red rash to vesicles, fatigue, headache, malaise, vesicular rash confined to one dermatome.	Acyclovir or famciclovir or ganciclovir or foscarnet; pain management
• Molluscum Contagiosum	Cutaneous poxvirus infection, sexually transmitted; flesh-colored umbilicated papules along face, neck, scalp and trunk	Removal, Retin-A®
• PML (progressive multifocal leuko-encephalopathy)	Progressive weakness, abnormal gait, ataxia, focal neurological deficits, speech problems, dementia, forgetfulness, incontinence	Experimental treatments only
Common Cancers		
• Kaposi's Sarcoma	Cause[5] symptoms dependent on organ system affected; pigmented purple, red or brownish lesions on skin, in gastrointestinal tract, lung	Small lesions treated only if painful or causing cosmetic problems; KS lesions highly sensitive to radiation therapy. Isolated lesions can be treated with cryotherapy or laser surgery. Interferon alpha with antiretroviral agents may help, as well as single agent or combination chemotherapy
• CNS Lymphoma	One of first malignancies associated with HIV; aphasia, confusion, cranial nerve palsy, headache, hemiparesis, lethargy, memory loss, seizures	Radiation therapy, usually whole brain
• Non-Hodgkin's Lymphoma	Incidence 10%; anorectal abscess, fever, lymphadenopathy, night sweats, weight loss	Chemotherapy, antiretroviral agents may enhance clinical response to chemotherapy

(continued)

Condition	General Information Signs and Symptoms	Treatments[6]
Other Conditions		
• HIV-associated dementia (also called AIDS dementia complex (ADC)	Most common CNS complication in patients with AIDS; *early S & S:* apathy, reduced spontaneity, social withdrawal, agitation, confusion, hallucinations, short term memory loss (long term memory usually preserved), ataxia, leg weakness, tremors, decreased coordination, impaired handwriting; *late S & S:* global dementia, confusion, delayed verbal responses, vacant stare, restlessness, disinhibition, organic psychosis, motor slowing, truncal ataxia, leg weakness greater than arm weakness; long term prognosis is poor with death following a vegetative state within weeks or months	Zidovudine; palliative management
• Wasting Syndrome	Weight loss greater than 10% of usual weight in ≤ 6 months, chronic diarrhea, chronic weakness, anorexia and fever in the absence of other conditions which cause similar symptoms	Management of symptoms, nutritional counseling and emotional issues related to body image; appetite stimulation may also be tried

[a] Prepared by Susan Corrado, RN, HospiceCare Inc., Madison, WI, 1996; Reviewed and revised, 2001.

K. Other Symptom Management Issues Particular to AIDS

1. AIDS-related diarrhea

   a) One of the most common symptoms seen in AIDS patients; contributes significantly to morbidity and cachexia and wasting syndrome

   b) Small bowel—profuse, non-bloody, related to food intake

   c) Large bowel—frequent, small, mucoid, bloody, left lower quadrant cramps, tenesmus, less related to food intake

   d) Causes—cryptosporidium (protozoal infection) is the cause in 1 of 3 cases; other causes include salmonella, Shigella, campylobacter, clostridium difficile and Giardia

   e) Treatment—treat the cause; use bulk forming agents; diphenoxlate/atropine, loperamide, octreotide

2. Pain

   a) Peripheral neuropathies are common

   b) Rectal pain should be considered due to herpes until proven otherwise; squamous cell carcinoma of the anus is a very treatable cancer seen in these patients

   c) Headache from opportunistic infections also common

   d) Dysphagia—pain in the mouth or throat that causes difficulty in swallowing; usually related to fungal infections, herpes simplex, T-cell lymphomas or Kaposi's sarcoma; treat the underlying cause and provide symptomatic support

e) Dermatologic problems—psoriasis, rashes and dry skin are common

f) Cardiac disease—an infrequent clinical problem in HIV, but abnormalities have been found on a majority of patients either upon autopsy or invasive exploration; as persons with AIDS live longer, symptoms related to myocarditis and cardiomyopathy may appear. In addition, lipid and other metabolic abnormalities related to anti-retroviral therapy may affect development of CAD

II. Neoplastic Conditions

A. Pathophysiology

1. Cancer is a mass of abnormal cells characterized by dysplasia (dissimilar growth), hyperplasia (increased number of cells). The basic features of the cells include

   a) Unregulated cell growth

   b) Poor cell differentiation

   c) Ability of cells to invade other tissues

   d) Ability to initiate new growth at distant sites

   e) Ability to evade immune system

2. Cancer is second leading cause of death

   a) The American Cancer Society estimates that over 1.3 million new cases of cancer are diagnosed each year

   b) Approximately 500,000 deaths annually

   c) Since 1990, > 17 million new cancer diagnoses[1]

   d) Much confusion in the general public exists over the definition of cure with cancer. Many people believe that once the five year disease free mark is passed the cancer is cured; this is not true, however, with many cancers

B. Patterns of Disease Progression

1. Metastatic Process

   a) Angiogenesis—the generation of blood vessels around the primary tumor that increases the chance for tumor cells to reach the bloodstream and, ultimately colonize into secondary sites

   b) Attachment or adhesion—tumor cells need to attach themselves to other cells and/or cell matrix proteins

   c) Invasion—tumor cells move across the normal barriers imposed by extracellular matrix

   d) Tumor cell proliferation—a new colony of tumor cells is stimulated to grow at the secondary site

2. Patterns historically predicted by basis of the pattern of lymphatic and venous drainage in the area surrounding the tumor

C.   The Signs and Symptoms of Advanced Cancer May Include

1.   Asthenia defined as debility, loss of strength, weakness

2.   Anorexia and accompanying weight loss and cachexia

3.   Pain

4.   Nausea

5.   Constipation/obstipation/diarrhea

6.   Sedation/confusion/agitation

7.   Dyspnea

8.   Edema/swelling

9.   Bleeding

10. Infections

D.   Treatment Modalities

1.   Surgery

a)   Removal of tissue to treat cancer locally

b)   Prophylactic—excision, laser or cryotherapy to prevent cancer such as for polyps or breast cancer or cervical cancer

c)   Diagnostic—obtain tissue to confirm the diagnosis and identify the specific type of cancer (e.g., incisional, excisional and needle biopsies)

d)   Staging—determine the extent of disease

e)   Definitive or curative—curative procedure to remove all of the malignant tumor and a margin of surrounding tissue or removal of tissues to decrease the risk of cancer development, progression or recurrence

f)   Palliative—prolongs life, promotes comfort and quality of life without the goal of curing the illness (e.g., bone stabilization, relief of obstruction, treatment for oncologic emergency, pain management, tumor debulking)

g)   Adjuvant or supportive—surgery is used with other treatment modalities to assess response to treatment or improve cosmetic and/or functional outcomes (e.g., gastrostomy tube, venous access devices, radioactive implants, implantable pumps)

h)   Reconstructive or rehabilitative—minimize deformity and improve quality of life

2.   Radiation Therapy

a)   The use of high-energy radiation (particles or waves) to eradicate cancer cells in local treatment

i.   Delivered by either external beam, referred to as teletherapy (where the source of the ionizing radiation is outside the body)

ii.   Internal radiation, referred to as brachytherapy (where the radioactive source is placed directly into a body cavity or directly on the body)

b)   Primary therapy—radiation given to eradicate disease

    c) Combined modality therapy

        i. Decrease the risk of local recurrence, in conjunction with surgery and chemotherapy

        ii. Increase tumor destruction, in conjunction with chemotherapy

    d) Prophylaxis—radiation is used to treat tissues or organs before the disease is clinically evident, as with central nervous system prophylaxis

    e) Palliative therapy

        i. Radiation therapy is used to relieve symptoms in patients with advanced disease, including pain, bleeding, compression of vital organ systems, ulcerating skin lesions, skeletal and brain metastases

        ii. While external beam radiation is the modality commonly used for palliative radiation therapy, an intravenous radioactive medication such as strontium-89, phosphorus 32 or samarium 153 may also be used for bone disease if indicated to improve quality of life (cost versus benefit/burden)

    f) Oncologic emergencies—radiation therapy is the treatment of choice for spinal cord compression and frequently in superior vena cava syndrome and symptomatic brain metastases when these are not terminal events

3. Chemotherapy

    a) Definition: the systemic treatment of disease by medication

        i. Initially used in the treatment of infectious disease and currently is most commonly used in the context of cancer treatment

        ii. The use of chemotherapy for cancer treatment is based on cellular kinetics, which include cell life cycle, cell cycle time, growth fraction and overall tumor burden

        iii. There are over 50 chemotherapeutic agents in current use with more in the development phases

        iv. Often used in combination to achieve better response by affecting various phases of cellular growth and to reduce toxic effects

    b) Chemotherapy is used to treat cancer in three ways

        i. Cure—either by chemotherapy alone or in combination with other cancer treatment modalities, such as surgery, radiation

        ii. Control—to extend the length and quality of life when cure is not a realistic goal

        iii. Palliation—to improve or enhance comfort when neither cure nor control are possible. Examples include relief of pressure on nerves, lymphatics and blood vessels and reduction in organ obstruction

    c) Side effects of chemotherapy; vary from one drug to another and most can be prevented[2]

        i. Short-term side effects, generally lasting a few days

            (a) Nausea and vomiting—from denuded GI epithelium and stimulation of Chemoreceptor Trigger Zone (CTZ) in the emetic center of the brain. Effects of tumor destruction may also include nausea and vomiting

    (b)   Diarrhea—resulting from denuded epithelium in the bowel and subsequent inflammation

    (c)   Anorexia, taste changes and stomatitis—from denuded epithelium and subsequent inflammation; anorexia may have already existed from the cancer itself

    (d)   Bone marrow suppression

        (i)   Neutropenia—making the patient susceptible to infection

        (ii)   Thrombocytopenia—making the patient susceptible to bleeding problems

        (iii)   Anemia usually results after several cycles of chemotherapy because of the long life-span of red blood cells (120 days). These same patients also frequently develop anemia as a chronic disease

  ii.   Long-term side effects

    (a)   Neurotoxicity—from drugs such as plant alkaloids, etoposide, taxanes, platinum compounds

        (i)   Peripheral nerve damage can result in varying degrees of numbness in toes and legs first, which may lead to stumbling causing inadvertent injury, then progress to fingers affecting ADLs

        (ii)   Constipation can result when nerve endings in the bowel are affected

    (b)   Nephrotoxicity (acute tubular necrosis)—from drugs such as cisplatin, high dose methotrexate or streptozocin

        (i)   Usually prevented by adequate hydration

        (ii)   Once tubular necrosis occurs, some degree of renal failure will persist

    (c)   Cardiotoxicity resulting in irreversible cardiomyopathy—from drugs such as doxorubicin and daunomycin

    (d)   Hemorrhagic cystitis—usually from cyclophosphamide

        (i)   Usually prevented by adequate fluid intake and frequent bladder emptying

        (ii)   Once it occurs, patient will have chronic flair-ups of cystitis (dysuria, frequency, urgency and/or hematuria)

    (e)   Pulmonary fibrosis—long term effects of bleomycin

E. Supportive Treatments

1.   Blood component therapy, antimicrobial therapy, nutritional support (parenteral or enteral), hydration and supplementation for metabolic and chemistry abnormalities

2.   Complementary therapies—psychological techniques, supplements and herbs, support groups

3.   Unproven therapies—unproven in animal or human trials, usually expensive to the patient because they are not covered by insurance

4.   Alternative therapies—massage, healing touch, imagery, reflexology, acupressure, etc.

F. The Major Cancer Diagnoses[b]

1. Lung cancer (11% of new cancer diagnoses; lung cancer is the leading cause of cancer death—28% of all cancer deaths)

    a) Indications of advanced disease: cough, hemoptysis, dyspnea, pneumonia, shoulder pain, arm pain, superior vena cava syndrome, Syndrome of Inappropriate Diuretic Hormone (SIADH)

    b) Unique issues: cures are very rare (13% long term survival greater than 5 years), often advanced at diagnosis; association with smoking and tobacco use, small cell variety may present with brain metastasis

    c) Social/psychological issues: social isolation, limited survival, rapid family role changes and disruptions, guilt over smoking

2. Breast cancer (15% of new cancer diagnoses; 7% of cancer deaths)

    a) Indications of advanced disease

        i. Local—painless mass, dimpling of skin, nipple retraction or deviation, asymmetry of breasts, scaling of skin on nipple or areola, peau d'orange skin (skin takes on a porous thickening, similar to the skin of an orange), bloody or serous discharge from nipple, ulceration of the breast

        ii. Metastatic—bone, brain, liver

    b) Unique issues—sexuality, femininity; body image changes, genetic susceptibility

3. Genitourinary cancers

    a) Prostate cancer (16% of new cancer diagnoses; 5% of cancer deaths)

        i. Indications of advanced disease

            (a) Local: hematuria, painful defecation, obstructive urinary symptoms, weight loss

            (b) Metastatic: appear generally debilitated, older than chronological age and may present with bone and neuropathic pain from bone involvement or nerve compression, weight loss, lethargy and secondary disease (pneumonia, etc.)

        ii. Unique issues: sexual dysfunction after resection, age at onset

    b) Bladder cancer (4% of new cancer diagnoses; 2% of cancer deaths)

        i. Indications of advanced disease: hematuria, decrease in force or caliber of urine stream, flank pain, hydronephrosis, renal failure

        ii. Unique issues: surgical resection in males may cause impotence, in females the anterior wall of the vagina may be removed; body image changes if stomas are present, sexuality

    c) Kidney cancer (2% of new cancer diagnoses; 2% of cancer deaths)

        i. Indications of advanced disease: gross hematuria, pain (dull aching), palpable abdominal mass, fever, weight loss, elevated erythrocyte sedimentation rate (ESR) and/or anemia, dyspnea

---

[b] Estimates of new cases and deaths for the cancer diagnoses listed below are from the American Cancer Society's publication, *Cancer Facts and Figures—2003.*

ii.   Unique issues: approximately 30–50% of patients have metastatic disease at diagnosis; associated with cigarette smoking and occupational exposure to asbestos, cadmium and lead

iii.   Unique issues: some patients exhibit signs and symptoms of bone marrow involvement, anemia, blood loss and tendency to hemorrhage, sexual dysfunction, surgical or medical castration may cause psychological sequelae

4.   Reproductive cancers

a)   Ovarian cancer (2% of new cancer diagnoses; 2.5% of cancer deaths)

i.   Indications of advanced disease: palpable abdominal or pelvic mass, ascites, increased abdominal girth, pleural effusions, intestinal obstruction, weight loss

ii.   Unique issues: majority of cases are diagnosed at later stages

b)   Endometrial cancer (3% of new cancer diagnoses; 1% of cancer deaths)

i.   Indications of advanced disease: hemorrhage, ascites, jaundice, bowel obstruction, dyspnea

ii.   Unique issues: sexual dysfunction; disease difficult to treat with distant metastasis

c)   Cervical cancer (1% of new cancer diagnoses; less than 1% of cancer deaths)

i.   Indications of advanced disease: dyspareunia, urinary symptoms (dysuria, urinary retention, urinary frequency, hematuria), bowel symptoms (rectal bleeding, constipation, bowel obstruction), abdominal or pelvic pain referred to flank or leg, lower extremity edema

ii.   Unique issues: advanced disease upon diagnosis, sexuality; body image, guilt if not doing regular PAP smears

d)   Testicular cancer (less than 1% of new cancer diagnoses; less than 1% of cancer deaths)

i.   Indications of advanced disease: back pain, bone pain, dyspnea, seizures, headache, cough

ii.   Unique issues: early signs and symptoms are usually absent; because testicular cancer is often curable even in later stages, patients and families may have issues associated with treatment failure

5.   Gastrointestinal cancers

a)   Colon, rectal and anal cancers (11% of new cancer diagnoses; 10% of cancer deaths)

i.   Indications of advanced disease: constipation, incontinence, weight loss, sensation of rectal fullness, dull or aching perineal or sacral pain often radiating down the legs; cutaneous manifestations, rectal-vaginal fistula, rectal bleeding

ii.   Symptoms of metastatic disease: pulmonary (cough, chest pain, dyspnea, hemoptysis, wheezing, dysphagia), hepatic (ascites, abdominal distention, nausea, anorexia, increasing abdominal girth, changes in color of urine and stool, pruritus)

iii.   Unique issues: common cancer site; may be perceived as preventable; body image secondary to colostomy or ileul conduits

b) Esophagus (1% of new cancer diagnoses; 2% of cancer deaths)

  i. Indications of advanced disease: progressive dysphagia or airway obstruction (often with need for gastrostomy or jejunostomy), dehydration, general debilitation, larger tumors can cause aspiration

  ii. Unique issues: grows and disseminates rapidly, advanced disease upon diagnosis, nutritional issues

c) Liver (1% of new cancer diagnoses; 2% of cancer deaths)

  i. Indications of advanced disease: hepatic failure, severe ascites, infection, predisposition to bleeding, pain, weight loss, weakness, pneumonia, anorexia, nausea, vomiting, muscle atrophy, confusion, dyspnea, pruritis, jaundice, peripheral edema, immobility with its sequelae

  ii. Unique issues: frequently associated with cirrhosis, aggressive disease course

d) Stomach (2% of new cancer diagnoses; 2% of cancer deaths)

  i. Indications of advanced disease: enzyme and nutritional deficiencies, malnutrition, weakness, immobility

  ii. Unique issues: most patients die of bronchopneumonia or lung abscess secondary to immobility and malnutrition; deep vein thrombosis and pulmonary embolism secondary to immobility are also common causes of death; nutritional concerns

e) Pancreas (2% of new cancer diagnoses; 5% of cancer deaths)

  i. Indications of advanced disease: hepatic failure, ascites, severe jaundice, hemorrhage, nausea, infection, abdominal pain, especially neuropathic pain related to invasion of the celiac plexus, anorexia, nausea, vomiting, diarrhea, early satiety

  ii. Unique issues: early symptoms are vague and mimic common gastrointestinal illnesses, advanced disease upon diagnosis

6. Leukemias/hematological malignancies

  a) Leukemia (2% of new cancer diagnoses; 4% of cancer deaths)

    i. Indications of advanced disease: bruising, bleeding from nose, gums, bladder or bowel, fatigue, recurrent or persistent infection, fevers, disseminated intravascular coagulation

    ii. Unique issues: emotional ups and down related to multiple remission inductions and relapses, necessity for long periods of treatment, possible failure of bone marrow transplantation

  b) Multiple Myeloma (1% of new cancer diagnoses; 2% of cancer deaths)

    i. Indications of advanced disease: infections, pain, hypercalcemia, pathologic fractures, decreased mobility, anemia, decreased platelets, bleeding tendencies, renal insufficiency, hyperuricemia, constipation

    ii. Unique issues: leading cause of death is bone marrow failures, infections, respiratory and renal failure; patients may experience long periods of latent disease

      c)   Lymphomas (4% of new cancer diagnoses; 4% of cancer deaths)

          i.   Indications of advanced disease: fever, night sweats, weight loss, decrease in urinary output, itching, lower back pain, shortness of breath, pruritis, adenopathy

          ii.   Unique issues: some types are highly treatable and curable

  7.   Melanoma (4% of new cancer diagnoses; 1% of cancer deaths; incidence has doubled in last 20 years)

      a)   Indications of advanced disease: depend on site of distant metastasis (most common sites are liver, lung, bone and brain)

      b)   Unique issues: metastatic disease is highly resistant to systemic chemotherapy; patient and family may have issues regarding prevention, diagnosis

  8.   Head and Neck cancers (4% of new cancer diagnoses; 3% of cancer deaths)

      a)   Indications of advanced disease: local extension, formation of fistulas, wound breakdown, potential for carotid artery rupture (occurs in approx. 3.5% of patients with head and neck cancer, pain (described often as throbbing, pounding, pressure-like), dysphagia, increase in neck lymph nodes, ulceration, airway obstruction, bone pain

      b)   Unique issues: disfigurement, self image, depression, social isolation, many patients have reconstructive surgery; presence of tracheostomy, inability to speak

  9.   Brain tumors (1% of new cancer diagnoses; 2% of cancer deaths)

      a)   Indications of advanced disease: increased intracranial pressure

          i.   *Beginning late-stage signs:* drowsiness, decreased attention span, mood changes, poor judgment, impaired cognitive skills, short term memory, agitation

          ii.   *End-stage signs and symptoms:* headache, vomiting, papilledema, decreased level of consciousness, changes in vital signs, including widening of pulse pressure, bradycardia, slowed, irregular pulse, displacement of brain structures (herniation), seizures, personality changes, loss of sensation, disturbances in coordination, malnutrition and dehydration

      b)   Unique issues: prognosis has not changed in last 10 years; many symptoms/ treatments drastically affect normal functioning

G. Oncologic Emergencies and Complications

  1.   For any of these life-threatening complications, interventions should be determined only after

      a)   Considering where the patient is along the disease trajectory

      b)   Clarifying goals of treatment with patient and family

      c)   Helping patient and family to arrive at attainable goals

      d)   Considering how likely it is that the treatment will result in hoped-for outcomes

      e)   Considering underlying cause(s)

2.   Central Nervous System

    a)   Spinal Cord Compression

        i.   Pressure on cord resulting in loss of nerve function

        ii.   Caused by neoplastic invasion or cord ischemia secondary to collapse of vertebra

        iii.   Signs and Symptoms

            (a)   Localized back pain may be only symptom prior to complete paralysis

            (b)   Motor deficits—hypotonicity, hyperflexia, paralysis

            (c)   Sensory deficits—paresthesia, bowel and bladder incontinence, urinary retention

        iv.   Requires emergent treatment (unless contraindicated by patient condition or preferences)

            (a)   High dose corticosteroids

            (b)   MRI or CT scan

            (c)   Radiation

            (d)   Surgical consult for decompression and stabilization

    b)   Intracerebral Metastases

        i.   Causes increased intracranial pressure

        ii.   Signs and symptoms

            (a)   Early morning headache

            (b)   Cognitive dysfunction

            (c)   Confusion and agitation

            (d)   Projectile vomiting

        iii.   Treatment

            (a)   Corticosteroids

            (b)   Whole brain radiation

            (c)   Sometimes surgical removal of single lesion

3.   Metabolic/Endocrine

    a)   SIADH (Syndrome of Inappropriate Diuretic Hormone)

        i.   Caused by excessive antidiuretic hormone from the posterior pituitary gland. Can be medication induced

        ii.   Signs and symptoms include hyponatremia, weight gain, nausea, vomiting, CNS changes, weakness, lethargy, irritability, confusion, diarrhea, muscle cramps, convulsions

        iii.   Treatment (if patient can tolerate and desirable effects can be obtained)

            (a)   Fluid restriction

            (b)   Hypertonic saline

(c) Furosemide

(d) Demeclocycline

b) Hypercalcemia

    i. Caused by increased calcium levels from cancer involvement of the bone; serum calcium greater than 11 (may be lower if albumin is low as calcium is bound to protein)

    ii. Signs and symptoms nausea, vomiting, anorexia, constipation, lethargy, confusion, polyuria, stupor, coma, mental status changes, polydipsia

    iii. Treatment may include

        (a) Hydration

        (b) Furosemide if indicated to manage fluid retention

        (c) Steroids

4. Cardiovascular/Hematologic

a) Carotid Arterial Rupture—most often a terminal event

    i. Caused by tumor invasion or erosion of arterial wall due to neoplastic tumor, radiation necrosis, infection or poor wound healing

    ii. Signs and symptoms include tumor involvement around the artery, pulsating tumor, exposure of artery, minor oozing to major hemorrhage, anxiety, decreased blood pressure, respiratory distress

    iii. Treatment focuses on supporting patient and family

        (a) Patient/family education to potential terminal event—dark towels should be available to apply to site and manage bleeding if needed

        (b) Pre-filled syringes of pain medications and benzodiazepines available to sedate patient if time allows

        (c) Treat areas of oozing with topical epinephrine

        (d) Bleeding may not be evident externally

b) Cardiac Tamponade

    i. Caused by excessive accumulation of blood or fluid around pericardium, which prevents adequate pumping of ventricles due to tumor spread

    ii. Signs and symptoms include retrosternal chest pain, dysphagia, cough, dyspnea, hoarseness, increased jugular venous pressure, muffled heart sounds, pericardial friction rub, tachycardia and pulsus paradoxus

    iii. Requires emergent treatment (unless contraindicated by patient condition or preferences)

        (a) Pericardiocentesis

        (b) Anxiolytics

        (c) Oxygen

        (d) Radiation

c) SVCS (superior vena cava syndrome)

    i. Caused by venous congestion secondary to obstruction in upper thorax, common in lung and breast cancer, lymphomas, brain tumors and tumors compressing on chest wall

    ii. Signs and symptoms include dyspnea, headache, visual disturbances, facial edema, jugular distention, swelling of trunk and upper extremities, chest pain, hoarseness and cough

    iii. Treatment (depending on disease trajectory and patient goals)

        (a) Steroids

        (b) Diuretics

        (c) Thrombolytic therapy

        (d) Radiation

        (e) Chemotherapy

        (f) Elevate head of bed

d) DIC (disseminated intravascular coagulation)

    i. Caused by the process of generalized activation of hemostatis, which results in widespread fibrin formation, followed by lysis within the vascular system

    ii. Signs and symptoms include bleeding and clotting, ecchymosis, petechiae and purpura, dyspnea, restlessness, altered LOC, tachycardia

    iii. Treatment is controversial since clotting and bleeding must be treated simultaneously; best managed by treating underlying malignancy. Can also present as a low level, chronic disease

        (a) Blood component therapy

        (b) Antiembolic medications including heparin, antithrombin II and fibrinolytic inhibitors

        (c) Hydration

        (d) Oxygen

        (e) Anxiolytics

5. Gastrointestinal: bowel obstruction

a) Caused by tumor blocking bowel causing normal transit in the intestinal tract to be delayed or prevented

b) Signs and symptoms include pain, nausea, vomiting, constipation, diarrhea, abdominal distention, abnormal bowel sounds (hyperactive in small bowel obstruction; borborygmi in large bowel obstruction)

c) Treatment

    i. Surgery if consistent with overall goals of care

    ii. Nasogastric suction or venting gastrostomy

    iii. IV fluids, if appropriate

      iv.   Pain medications

      v.   Steroids

      vi.   Octreotide 100–600 mcg/day by subcutaneous injection

      vii.   Anxiolytics

6.   **Other**

   a)   Tumor Lysis Syndrome

      i.   Caused by rapid release of intracellular potassium, phosphate and nucleic acid into the blood stream, resulting in electrolyte imbalance

      ii.   Signs and symptoms are hyperkalemia, hyperphosphatemia, hyperuricemia, hypocalcemia, neuromuscular changes, twitching, renal failure

      iii.   Treatment/prevention (if patient can tolerate and desirable effects can be obtained)

         (a)   Hydration

         (b)   Diuretics

         (c)   Allopurinol

   b)   Septic Shock

      i.   Caused by cardiovascular collapse in response to toxins in the blood

      ii.   Signs and symptoms include fever, chills, warm skin progressing to cold, clammy skin, hypotension, mental status changes, oliguria

      iii.   Treatment (if patient can tolerate and desirable effects can be obtained)

         (a)   Fluid replacement

         (b)   Antibiotics

         (c)   Vasoconstrictive medications

         (d)   Oxygen

   c)   Anaphylaxis

      i.   Caused by immediate sensitivity reaction caused by chemotherapy, biological response modifiers and some medications

      ii.   Signs and symptoms include respiratory distress, hypertension, fainting, itching bradycardia, tachycardia and respiratory arrest

      iii.   Treatment is emergent

         (a)   Epinephrine

         (b)   DiphenhydrAMINE

         (c)   Hydrocortisone

         (d)   Airway maintenance

PATTERNS OF METASTATIC SPREAD[3]
Common Sites of Metastases

Primary Disease	Bone	Marrow	Skin	Lung	Liver	Bowel Rectum	Nodes	Kidney GU	Brain Meninges	Perito-neal	Adrenal Glands
Bladder							X	X		X	
Brain											
Breast	X*	X		X*	X*		X*		X*		
Cervix	X			X	X	X	X*	X			
Colon				X*	X*		X*	X			
Esophagus	X			X	X		X*				
Head/Neck			X	X*			X*				
Hepatoma	X			X			X				
Kidney	X			X	X		X		X		
Leukemia/Lymphoma		X*	X	X	X*		X*	X			
Lung	X*	X			X*		X*		X*		X
Melanoma	X*	X	X	X*	X*		X*		X		
Ovary				X	X	X	X*			X*	
Pancreas				X	X	X	X				
Prostate	X	X		X*	X		X*				
Sarcoma				X*	X		X	X*			
Stomach	X			X	X		X				
Testes	X			X	X		X				
Thyroid	X			X			X				
Uterus							X			X	

*Most common sites of metastasis

Cancers that spread to *brain*: breast, kidney, lung, melanoma

Cancers that spread to *bone*: breast, cervix, esophagus, liver, kidney, lung, melanoma, prostate, stomach, testes, thyroid

All spread to *lung* except: bladder, brain and uterus

INTRODUCTION TO NON CANCER CONDITIONS

Diseases other than cancer enter the terminal phase with varying and less predictable trajectories and outcomes. Chronic illness often follows a course of multiple exacerbations and remissions over months or years. The terminal phase may be a slow deterioration or an acute episode that cannot be reversed. Death usually occurs when a vital organ fails or as a result of increasing debility and multi-organ failure. Major systems involved are neurological, cardiovascular, respiratory and renal.

In 1996, The National Hospice and Palliative Care Organization's (NHPCO) Standards and Accreditation Committee, Medical Guidelines Taskforce, released the Medical Guidelines for Determining Prognosis in Selected Non-cancer Diseases.[4] These guidelines are by no means absolute, but they do represent, in general, disease markers indicating a significantly decreased prognosis should the illness run its usual course. You should be aware these guidelines exist as they are often used as a basis for beginning discussions about the appropriateness of a referral to palliative care or hospice. They are scheduled to be reviewed and updated by NHPCO.

III. Neurological Conditions

  A. **Pathophysiology**[c]

  1. Injury

   a) Cerebrovascular Accident (CVA) (Leading cause of serious long-term disability and third leading cause of death in the United States)

   b) Cerebral cell death occurs in localized areas due to embolic materials clogging a vessel, vessel rupture from aneurysm or hypertension, infections or plaques in cerebral blood vessels that diminish blood flow

   c) Damage depends on size and location; sequelae range from none to irreversible comatose state and/or brain death

   d) Cerebral hemorrhage may cause more diffuse damage and death

  2. Trauma

   a) Injury to skull, with intracranial or subdural bleeding and prolonged high ICP (intracranial pressure), leads to damage in patterns similar to CVAs

   b) Central Nervous System Anoxia: Global CNS anoxia following cardiopulmonary arrest can result in a persistent vegetative state

  3. Degenerative Diseases

   a) Motor neuron disease: amyotrophic lateral sclerosis (ALS)[2]—a degenerative disease of the motor neurons in the cerebral cortex, brainstem and spinal cord, resulting in progressive weakness and atrophy of striated muscles. Usually there is no change in intellectual function

   b) Dementia: dementia of the Alzheimer's Type (DAT)—an irreversible and progressive dementia characterized by intellectual deterioration, disorganization of the personality and inability to carry out the tasks of daily living. Multi-infarct dementia can mimic some aspects of Alzheimer's disease. The end result is a progressive decline in physical and mental function leading to immobility, debility and death

---

[c] With thanks to Kathy Roelke, RN, Nurse Clinician-3, Neurology and ALS Clinic, University of Wisconsin Hospitals and Clinics, Madison, WI

B.   Primary Treatment of Disease

    1.   Pharmacologic

        a)   CVA: anticoagulants during the acute phase; diuretics to reduce cerebral edema, anticonvulsants for seizure control; antihypertensives and ASA for subsequent CVA prevention. ASA may be used daily if thrombotic CVA, steroids are appropriate

        b)   Trauma: management of increased ICP with corticosteroids and mannitol in acute phases

        c)   CNS anoxia: no treatment available

        d)   ALS: none have been identified effective; experimental trials are ongoing

        e)   Alzheimer's: drugs include cholinergic, dopamine and serotonin precursors; neuropeptides; and transcerebral dilators; haloperidol and anxiolytics help control agitation

    2.   Functional

        a)   Re-establish or maintain simple and routine ADLs

        b)   Build on or adapt ADLs as possible and necessary

        c)   Nutritional support

        d)   Prevention of complications related to immobility

        e)   Safety issues and constant surveillance

    3.   Psychological/social

        a)   Structured environment

        b)   Consistency of caregivers

        c)   Close observation

        d)   Reorientation may not be possible and may increase agitation

C.   Indications of Advanced Disease

    1.   Injury: CVA, Trauma and CNS anoxia result in permanent neurological deficits that predispose the patient to complications, particularly impaired mobility, dysphagia and incontinence; death usually results from untreated or refractory infection or from general malnutrition even with the use of feeding tubes; in the case of post-CVA patients, subsequent CVAs may cause death

    2.   Degenerative diseases

        a)   ALS: progressive muscle weakness eventually affects all striated muscles except sphincters and extraocular muscles

            i.   Common symptoms include cramps, atrophy of one or more extremities, fasciculations, hyperreflexia, dysphagia, dyspnea and impaired speech

            ii.   Although choking spells are common and distressing in the last stages of ALS, it is rarely the cause of death

            iii.   Involvement of respiratory muscles and subsequent upper respiratory infections generally leads to sudden deterioration and death; most predictable indicator of end of life

            iv.   Treat with aggressive psychological support

b) Alzheimer's disease: with disease progression, performance of ADLs becomes impossible and the patient eventually becomes bed bound

   i. Problems in late disease include incontinence, loss of speech, myoclonic jerking, seizure activity and loss of consciousness

   ii. Death is usually a result of complications related to immobility

IV. Cardiac Conditions

A. Pathophysiology

1. Cardiovascular disease is the single leading cause of death in the United States today

2. Cardiomyopathies: a diverse group of primary myocardial diseases

   a) About half of the cases are idiopathic

   b) Others can be attributed to chronic, high alcohol intake, auto-immune processes, viral infections, inherited tendencies, inflammatory processes, metabolic and endocrine diseases, exposure to toxins and selected medications (including some chemotherapeutic agents), infiltrative diseases (amyloidosis, sarcoidosis), fibroplastic diseases, hypersensitivity to selected medications and coronary artery disease

   c) Presents as either diffuse degeneration of myocardial fibers, hypertrophy of the myocardium or infiltration of the myocardium with fibrous tissue, resulting in decreased cardiac output

3. Coronary artery disease (CAD): also referred to as heart disease

   a) A state in which one or more of the coronary arteries has a narrowing of the lumen resulting in loss of oxygen to the myocardium and causing the symptoms of ischemia, angina or myocardial infarction

   b) Underlying pathology of CAD is accumulation of atherosclerotic lesions which adhere to the smooth muscle of the coronary artery and are made up of connective tissue and intracellular and extracellular lipids

B. Treatment

1. Surgical

   a) For cardiomyopathies, only surgical treatment is heart transplant. Hospice and palliative care programs will occasionally care for persons with rejected or failed heart transplants

   b) For CAD, angioplasty or bypass surgery attempt to permanently increase coronary blood flow. In some cases agents are tried

2. Pharmacologic

   a) For cardiomyopathy, drug therapies include cardiac glycosides to increase cardiac contractility (digitalis); pre-load reducers (diuretics, nitrates, morphine); after-load reducers (ACE inhibitors and calcium channel blockers)

   b) For CAD, drug therapies are nitrates for vasodilation and improved blood flow; calcium channel blockers to reduce cardiac afterload; ACE inhibitors which also reduce left cardiac afterload; beta blockers to decrease heart rate and oxygen demand

3. Other treatment modalities

   a) Stress management programs

   b) Lifestyle adaptation

4. Poor prognosis if

   a) Previous cardiac arrest and resuscitation

   b) Unexplained syncope

   c) Embolic CVA of cardiac origin

C. Indications of Advanced Disease

1. Congestive heart failure (CHF) is defined as the inability of the heart to supply the heart muscle itself and the rest of the body with adequate arterial pressure and circulatory volume. Initially, it may occur on the right or left side of the heart, but eventually both sides are affected

2. CHF also activates the renin-angiotensin-aldosterone system causing salt and water retention, arteriolar vasoconstriction and increased cardiac afterload. Sodium retention is a chief feature in the pathology of CHF

3. Left-sided congestive heart failure initially causes congestion in the lungs and has the following signs and symptoms

   a) Anxiety and restlessness

   b) Dyspnea

   c) Orthopnea, paroxysmal nocturnal dyspnea

   d) Cough, hemoptysis

   e) Tachycardia, palpitations

   f) Basilar rales, bronchial wheezes

   g) Fatigue, decreased exercise tolerance

   h) Cyanosis (a late sign of hypoxia in adults) or pallor

4. Right-sided congestive heart failure causes congestion in the systemic circulation, most notable in the lower extremities and liver and has the following signs and symptoms

   a) Anorexia, nausea

   b) Weight gain

   c) Nocturia, oliguria

   d) Dependent peripheral edema

   e) Weakness

D. Unique Issues

1. Perception that with heart disease there is always something more that can be done

2. Symptom management can and likely will prolong the patient's life

3. The "ups and downs" of the disease (exacerbations) keep patient and family thinking that the patient will "recover" again

V. **Pulmonary Conditions**

A. **Pathophysiology**

1. Obstructive pulmonary diseases: chronic spasm of small airways due to chronic disease, toxin and tobacco exposure; forced expiratory volume (FEV1) is reduced < 30% and chest is chronically hyperinflated; Pco_2 increased; Po_2 drops

2. There are two types of obstructive lung disease, each with its own unique presentation

   a) Type A COPD (emphysema)

      i. Patient is typically thin; muscle wasting

      ii. Absence of central cyanosis

      iii. Use of accessory muscles for breathing

      iv. "Barrel chest" appearance

      v. Decreased ability to cough effectively

      vi. Hyper-resonance on percussion

      vii. Distant, diminished breath sounds

   b) Type B COPD (chronic bronchitis)

      i. Patient is typically overweight

      ii. Central cyanosis is present

      iii. Minimal use of accessory muscles

      iv. Resonance on percussion

      v. Adventitious breath sounds, typically wheezes

3. Restrictive pulmonary diseases

   a) Defined as loss of lung tissue or limited lung expansion due to decreased compliance of the lung or muscle weakness; forced vital capacity (FVC) and vital capacity are less than 80% of normal predicted value

   b) Examples: pectus excavatum, myasthenia gravis, diffuse idiopathic interstitial fibrosis and space occupying lesions (effusions, tumors)

B. **Treatment Modalities**

1. Pharmacologic

   a) For obstructive lung disease: xanthines and other bronchodilators, corticosteroids, anticholinergics by IV, oral, topical routes; nebulizer treatments; oxygen is less helpful, but can provide comfort; antibiotic therapy may be used to treat infections if appropriate

   b) For restrictive lung disease: corticosteroids, oxygen; respiratory therapies/nebulizers/ IPPB; antibiotic therapy may be used to treat infections if appropriate

C. **Indications of Advanced Disease**

1. Cor pulmonale

a) Both types of lung failure cause an increase in pulmonary pressure, which can lead first to right ventricular failure (cor pulmonale), then to left ventricular failure

b) Can present as acute or chronic

2. Respiratory Failure

a) Both types of lung disease eventually result in lungs that are unable to meet the needs of life

b) Low Po_2 and high Pco_2 leads to chronic fatigue, very limited tolerance to physical exertion, profound feeling of breathlessness and poor quality of life

3. Weight loss >10% over six months

4. Tachycardia > 100 bpm

VI. **Renal Conditions**

A. **Pathophysiology**

1. Renal Failure: the causes of acute and chronic renal failure are the same; the onset of chronic is slower and more insidious

a) Can be oliguric or non-oliguric

b) BUN and creatinine rise

2. Causes include: toxins; nephrotoxic medications (e.g., cisplatinum, gentamicin); infiltrative malignant processes (e.g., metastatic tumor); metabolic ion overload (e.g., hypercalcemia or uricemia); infectious processes (e.g., glomerulonephritis); collagen vascular disease (e.g., lupus, scleroderma); diabetes, hypertension

B. **Treatment Modalities**

1. Dialysis: peritoneal or hemodialysis

a) Useful short term in acute renal failure

b) Provides renal cells a chance to regenerate

c) May also be required long term with permanent kidney damage

2. Surgical intervention

a) Many surgical procedures available to relieve obstruction, ranging from simple nephrostomy tubes to major tumor debulking with ostomies

b) Procedures chosen, if any, depend on goals of the patient and family, goals of treatment based on the disease trajectory and quality of life

3. Pharmacologic interventions: for chronic renal failure, diuretics are often prescribed; high phosphate levels are often treated with aluminum gels such as aluminum hydroxide, as well as phosphate binders such as calcium acetate

4. Nutritional interventions: low sodium, low protein, low potassium and/or low phosphate diet, if applicable based on the course of the disease trajectory

C.   Indications of Advanced Disease

1.   Fluid and electrolyte imbalances

    a)   With increasing renal insufficiency, patients may become oliguric requiring fluid restriction with increased doses of diuretics; most patients require sodium restriction

    b)   Potassium restriction is usually necessary; hyperkalemia is frequent and can be life threatening; patients who choose to allow potassium to rise to lethal levels usually experience profound muscle weakness and death from arrhythmia

    c)   Anemias: with associated dyspnea, chest pain, weakness

    d)   Uremia: symptoms of end-stage uremia include renal osteodystrophy (bone pain, fractures, skeletal deformity, proximal muscle), severe pruritis, CHF and coronary insufficiency; hypertension; uremic encephalopathy develops as condition worsens and as death approaches. May be due to end-of-life decision to discontinue dialysis

VII. Gastrointestinal Conditions

A.   Pathophysiology

1.   Hepatic failure: a number of liver diseases can lead to hepatocellular injury and cirrhosis, including alcoholic liver disease, chronic hepatitis, viral infections, autoimmune diseases, drug toxicities, metabolic causes

B.   Treatment

1.   Treat underlying disease to extent possible

2.   Manage symptoms for comfort only

C.   Indications of Advanced Disease

1.   Esophageal varices (along with portal hypertension and abnormal coagulation); this is a major risk for hemorrhage

2.   Ascites (major risk is spontaneous bacterial peritonitis and respiratory compromise)

3.   Hepatic encephalopathy

4.   Other symptoms may include jaundice, pruritis, anorexia, nausea and liver capsule pain

VIII. General Debility

A.   Pathophysiology

1.   Debility, unspecified, is a diagnostic category for elderly, debilitated patients with functional disabilities and progressive multiple organ failure who do not meet criteria for a specific terminal illness

    a)   In the past, the pediatric diagnosis "failure to thrive" has been used for this condition

    b)   There is now an ICD-9 Code (783.7) for use with adult patients[5]

2.   Severe functional deficits in activities of daily living (ADLs)

3.   Low Karnofsky performance scores

4.   Signs and symptoms of multiple organ impairment and impending failure

5.   Progressive physical deterioration

B.   Treatment

1.   Symptom management

2.   Appropriate nutritional support

3.   Prevention of complications related to immobility

C.   Indications of Advanced Disease: Terminal phase consistent with organ failure and complications of immobility

IX.   **Endocrine Disorders**

A.   **Pathophysiology**

1.   Diabetes mellitus (DM): leading cause of chronic renal failure

2.   Persistent hyperglycemia related to an inability to produce or utilize insulin to meet metabolic demand

   a)   Insulin Dependent (Type I) DM

   i.   Usual onset in children and young adults, but can occur at any age

   ii.   Research suggests an autoimmune process that progressively destroys pancreatic beta cells causes Type I DM; the body is unable to produce insulin and exogenous insulin is necessary for survival

   b)   Non-insulin dependent (Type II) DM

   i.   Usual onset after age 30

   ii.   Type II DM is caused by impairment in the pancreatic insulin release sites or a diminished number of peripheral receptor sites, leading to insulin resistance; exogenous insulin is not necessary to sustain life, but may be given to treat hyperglycemia

   c)   Other (secondary) DM: hyperglycemia related to another cause, such as pancreatic disease or medication effects

B.   **Treatment: Directed to maintaining glycemic control through insulin or oral anti-diabetic drugs, dietary modifications, blood glucose monitoring and patient teaching**

C.   **Indications of Advanced Disease**

1.   Diabetic ketoacidosis in Type I DM or non-ketotic hyperglycemic-hyperosmolar coma in Type II DM can result in death at any time in the disease process

2.   Chronic, life-limiting complications can occur in all types of DM and there is strong evidence that poor glycemic control is directly related to their development

3. Complications include

a) Diabetic retinopathy

b) Peripheral vascular and coronary artery disease

c) Diabetic enteropathy with impaired GI motility

d) Diabetic neuropathy

e) Autonomic neuropathy, which can cause postural hypotension, persistent tachycardia, neurogenic bladder, incontinence of urine or feces, diabetic nephropathy, resulting in hypertension and ultimately, renal failure

f) Recurrent infections and impaired wound healing

g) Multi-organ failure

CITED REFERENCES

1. American Cancer Society. Cancer facts and figures 2003: *American Center Society.* 2002.

2. Yarbro CH, Frogge MH, Goodman M, Groenwald S. *Cancer Nursing: Principles and Practice.* Sudbury, MA: Jones and Bartlett; 2000.

3. Volker B. *Hospice and Palliative Nurses Practice Review.* Dubuque, IA: Kendall/Hunt Publishing; 1999.

4. American Medical Association. *International Classification of Disease.* Chicago, IL: AMA Press; 2001.

5. Sherman DW. Patients with acquired immune deficiency syndrome. In: Ferrell BR, Coyle N, eds. Textbook of Palliative Nursing. New York, NY: Oxford University Press; 2001.

6. Standards and Accreditation Committee, Medical Guidelines Task Force. *Medical Guidelines for Determining Prognosis in Selected Non-cancer Disease.* 2nd ed. Arlington, VA: National Hospice and Palliative Care Organization; 1996.

ADDITIONAL REFERENCES AND RESOURCES

Ahya SN, Flood L, Paranjothi S, eds. *The Washington Manual of Medical Therapeutics.* St. Louis, MO: Washington University School of Medicine; 2001.

Berger AM, Portenoy RK, Weissman DE, eds. *Principles and Practice of Supportive Oncology.* Philadelphia, PA: Lippincott, Williams and Wilkins; 1998.

Borasio GD, Voltz R. Palliative care in amyotrophic lateral sclerosis. *Journal of Neurology.* 1997;October Suppl. 4:S11–17.

Borasio GD, Voltz R. Palliative therapy in the terminal stage of neurological disease. *Journal of Neurology.* 1997;October Suppl. 4;S2–10.

Boswell SL. Outpatient management of HIV infection in the adult: an update. *Current Clinical Topics in Infectious Diseases.* 1995;15:30–43.

Ciezki JP, Komurcu S, Macklis R. Palliative radiotherapy. *Seminars in Oncology.* 2000;Vol 27(1):90–93.

Dow KH, Bucholtz JD, Iwamoto R, Fieler V, Hilderly L. *Nursing Care in Radiation Oncology.* 2nd ed. Philadelphia, PA: W. B. Saunders; 1997.

Doyle D, Hanks GWC, MacDonald N, eds. *Oxford Textbook of Palliative Medicine.* 2nd ed. New York, NY: Oxford University Press; 1998.

Dressler D. DIC: coping with a coagulation crisis. *Nursing 2004.* 2004;34(5):58–64.

Dunne-Daly C. Principles of radiotherapy and radiobiology. *Seminars in Oncology Nursing.* 1999;15(4):250–259.

Ersek M. Artificial nutrition and hydration: clinical issues. *Journal of Hospice and Palliative Nursing.* 2002;5(4):221–230.

Evans BD. Improving palliative care in the nursing home: from a dementia perspective. *Journal of Hospice and Palliative Nursing.* 2002;4(2):91–99.

Ferrera-Reid R. Access barriers to hospice care for noncancer conditions. *Journal of Hospice and Palliative Nursing.* 2002;6(2):103–107.

Haylock PJ. Cancer metastasis: An update. *Seminars in Oncology Nursing.* 1998;14(3):172–177.

Jablonski A, Wyatt GK. A model for identifying barriers to effective symptom management at the end of life. *Journal of Hospice and Palliative Nursing.* 2002:23–36.

Kenny P. The changing face of AIDS. *Nursing 2004*. 2004;34(8):56–62.

Kirton CA, Ferri RS, Eleftherakis V. Primary care and case management of the patient with AIDS. *Nursing Clinics of North America*. 1999;34(1):71–93.

Kolcaba K, Dowd T, Steiner R, Mitzer A. Efficacy of hand massage for enhancing the comfort of hospice patients. *Journal of Hospice and Palliative Nursing*. 2002:6(2):91–102.

Langford R, Thompson J, eds. *Mosby's Handbook of Diseases*. St. Louis, MO: Mosby; 2000.

Lentz L. Daily baths: torment or comfort at end of life. *Journal of Hospice and Palliative Nursing*. 2002:5(1):34–39.

Letizia M, Norton E. Successful management of malignant bowel obstruction. *Journal of Hospice and Palliative Nursing*. 2002;5(3):152–158.

Miller K, Miller M. Managing common gastrointestinal symptoms at the end of life. *Journal of Hospice and Palliative Nursing*. 2002;4(1):34–42.

National Hospice Organization. *Medical Guidelines for Determining Prognosis in Selected Non-cancer Diseases*. 2nd ed. Arlington, VA: Author; 1996.

Nelson KA, Walsh D, Abdullan O, McDonnell F, Homsi J, Komucurcu S, LeGrand SB, Zhuovsky D. Common complications of advanced cancer. *Seminars in Oncology*. 2000;27(1):34–44.

Newshan G, Sherman DW. Palliative care—pain symptom management in persons with HIV/AIDS. *Nursing Clinics of North America*. 1999;34(1): 131–145.

Oliver D, Borasio GD, Walsh D, eds. *Palliative Care in Amyotrophic Lateral Sclerosis*. Oxford: Oxford University Press; 2000.

O'Mahony S, Coyle N, Payne R. Multidisciplinary care of the terminally ill patient. *Surgical Clinics of North America*. 2000;80(2):729–744.

Panke JA, Volicer L. Caring for persons with dementia: a palliative approach. *Journal of Hospice and Palliative Nursing*. 2002;4(3):143–149.

Story P, Knight C, Schonwetter R. *Pocket Guide to Hospice/Palliative Medicine*. Glenview, IL: American Academy of Hospice and Palliative Medicine; 2003.

Welsby PD, Richardson A, Brettle RP. AIDS: aspects in adults. In: Doyle D, Hanks GWC, MacDonald N, eds. *Oxford Textbook of Palliative Medicine*. 2nd ed. New York, NY: Oxford University Press; 1998:1121–1148.

CHAPTER IV

PAIN MANAGEMENT

Patricia H. Berry, PhD, APRN, BC-PCM
Judith A. Paice, PHD, RN, FAAN

I. Introduction

    A. Overview

        1. Prevalence

            a) Pain is experienced by 70 to 90 percent of patients with advanced disease, with 40–50% of patients experiencing moderate pain and 25–30% have severe pain

            b) Pain scores (on a 0–10 scale) greater than or equal to "5" greatly impact on quality of life

        2. It is estimated that almost all patients (85–90%) could be free of pain and 98–99% pain controlled using the knowledge and tools currently available; the remaining 1–2% of patients at end of life can be offered palliative sedation in addition to analgesics (defined as providing relief of refractory and intolerable symptoms with the use of sedatives at the end of life)

            a) This practice is within the realm of good supportive palliative care and is *not* euthanasia. The goal of sedation is to relieve distress from unrelenting physical, psychological or spiritual symptoms.

            b) This was formerly referred to as "terminal sedation," however this term led to confusion, suggesting assisted suicide and the preferred terminology is palliative sedation

    B. Barriers to Both the Assessment and the Treatment of Pain

        1. Barriers from the patient/family perspective

            a) "Good" patients don't complain

            b) Pain is inevitable with aging

             c) Strong medicine only comes in injectable form

            d) Bearing the pain is better than bearing the side effects of pain medicine

            e) Misconception that addiction to pain medicine is common

            f) Strong pain medicine should only be used for very severe pain

            g) Morphine is a "last ditch drug" used only when one is imminently dying

2. Barriers from the healthcare provider perspective

   a) The patient's self report of pain is not believed—healthcare professionals are the best judge of pain

   b) In the hospital setting, pain is often not seen as important as other indicators

   c) Only opioids are effective in severe pain

   d) Opioids cause respiratory depression

   e) Double effect—an ethical principle that permits an action, intended to have a good effect, when there is a risk of also causing a harmful effect, ONLY when the intention was to produce the good effect

      i. Double effect, as a principle guiding care, is complex, but nonetheless erroneously applied to end-of-life care, especially pain and symptom management

      ii. Adequately controlling symptoms at end of life is not known to shorten life; opioids are not associated with a shortened survival period in people at end of life[1,2]

      iii. An analysis of the potential benefits of a therapy weighed against the possible risks should be conducted when considering any therapy

   f) The confusion over addiction/tolerance/physical dependence (see below)

   g) General lack of education relating to pain assessment, treatment and pharmacology in basic and graduate education programs

      i. There are still physicians and nurses who believe that morphine hastens death when used for pain management at end of life

      ii. There is a lack of knowledge regarding the treatment of chronic versus acute pain

3. Other barriers that impact on reporting pain and using analgesics

   a) Anti-drug, "opio-phobic" culture—"Just say 'no' to drugs"

   b) Restrictions that vary by state, including prescription laws or other programs that monitor provider prescribing patterns, lack of laws facilitating pain management in end-stage illness, including partial filling of scheduled medications (fractioning) and third party payer limitations on the number of tablets that can be dispensed

   c) Access to medication (i.e., pharmacies that do not stock medications, patients who live in rural areas, etc.)

C. Important Definitions

1. Pain is whatever the experiencing person says it is, existing whenever he/she says it does.[3] History is 80% of the diagnosis—the patient's subjective report of pain is even more important to an accurate diagnosis, as there are no physical exam techniques or diagnostic tests to confirm pain history—*the patient's report must be accepted!*

2. Pain, according to the IASP (International Association for the Study of Pain), is defined as an unpleasant sensory and emotional experience associated with actual or potential tissue damage or described in terms of such damage. In 2001, the following was added: The inability to communicate verbally does not negate the possibility that an individual is experiencing pain and is in need of appropriate pain-relieving treatment[4]

3. *Addiction:* addiction is a primary, chronic, neurobiologic disease with genetic, psychosocial and environmental factors influencing its development and manifestations. It is characterized by behaviors that include one or more of the following: impaired control over drug use, compulsive use, continued use despite harm and craving[5]

4. *Tolerance:* tolerance is a state of adaptation in which exposure to a drug induces changes that result in a diminution of one or more of the drug's effects over time[5]

5. *Physical Dependence:* physical dependence is a state of adaptation that is manifested by a drug class specific withdrawal syndrome that can be produced by abrupt cessation, rapid dose reduction, decreasing blood level of the drug and/or administration of an antagonist[5]

   a) Signs and symptoms of abstinence syndrome (withdrawal) include: anxiety, irritability, lacrimation, rhinorrhea, sweating, nausea, vomiting, diarrhea, abdominal cramps, insomnia, tachycardia, elevated blood pressure and *rarely* multifocal myoclonus

      i. Appearance of abstinence syndrome is a function of the elimination half-life of the opioid; for example, abstinence symptoms appear between 6–12 hours and peak between 24–72 hours following the last dose of a medication with a short half-life (morphine is an example)

      ii. Conversely, with medications with a longer half-life, the appearance of abstinence symptoms are delayed, for example, with methadone, as much as 36 to 48 hours, although this can be quite variable

   b) *Opioid "pseudo-addiction:"* An iatrogenic syndrome in which patients develop certain behavioral characteristics of psychological dependence as a consequence of inadequate pain treatment. Patients with this syndrome must continually demonstrate their need for analgesics and are often described as difficult patients, chronic complainers, drug seekers and/or "addicts." Patients will often resort to bizarre or dramatic behavior (acting out) in an attempt to prove their pain is real so analgesics are provided[6]

II. Assessment of Pain—effectiveness of pain management is directly related to assessment

A. Assessment Parameters (note: there are several tools available for clinical practice that include all of these parameters)

1. *Site:* have patient point on self or diagram, identify and assess all sites as well as sites of radiation; remember, also, the patient may have more than one site of pain; in that case, it would be helpful to number pains to organize assessment, interventions and evaluations

2. *Character:* use the patient's *own* words; a careful description will lead to the diagnosis of pain type and therefore use of appropriate adjuvant analgesics (i.e., sharp, shooting describes neuropathic pain syndromes); refer to the section, "Types of Pain," for additional, in depth descriptions

3. *Onset:* when did it start? Did (or does) a specific event trigger the pain?

   a) Carefully distinguish between new and pre-existing pain (i.e., arthritis, chronic low back pain syndromes, etc.)

   b) Also assess for breakthrough pain

      i. Transient flares of pain in patients with chronic pain syndromes are referred to as breakthrough pain

       ii.   Breakthrough pain can be incidental (e.g., associated with movement), idiopathic (i.e., the cause is not known) or can occur as end-of-dose failure (e.g., the pain recurs prior to the next dose of pain medication)

4. *Duration and frequency:* How long has the pain persisted? Is it constant or does it come and go (intermittent)?

5. *Intensity:* ***Important note: ratings of pain intensity are the most important piece of pain assessment data to obtain if time is short; pain intensity directly correlates with interference with the patient's quality of life.*** Commonly defined on a scale, most frequently 0–10, intensity rating method must be adapted to patient. Record pain intensity "now," at its "worst," at its "least" and on an average. Pain rating scales for cognitively impaired or nonverbal patients are available, but caregivers (be they family or staff in a care facility) can often give valuable information to add to the pain assessment

    a)   A change in the patient's behavior, however, is considered the "gold standard"

    b)   One indicator of the presence of pain in patients who are unable to respond is the furrowed brow

    c)   Relief of the furrowing is often seen when pain is relieved; likewise, response to treatment can be considered part of the assessment

6. *Exacerbating factors*: what times, activities or other circumstances make the pain worse?

7. *Associated symptoms:* what other symptoms occur before, with or after the pain?

8. *Alleviating factors:* what makes the pain better? What treatments (including non-pharmacologic interventions) have been successful in the past and what have been unsuccessful? Include a thorough medication history

9. *Medication History:* what medications have been ordered? What medications is the patient currently taking? If there is a disparity, examine the underlying reasons (e.g., cost, adverse effects, fears of addiction or tolerance). What medications worked in the past for unrelated pain episodes? What are the patient/family/caregivers' beliefs about opioids?

10. *Impact on quality of life:* what does the pain mean to the patient and family? How has this pain affected them and their quality of life? Does it keep the patient from doing things he/she wants to do? How much do the patient and the family know about pain? Do they have the expectation that it can be relieved? Are there emotional or spiritual components to the pain? Does unrelieved pain lead to increased fear or anxiety or to fears that death is imminent?

11. *Physical examination:* observe the site of the pain and validate with the patient the pain's location; note skin color, warmth, irritation, integrity and any other unusual findings; utilize other physical assessment techniques, for example, percussion and auscultation, as appropriate; be mindful that persons with chronic pain often have no changes in vital signs or facial expression

B.   Etiology of Pain

   1.   Cancer Pain Syndromes

      a)   Pain associated with direct tumor involvement

         i.   Direct tumor involvement accounts for approximately 78% of pain problems among cancer inpatients and 62% among cancer outpatients

  ii. Examples include metastatic bone disease, nerve compression or infiltration, hollow viscus involvement, among others

 b) Pain associated with cancer therapy

  i. Cancer therapy accounts for approximately 19% of pain problems among cancer inpatients and 25% among cancer outpatients

  ii. Examples include any pain that occurs in the course of or as a result of surgery, chemotherapy or radiation therapy (specific examples are mucositis, peripheral neuropathy, phantom pain syndromes, extravasation of vesicant chemotherapy)

 c) Pain unrelated to cancer or cancer therapy (Important note: many patients have more than one site of pain; some unrelated to their end stage diagnosis)

  i. Incident pain accounts for approximately 3% of pain problems among cancer inpatients and 10% of pain problems among cancer outpatients

  ii. Examples include arthritis, osteoporosis, migraine headache, low back pain, fibromyalgia or any other pain syndromes present among the general population

2. Pain syndromes common in the terminal phase of other medical conditions

 a) HIV infection and AIDS

  i. Statistics on the prevalence of pain in AIDS range from 30 to 97%, with an estimate of 50% relating directly to the HIV infection and 30% to the therapy for AIDS

  ii. HIV pain is often categorized in a manner similar to cancer: pain associated with the virus (e.g., direct involvement of the virus in the sensory neurons that transmit pain), pain associated with the treatment (e.g., neuropathy due to antiretroviral drugs) or pain unrelated to HIV or its treatment (e.g., musculoskeletal pains after exercise)

  iii. Examples of HIV/AIDS related pain include neuropathies (specifically peripheral neuropathy, acute and chronic polyneuropathy, symmetric distal sensory neuropathy, brachial plexopathy, herpetic neuralgia, cranial neuropathy and headaches from acute and chronic meningitis), central pain from cerebral abscesses, esophagitis and abdominal pain from infectious gastrointestinal disease, chest pain from pneumocystis pneumonia and generalized myalgias

 b) Sickle cell disease

  i. Three or more vascular occlusive episodes are a poor prognostic sign (less than 50% of those patients live beyond age 40). Hydroxyurea may decrease frequency of vaso-occlusive crises

  ii. Pain is severe and acute; focal (bone, joint and muscle) and visceral pain from ischemia and infarction

  iii. There are multiple myths and mistaken beliefs about sickle cell disease and sickle cell pain on the part of patients, their families and the healthcare professions

  iv. Factors related to race, ethnic and class stereotyping in our culture further complicate this issue and serve as additional impediments to the control of pain in sickle cell disease[7]

 c) Multiple sclerosis (MS)

  i. Pain is an issue in 55 to 82% of persons with MS

   (a) Neurological (paroxysmal trigeminal neuralgia, optic neuritis and periorbital pain, extremity pain, including dysthesia, allodynia and painful electric-shock sensations)

        (b)   Musculoskeletal—low back pain and extremity pain. Refer to Table 1 for definitions of the pain terms associated with neuropathic pain states

    d)   Cerebral vascular disease

        i.   Post stroke pain is a problem in 1–2% of patients

            (a)   Often delayed for several years after the stroke; accompanied by decreased temperature sensation; may be superficial or deep; often severe in intensity and accompanied by hyperalgesia and allodynia; may be elicited by emotional episodes and movement

            (b)   Another common post-stroke pain syndrome is mechanical shoulder pain unrelated to the central injury

    e)   Spinal cord injury: central pain may occur from an injury at any level of the spinal cord

C. Types of Pain

1. Acute pain: usually clear cause; meaningful; perceived as reversible; observable signs (such as increased pulse rate, increase in blood pressure; nonverbal signs and symptoms, such as facial expressions, tense muscles); examples: myocardial infarction, acute appendicitis

2. Chronic pain: often not a clear cause; does not fulfill a useful purpose; perceived as irreversible; cyclical (aching—agony); decreased social interaction, insomnia, depressed affect; few observable or behavioral signs; examples: cancer pain, chronic back pain

3. Nociceptive pain (or somatic and visceral pain) arises from direct stimulation of the afferent nerves due to tumor infiltration, of skin, soft tissue or viscera

    a)   Somatic pain: well-localized; often described as deep, dull ache; musculoskeletal in nature

        i.   Examples: bone metastasis, inflammation of soft tissue, tumor invasion of soft tissue

        ii.   Can be controlled with conventional analgesics, (including NSAIDs if mild and opioids, if moderate to severe) and in some cases, radiation therapy

    b)   Visceral pain: poorly localized; cramping, deep ache, pressure, often referred to distant dermatomal sites

        i.   Examples: bowel obstruction resulting in bowel spasms; cholecystitis; metastatic tumors in the lung

        ii.   Can be controlled with conventional analgesics, anti-spasmotics and in some cases, antineoplastic treatments

4. Neuropathic pain results from actual injury to nerves rather than stimulation of nerve endings (Refer to Table 1 for definitions of pain terms associated with neuropathic pain states)

    a)   Characteristics: sharp, burning, shooting, shock-like. (Refer to the table entitled Pain Terms Associated with Neuropathic Pain States)

    b)   Examples: spinal nerve root compression, tumor invasion of nerves, post-herpetic neuralgia, surgical interruption of nerves, central pain syndromes occurring after stroke

       c) Opioids relieve neuropathic pain, as do adjuvants. But antidepressants, (e.g., nortriptyline) anticonvulsants (e.g., gabapentin, carbamazepine), corticosteroids and non-drug therapies may be beneficial as adjuvant analgesics to the opioids or in some cases as the primary analgesic

   5. Mixed nociceptive and neuropathic pain syndrome

       a) Common in life-threatening illnesses

       b) Thorough assessment is indicated

           i. Pharmacological therapy is based upon these different pain syndromes

           ii. Occur concomitantly so patients may require agents from more than one category of analgesics (e.g., non-opioids, opioids and adjuvants)

   6. Referred pain is usually a visceral pain referred to skin, bone and muscle, often distant from the site of origin

       a) Pain from tumor involvement of the pancreas, lower esophagus, stomach or retroperitoneal area may be referred to the back

       b) Gallbladder or liver disease may produce referred pain in the back or right shoulder (suprascapular)

       c) Rectosigmoid involvement may result in pain to sacrum or rectal area

D. Factors that may influence the experience of pain: pain is experienced by the patient *and* family in keeping with the model of "total pain" and includes physical, psychological, social and spiritual effects; when adequate assessment and management of controllable symptoms precede psychological, social and spiritual assessment and intervention, overall outcomes often improve (Remember the lesson in Maslow's Hierarchy of needs); common effects of pain include

   1. Physical effects: decreased functional ability, including ability to walk and perform other basic ADLs, decreased strength and endurance, nausea, anorexia, insomnia and impaired immune response

   2. Psychosocial effects: alteration in social and close relationships, isolation, inability to work; loss of self-esteem, self-worth; increased caregiver burden, further disruption of important social supports for both patient and family

   3. Emotional effects: diminished leisure, increased fear and anxiety, depression, hopelessness, despair, loss of control; if pain uncontrolled, consideration of suicide or physician assisted suicide

   4. Spiritual issues: increased suffering, re-evaluation and perhaps doubt regarding past religious foundations and beliefs; questioning the meaning of suffering

   5. Financial effects: inability to work and earn income, loss of caregiver income, issues of workplace discrimination and having to apply for governmental assistance leading to decreased income and loss of health insurance coverage

   6. Cultural issues: ethnic minority, female and elderly persons often receive less than optimal pain management in all settings[8]

       a) Consider the patient's family of origin, their manner of expressing pain and how suffering is valued

    b) Perceptions of pain, end of life, afterlife, bereavement and other aspects of palliative care vary widely by ethnicity and within ethnicities

    c) Be careful of "stereotyping," and do everything possible to learn about the patient and family's unique situation

    d) Specific aspects of culture to assess when caring for patients in pain include ethnic identity, gender, age, differing abilities, sexual orientation, religion and spirituality, financial status, place of residency, employment and educational level

III. Pharmacologic Intervention

A. Recommend medications according to severity and specific type of pain

1. World Health Organization (WHO) analgesic ladder

    a) Step one: mild pain (defined as a pain score of 1–3 on a 0–10 scale): non-opioids +/– adjuvants. Examples: aspirin, non-steroidal anti-inflammatory drug (NSAID) or acetaminophen

    b) Step two: moderate pain (defined as a pain score of 4–6 on a 0–10 scale): opioids+/– adjuvants. Examples: any opioid in combination products with acetaminophen or ibuprofen smaller doses, codeine, hydrocodone, oxycodone

    c) Step three: severe pain (defined as a pain score of 7–10 on a 0–10 scale): opioids+/- adjuvants. Examples: morphine, hydromorphone, methadone, fentanyl, oxycodone

2. While several guidelines still recommend the use of the WHO analgesic ladder, the most recent American Pain Society cancer pain guidelines[9] and the guideline developed jointly by the National Comprehensive Cancer Network and the American Cancer Society, recommend the use of algorithm approaches[10]

3. Drug actions and side effects

    a) Aspirin-like drugs (salicylates and non-salicylates [NSAIDs])

       i. Actions: analgesic, antipyretic, anti-inflammatory, anti-platelet

       ii. Adverse effects

         (a) GI distress: no relation between symptoms and seriousness of GI effects; concomitant administration of misoprostol or omeprazole (or another proton pump inhibiter) can prevent gastropathy

         (b) Renal insufficiency: elderly and dehydrated are at increased risk

         (c) Inhibiting of platelet aggregation with the exception of non-acetylated salicylates

         (d) Hypersensitivity reactions (not allergic reactions); symptoms include urticaria, bronchospasm, severe rhinitis and shock.

            (i) Adverse effects are often labeled by patients/caregivers as "allergies" (e.g., nausea and vomiting)

            (ii) These are not absolute contraindications to using the drug

         (e) CNS effects: dizziness, tinnitus, decreased hearing, headache

       iii. Dose escalation is limited by analgesic ceiling and the appearance of side effects

b)   The selective cyclooxygenase (COX-2) inhibitors

   i.   In Fall, 2004, rofecoxib (Vioxx®) was voluntarily withdrawn from the market due to increased cardiovascular events, including myocardial infarction and stroke, particularly for those patients who had been taking the drug for more than 18 months[11]

   ii.   Other COX-2s have remained on the market with boxed warnings regarding the increased risk of cardiovascular events and gastrointestinal bleeds[12]

c)   Acetaminophen

   i.   Actions: analgesic, antipyretic, *not anti-inflammatory*

   ii.   Adverse effects: far fewer than with NSAIDs; hepatotoxic in large doses; ceiling is 4 grams a day; ceiling is 2.4 to 3 gm/day in older/debilitated or in protracted use, alcoholic patients, AIDS patients, patients with liver metastasis or those with active liver disease. Dose escalation is limited by analgesic ceiling—consider quantity of acetaminophen in combination medications (see Table 2)

d)   Opioid medications

   i.   Pure agonists

   ii.   Partial agonists (buprenorphine) (same precaution below)

   iii.   Mixed agonist-antagonists (pentazocine, butorphanol, nalbuphine); not recommended for the treatment of cancer pain due to analgesic ceiling, psychomimetic actions, precipitation of withdrawal when given to patients on pure mu opioid agonists such as morphine, oxycodone, hydromorphone.

   iv.   Action: bind to receptors in the brain, spinal cord and in periphery

   v.   Side effects of opioids

      (a)   Tolerance develops rapidly to the sedative, emetic and respiratory depressant effects of opioids with consistent dosing; however it does not develop to constipation

      (b)   Sedation, sometimes, but rarely confusion

      (c)   Dizziness, dysphoria

      (d)   Nausea

      (e)   Constipation; tolerance *does not* develop—*must be prevented and treated aggressively*

      (f)   Itching and urticaria

      (g)   Respiratory depression

         (i)   Feared and misunderstood

         (ii)   Clinically significant respiratory depression is extremely rare when patients in severe pain receive opioids, especially in patients who are currently receiving opioids and when doses are titrated upward in appropriate steps; there is not good data to support the prevalence of respiratory depression due to opioids, however, there is general agreement that patients who are at risk are those who are opioid naïve and concomitantly taking other sedating drugs

(iii) Respiratory rate alone is not an indicator of respiratory depression; some patients may have a respiratory rate of 7, while alert and well perfused; other factors that must be considered are the level of sedation, the depth of respiration and the adequacy of perfusion of oxygen in the tissues as determined by examining nail beds for changes in color or obtaining an oxygen saturation level or pulse oximmetry

(iv) How opioids cause respiratory depression: opioids render the CO_2 receptors gradually less sensitive to increasing CO_2 levels

(v) True respiratory depression (remember it is rare!) is best treated by slow infusion of *dilute* naloxone

vi. Some other drug adverse effects include

   (a) Meperidine

   (i) Converted to a long-lived centrally acting excitatory metabolite (normeperidine) causing shaky feelings, tremors/twitches and myoclonus/grand mal seizures; should not be used in cancer pain management

   (ii) Poor oral bioavailability

   (b) Propoxyphene, the opioid in Darvon® and Darvocet® is, although widely prescribed, an

   (i) Ineffective analgesic; should not be used pain management especially with the elderly

   (ii) Long-lived metabolite toxic to the central nervous system and cardiovascular system

   (iii) Includes a large amount of acetaminophen; not recommended for long-term use or use in the elderly

   (c) Morphine

   (i) Active metabolites (morphine-6-glucuronide, morphine-3-glucuronide), excreted by the kidneys that will be retained by elderly patients and by those with diminished renal function; has strong analgesic and respiratory depressant properties; M3G may produce central nervous system hyperexcitablilty and possibly myoclonus, while elevated M6G levels appear to cause sedation

   (ii) Small amounts of hydration (IV fluids at 30–50cc/hr) helps to clear it through the kidneys

vii. No dosage ceiling for most opioids—so are able to titrate to effect (Important note: codeine, hydrocodone and all partial agonists and mixed agonist/antagonists do have dosage ceilings and thus, cannot be titrated to effect)

viii. Choosing delivery routes

   (a) Oral: most preferred for comfort, convenience and cost effectiveness; many forms available, immediate release tablets, sustained release tablets, liquids; transmucosal oral fentanyl

   (i) Sublingual is similar to oral route, as 50% dose absorbed across transmucosal membrane and 50% via the gastrointestinal tract after swallowing

(b) Rectal: useful for patients who are NPO or have nausea and vomiting; contraindicated with anal lesions, diarrhea, constipation or leukopenia; varying comfort levels with family caregivers and some cultures

(c) Subcutaneous or intravenous infusion: rarely required, but useful for pain requiring rapid titration of medication; while subcutaneous infusion is useful in most cases, impaired circulation or the presence of fibrosis can compromise absorption; used extensively at home for patients who are obstructed or who can no longer swallow and have severe pain. Can be managed within home setting; especially useful if parenteral route required and reliable or intravenous access not possible. Expense of home parenteral infusions to hospice programs are a barrier to use. Subcutaneous delivery is a reasonable alternative although absorption may be erratic in patients with third-space fluid retention and generalized edema

(d) Intramuscular injections should be avoided, injections are painful, unnecessary and absorption is not reliable

(e) Transmucosal: easily accessible route, provides rapid onset of action and is much faster if used with lipophilic drugs such as fentanyl

(f) Transdermal (e.g., fentanyl) for patients with stable pain (not good for rapid titration of medication); reservoir in subcutaneous tissue, delayed onset of action (12–24 hours), so patient must have an immediate release medication during the first several hours after the fentanyl patch is applied, some patients require a patch change every 48 hours; should not be given to opioid naïve patients; erratic absorption with patients who have edema, fever or are cachectic

(g) Spinal: via indwelling catheters into the epidural or intrathecal space; an implantable pump should be used in only carefully selected patients after appropriate consultation; cost, care issues and potential adverse effects should also be carefully weighed however can dramatically improve some patients quality of life especially with severe pain in lower extremities

e) Adjuvant analgesics

   i. For treatment of neuropathic pain

      (a) Tricyclic antidepressants

         (i) Desipramine and nortriptyline recommended over amitryiptyline, which has more anticholinergic effects (causing cardiovascular changes, dry mouth, constipation, cognitive changes, especially in older adults)

         (ii) Serotonin selective reuptake inhibitors (SSRIs) have not been well studied in neuropathic pain and may seem to have limited analgesic effect

         (iii) Guidelines for use

            a. Start with a low dose (e.g., desipramine 10–25 mg PO or nortriptyline 10–25 mg at bedtime (these drugs may cause sedation and enhance sleep)

            b. Increase dose by 10–25 mg increments every few days based upon the patient's response

c. Response may be delayed by 3–7 days

d. Monitor adverse effects

e. Maximum dose of nortriptyline and desipramine is 75–100 mg/day

f. Adverse effects: sedation, orthostatic hypotension, anticholinergic side effects (including urinary retention), cardiac effects

(b) Duloxetine, a newly approved serotonin-norepinephrine reuptake inhibitor for the management of diabetic peripheral neuropathic pain and major depression

(c) Anticonvulsants

(i) Because newer anticonvulsants do not have the severe adverse effects associated with earlier agents, these may be first line therapies for many people with neuropathic pain

(ii) Gabapentin: normal effective range 900–1800 mg/day in 2–3 divided dose; carbamazepine (100-800 mg BID or QID); phenytoin (100–200 mg TID); valproic acid (200–400 mg BID or TID); clonazepam (0.25–.5 mg TID); (all doses are oral)

(iii) Guidelines for use

a. Start low, go slow

b. Watch for side effects

c. Monitor patient for signs of toxicity use labs to guide decisions

(iv) Major adverse effects

a. Gabapentin: sedation, ataxia, dizziness, side effects generally less than with others; less costly now that generic form is available

b. Pregabalin (Lyrica®): newly approved, similar to gabapentin with similar mechanisms of action; may provide an effect equivalent to gabapentin at lower doses

c. Carbamazepine: bone marrow suppression, vertigo, confusion, sedation; requires serum monitoring; costly

d. Phenytoin: ataxia, rash, hepatotoxicity; requires serum monitoring

e. Valproic acid: nausea, vomiting, sedation, ataxia, tremor, thrombocytopenia, neutropenia, hepatotoxicity; requires serum monitoring

f. Clonazepam: sedation, physical dependence; not as effective as an analgesic; useful for anxiety associated with pain

(d) Local anesthetics

(i) Useful in refractory neuropathic pain; only indication is for postherpetic neuralgia, but clinically is used for many neuropathic pain conditions

(ii) Lidocaine

 a. Adverse effects include dizziness, lightheadedness, lowered blood pressure, sensory disturbances and tremor, seizures at high doses, nausea and vomiting

 b. Lidocaine 5% is also available in a patch for topical relief of postherpetic neuropathy, post-thoracotomy pain and other pain syndromes

  (i) The patches should be placed over intact skin only

  (ii) Up to three patches can be used to cover the painful area; package insert instructs to apply for 12 hours and then remove for 12 hours, but studies document it is safe to leave in place for 18–24 hours

  (iii) Adverse effects are uncommon and include pain with removal of the patch

  (iv) Patients with sensitivity to touch (also called allodynia) often report relief

ii. Corticosteroids: used in metastatic bone pain (triple effect of pain control, mood elevation and increased appetite). Also useful to relieve pain associated with liver metastases and other visceral pain syndromes.

iii. Topical capsaicin: used for diabetic neuropathy, postherpetic neuralgia, arthritis, Kaposi's sarcoma lesions

iv. Other medications used to treat side effects of opioids e.g., psychostimulants, phenothiazines, benzodiazepines (muscle spasms)

4. Opioid Equianalgesic conversions

Important Note: If converting from one drug to another AND the patient's pain is well controlled, many experts recommend reducing the dose by 25% to account for incomplete cross tolerance. However, if you are converting from one drug to another AND the patient is in severe pain, dose reduction is often not necessary

a) Process

i. Step 1: Add up the total amount of the current drug given in 24 hours; remember to add in both the scheduled and breakthrough or rescue doses; calculate separately if more than one drug used

ii. Step 2: Divide current 24-hour total by the equianalgesic value for the current drug and route of administration (see Table 1)

iii. Step 3: Multiply the above number by the equianalgesic value for the new drug and route; this will give you the new 24-hour dose

iv. Step 4: Determine how many doses the patient will take each day and divide this number into the total 24-hour dose; this gives the amount of medication needed per dose

b) Example

i. The patient is taking 2 tablets of acetaminophen in combination with hydrocodone 5 mg every 4 hours. Because each tablet contains 5 mg of hydrocodone, two contain 10 mg 6 doses × 10 mg = 60 mg/day of hydrocodone; convert to oral hydromorphone

ii.   60 mg of hydrocodone divided by 30 mg (equivalent value for hydrocodone) = 2

iii.   2 × 7.5 mg (equivalent value for oral hydromorphone) = 15 mg (or 15 mg of hydromorphone in 24 hours)

iv.   Hydromorphone can be given every 4 hours, which is 6 doses a day; divide the 24 hour dose by 6 doses; *(15 divided by 6 = 2.5)* 2.5 mg hydromorphone every 4 hours; since hydromorphone comes in 2, 4 and 8 mg tablets, round the dose down to 2 mg, order appropriate breakthrough medications and carefully monitor the patient for the need to increase the dose

5.   Calculating breakthrough or rescue doses

   a)   A rescue dose is always ordered with long-acting opioids; it is preferable to match the breakthrough medication with the long-acting opioid, e.g., immediate release morphine with sustained release morphine

   b)   Doses should increase commensurate with increases in the scheduled doses

   c)   The 2003, 5th edition the American Pain Society (APS) guidelines recommend using 10–15% of the 24-hour oral dose, given every 2 hours as needed

   d)   Other clinical reports suggest the breakthrough dose should be 10–20% of the 24-hour dose and since the peak effect is usually within one hour, doses can be repeated every hour

   e)   For parenteral administration (IV or SQ), the breakthrough dose is 50–100% of the hourly rate; since the peak effect is in 15 minutes, boluses may be given safely in the majority of patients every 15 minutes

   f)   Increase baseline dose of long-acting opioid if more than 3 rescue doses are used in 24 hours

   g)   Example: a patient is taking 120 mg MS Contin® (long acting morphine) every 12 hours; the appropriate breakthrough dose of MSIR® (immediate release morphine) is 24–36 mg (10–15%) every 2 hours as needed

B.   **Non-pharmacologic interventions can be used concurrently with medications and other modalities to relieve pain and can often be taught to patients and/or family members; there are some that believe that medications should never be given without the addition of *some* non-pharmacologic intervention. However, the use of non-pharmacologic interventions should *never* preclude appropriate use of medications, including opioids. The most common non-pharmacologic interventions are listed below**

1.   Physical modalities

   a)   Consider PT and OT consults (especially in the inpatient palliative care setting)

   b)   Cutaneous stimulation (heat, cold)

   c)   Exercise (with limitations based on physical condition)

   d)   Transcutaneous nerve stimulation (efficacy controversial may be useful in patients with mild pain); acupuncture

   e)   Massage; healing touch; therapeutic touch

2. Psychosocial and spiritual interventions (helpful in maintaining control in uncertain, dependent and anxiety-provoking situations)

   a) Relaxation and guided imagery

   b) Distraction

   c) Music

   d) Reframing

   e) Patient/family education

   f) Hypnosis

   g) Counseling

   h) Prayer

   i) Spiritual reflection or meditation

3. Other

   a) Biofeedback

   b) Aromatherapy

4. Palliative radiation therapy

   a) May be used to relieve symptoms of patients with advanced disease, (e.g., pain, bleeding), compression of vital organ systems, (e.g., the brain, ulcerating skin lesions) and metastasis to weight bearing bones susceptible to fracture

   b) Radiation therapy is the treatment of choice for spinal cord compression, bone pain and is frequently used in superior vena cava syndrome and symptomatic brain metastases

   c) While external beam radiation is the modality commonly used for palliative radiation therapy, strontium-89, an intravenous radionucleotide that emits beta radiation at the bony metastatic site, is sometimes used to treat areas of painful skeletal metastasis; newer radionucleotides are currently under study that may not produce the painful flair that occurs when strontium-89 is given

5. Palliative chemotherapy: may improve or enhance comfort when neither cure nor control is possible

   a) Antineoplastic therapy may produce tumor shrinkage, relief of pressure on nerves, lymphatics and blood vessels and reduction in organ obstruction, thus relieving pain

   b) Bisphosphonates are useful in treating pain related to multiple myeloma and metastatic bone disease[13]

IV. Pain During the Final Days of Life

A. Pain Assessment

1. Patients may become nonverbal in the final days of life

   a) A furrowed brow may indicate pain

   b) Guarding and vocalization during turning or dressing changes may suggest pain

   c) A therapeutic trial of an opioid should be strongly considered to determine if these behaviors change with the use of an analgesic

2. If the patient had pain prior to becoming unresponsive, assume pain is still present

B.   Pharmacologic Management

1.   As organ system dysfunction increases, particularly renal clearance, drugs or their metabolites are cleared from the body less efficiently and sedation may increase

    a)   Therefore, a therapeutic trial of opioid dose reduction may be indicated if sedation is not a desired effect

    b)   In some cases, patients may become more alert and responsive

    c)   If any signs of pain return, the dose should be returned to its previous level

2.   Rapid discontinuation of opioids, benzodiazepines or other agents can result in the abstinence syndrome; whenever possible, gradual reduction in dose of these drugs is indicated

3.   Sedation at the end of life is an option for patients with intractable pain and suffering[13]

    a)   There are numerous combinations of medications that are used to accomplish sedation

        i.   Opioids

        ii.   Barbiturates

        iii. Neuroleptics

        iv.   Benzodiazepines

    b)   Therapy is based on obtaining initial relief of symptoms followed by ongoing sedation to maintain the effect

    c)   Parenteral ketamine, given either as a continuous infusion or as bolus doses, may also be used to accomplish sedation at the end of life

C.   Non-Pharmacologic Management Should Continue

V.   Summary of Principles of Pain Management

A.   Pain assessment data is documented so the pain etiology or syndrome can be identified and appropriately treated

B.   The oral route is used whenever possible

1.   If the patient is unable to take oral medications, buccal, sublingual, rectal and transdermal routes are considered before parenteral routes

2.   IM route is avoided

3.   IV and subcutaneous route can be used for any patient that cannot tolerate above choices under oral route or when pain is rapidly escalating and severe. Subcutaneous route is a useful alternative in the home setting when reliable IV access is not possible

C.   Constant pain calls for treatment with an around-the-clock scheduled long acting opioid and a short acting medication for breakthrough pain

1.   Only one long-acting opioid is ordered for constant pain

2.   Doses of opioids are increased commensurate with the patient's report of pain

3. Equianalgesic conversions are used when changing medications and/or routes

4. Adjuvant medications are used for neuropathic pain, some visceral pain states and bone pain

D. Breakthrough pain

1. Only one opioid analgesic is ordered for breakthrough pain

2. Use an adequate rescue dose for breakthrough pain; APS rescue dose recommendation is 10–15% of the 24-hour dose q3h PRN; always increase the rescue dose when the baseline dose is increased

3. Increase the baseline dose if the patient needs more than 3 rescue doses in 24 hours unless pain is related to a specific activity or if patient becomes sedated with increased around the clock dose

4. A higher dosage of breakthrough or rescue medication, is sometimes necessary if the frequency of breakthrough pain and/or intensity are at higher levels

5. To calculate rescue dose when fentanyl is used, divide the total patch dose by 3—that is the appropriate dose of MSIR®; (immediate release morphine). All chronic pain requires the use of breakthrough pain medication

6. Patients and families need to be educated about taking the medication when the pain is first perceived—not when it has become severe or unbearable

E. Non-pharmacologic approaches are always a part of any pain management plan

F. An appropriate preventative bowel regimen is ordered with a stimulant laxative and stool softener to correct the effects of the opioid. Refer to the chapter on symptom management

VI. Evaluation—pain management is predicated by ongoing assessment of treatment efficacy and control of treatment side effects.

A. Evaluation of interventions is a basic nursing function and completes the nursing process

B. Nursing evaluation should be accomplished in a timely manner, in accordance with expected pharmacologic peak action or when the non- pharmacologic intervention is completed

C. At each nursing visit assess for

1. Pain intensity, type, duration, etc.

2. Medication side effects, interactions or complications

3. Patient's satisfaction with method of pain relief

D. In the inpatient setting

1. Pain assessment every shift or more frequently as indicated

2. Patient/family teaching and reinforcement of pain management

3. Monitor bowel status daily and document

E. **Evaluate efficacy of pain relief interventions with a thorough assessment**

1. At appropriate intervals after any change in medication, dosage, route of administration, etc.

2. At each nursing visit

Table 1: Opioid Dosing Equivalence[a]

Drug	Dose (mg) Parenteral	Dose (mg) Oral	Duration (hours)
Morphine (IR)	10	30	3–4
Morphine, Controlled Release (MS Contin®, Oramorph SR®)	—	30	8–12
Hydromorphone (Dilaudid®)	1.5	7.5	3–4
Codeine	130	200	3–4
Oxycodone, Controlled Release (Oxycontin®)	—	20	8–12
Oxycodone (Roxicodone®, Percocet®)	—	20	3–4
Hydrocodone (Vicodin®, Lortab®)	—	30	3–4
Meperidine (Demerol®)[b]	100	300+	2–3
Levorphanol (Levo-Dromoran®)	2	4	6–8
Methadone (Dolophine®)[c,13]	10 acute pain 2–4 chronic pain		8
Fentanyl (Duragesic®, generic)	0.1	Convert present medication to 24 hour oral MS equivalent; then divide in half; this is mcg/hr dose of fentanyl	48–72
Propoxyphene (Darvon®; Darvocet®)[d]	—	180	4

[a] Important Note: If converting from one drug to another AND the patient's pain is well controlled, many experts recommend reducing the dose by 25% to account for incomplete cross tolerance. However, if you are converting from one drug to another AND the patient is in severe pain, dose reduction is often not necessary.

[b] WARNING: Long-lived toxic metabolite; CNS stimulant, not recommended for long-term use

[c] Methadone should be used with caution in older adults. Dose methadone using the following guidelines:[9,14,15]

  1. If the total morphine or equivalent dose per day is less than 90 mg (oral) a methadone ratio of 1:4 (methadone to morphine) is used. The total methadone dose is divided by 3 and given at 8-hour intervals.

  2. If the morphine or equivalent dose per day is between 90 and 300 mg (oral), a dose ratio of 1:8 (methadone to morphine) is used. The total methadone dose is divided by 3 and given at 8-hour intervals.

  3. If the morphine or equivalent dose per day is greater than 300 mg (oral), a dose ratio of 1:12 (methadone to morphine) is used. The total methadone dose is divided by 3 and given at 8-hour intervals.

  4. Patient maintained on an 8-hour schedule of methadone may have 10% of the daily dose for breakthrough pain.

[d] WARNING: Long-lived metabolite that is toxic to the central nervous system and cardiovascular system, not recommended for long-term use and use in the elderly.

Table 2: Combination Products

Opioid	Proprietary name and combination drugs[e]
Hydrocodone	Vicodin® (5mg + 500mg acetaminophen) Vicodin ES® (7.5mg + 750mg acetaminophen Lorcet-10® (10mg + 650mg acetaminophen) Lortab® Vicodin HP® (10mg + 660mg acetaminophen) Norco® (10mg + 325mg acetaminophen) Anexsia® (5mg + 500mg acetaminophen) Zydone® (5mg + 400mg acetaminophen) Vicoprofen® (7.5mg + 200mg ibuprofen) Reprexain™ (5mg + 200mg ibuprofen)
Oxycodone	Percodan® (5mg + 325mg ASA) Percocet® (5mg + 325mg acetaminophen) Tylox® (5mg + 500mg acetaminophen) Roxicet® (5mg +325mg acetaminophen) Combunox™ (5mg + 400mg ibuprofen)
Codeine	Tylenol #2® (15mg + 325mg acetaminophen) Tylenol #3® (30mg + 325mg acetaminophen) Tylenol #4® (60mg + 325mg acetaminophen)
Propoxyphene[f]	Darvon® (65mg)Darvocet N® (100mg + 650mg acetaminophen) Darvon Compound® (65mg + 325mg ASA + caffeine) Darvon-N® or Darvon® with ASA (65mg + 325mg ASA)

[e] Twenty-four hour dose of acetaminophen should not exceed 4 grams for healthy adults.

[f] WARNING: Long-lived metabolite that is toxic to the central nervous system and cardiovascular system, not recommended for long-term use and use in the elderly.

Table 3: Pain Terms Associated with Neuropathic Pain States (modified from the International Association for the Study of Pain; McCaffery and Pasero)

Term	Definition	
Allodynia	Pain due to a stimulus, which does not normally provoke pain	
Dysesthesia	An unpleasant abnormal sensation, whether spontaneous or evoked	
Hyperalgesia	A painful syndrome characterized by an abnormally painful reaction to a normally non-painful stimulus, such as touch. (Sometimes referred hyperpathia)	
Paresthesia	An abnormal anesthetic sensation (often described as a painful numbness)	
Neuralgia	Pain in the distribution of a nerve or nerves	
Neuropathic pain	Pain initiated or caused by a primary lesion or dysfunction in the nervous system	
	Peripheral neuropathic pain	Pain initiated or caused by a primary lesion or dysfunction in the peripheral nervous system (e.g., postherpetic neuropathy).
	Central pain	Pain initiated or caused by a primary lesion or dysfunction in the central nervous system (e.g., post thalamic pain syndrome occurring after stroke)

CITED REFERENCES

1. Sykes N, Thorns A. The use of opioids and sedatives at the end of life. *Lancet Oncol.* 2003;May4(5):312–318.

2. Thorns A, Sykes N. Opioid use in last week of life and implications for end-of-life decision-making. *Lancet.* 2000;Jul 29-356(9227):398–399.

3. McCaffery M, Pasero C. *Pain: Clinical Manual.* St. Louis, MO: Mosby; 1999.

4. International Association for the Study of Pain. Pain terms: a list with definitions and notes on usage. *Pain.* 1979;6:249.

5. American Academy of Pain Medicine, American Pain Society, American Society of Addiction Medicine. *Definitions Related to the Use of Opioids for the Treatment of Pain: A Consensus Document.* Glenview, IL: Author; 2001.

6. Weissman DE, Dahl JL, Dinndorf PA. *Handbook of Cancer Pain Management.* Madison, WI: The Wisconsin Cancer Pain Initiative; 1996.

7. Benjamin LJ, Dampier, CD, Jacox A, et al. *Guideline for the Management of Acute and Chronic Pain in Sickle-Cell Disease.* Skokie, IL: American Pain Society; 1999.

8. Cleeland CS, Gonin R, Hatfield AK, Edmonson JH, Blum RH, Stewart JA, Pandya KJ. Pain and its treatment in outpatients with metastatic cancer. *New England Journal of Medicine.* 1994;330:592–596.

9. Miaskowski C, Cleary J, Burney R, Coyne P, Finley R, Foster R, Grossman S, Janjan N, Ray J, Syrjala K, Weisman S, Zahrbock C. *Guideline for the Management of Cancer Pain in Adults and Children, APS Clinical Practice Guideline Series, No 3.* Glenview, IL: American Pain Society; 2005.

10. National Comprehensive Cancer Network, The American Cancer Society. *Cancer Pain: Treatment Guidelines for Patients.* Author; 2001. Available at http://www.nccn.org/ or http://www.cancer.org. Accessed May 17, 2005.

11. FDA Public Health Advisory: Safety of Vioxx. Available at: http://www.fda.gov/cder/drug/infopage/vioxx/PHA_vioxx.htm. Accessed May 15, 2005.

12. FDA's COX-2 Safety Plan: Remove Bextra, Add Black Box to Celebrex. *"The Pink Sheet" Daily.* FDC Reports, An Elsevier Company; April 7, 2005.

13. Paice JA, Fine P. Pain at the end of life. In: Ferrell B, Coyle N, eds. *Textbook of Palliative Nursing.* New York, NY: Oxford University Press; 2001:76–90.

14. DeConno F, Groff L, Brunelle C, Zecca E, Ventafridda V, Ripamonit C. Clinical experience with oral methadone administration in the treatment of pain in 196 advanced cancer patients. *Journal of Clinical Oncology.* 1996;14:2836–2842.

15. Ripamonti C, Zecca E, Bruera E. An update on the clinical use of methadone for cancer pain. *Pain.* 1997;70:109–115.

ADDITIONAL REFERENCES AND RESOURCES

AGS Panel on Persistent Pain in Older Persons. The management of persistent pain in older persons. *Journal of the American Geriatrics Society.* 2002;50:S205–S224.

American Medical Directors Association (AMDA). *Pain Management in the Long-Term Care Setting.* Columbia, MD: Author; 2003.

American Pain Society. *Principles of Analgesic Use in the Treatment of Acute Pain and Cancer Pain.* 5th ed. Skokie, IL: Author; 2003.

Doyle D, Hanks G, Cherny N, Calman K, eds. *The Oxford Textbook of Palliative Medicine.* 3rd ed. New York, NY: Oxford University Press; 2004.

Ersek M, Wagner B, Ferrell B, Paice JA, Scanlon C. Providing opioids at the end of life. *Journal of Hospice and Palliative Nursing.* 2004:6(4):244–246.

Ferrell BR, Cohen MZ, Rhiner M, Rozek A. Pain as a metaphor for illness: part II: family caregivers management of pain. *Oncology Nursing Forum.* 1991;18:1315–1321.

Ferrell BR, Dean G. The meaning of cancer pain. *Seminars in Oncology Nursing.* 1995;1(1):17–22.

Ferrell BR, Rhiner M, Cohen MZ, Grant M. Pain as a metaphor for illness: part I: impact of pain on family caregivers. *Oncology Nursing Forum.* 1991;18:1303–1309.

Ferrell BR, Taylor EJ, Grant M, Fowler M, Corbisiero RM. Pain management at home: struggle, comfort and mission. *Cancer Nursing.* 1993;16:169–178.

Gordon DB, Dahl JL, Stevenson KK. *Building an Institutional Commitment to Pain Management: The Wisconsin Resource Manual.* 2nd ed. Madison, WI: University of Wisconsin-Madison Board of Regents; 2000.

Panke JT. Difficulties in managing pain at the end of life. *Journal of Hospice and Palliative Nursing.* 2002:5(2):83–90.

Shaver WA. Suffering and the role of abandonment of self. *Journal of Hospice and Palliative Nursing.* 2002:4(1):46–53.

Ward SE, Goldberg N, Miller-McCauley V, Mueller C, Nolan A, Pawlik-Plank D, Robbons A, Stormoen D, Weissman DE. Patient-related barriers to management of cancer pain. *Pain.* 1993;52:319–324.

Zerwekh J, Riddell S, Richard J. Fearing to comfort: a grounded theory of constraints to opioid use in hospice. *Journal of Hospice and Palliative Nursing.* 2002:4(2):83–90.

CHAPTER V

SYMPTOM MANAGEMENT

Sandy Muchka, RN, MS, CS, CHPN®

First Edition Authors
Cathleen A. Collins, RN, MSN
Margery A. Wilson, MSN, FNP, CHPN®, APRN, BC-PCM

I. **Principles**

   A. **The nursing process (using assessment, diagnosis, planning, for symptom management and care at the end of life)**

   B. **Care at the end of life is multidimensional with emphasis on quality-of-life as the patient and family define it, with respect for, support and education of patient and family**

   C. **Understanding of expectations, goals of treatment, end-of-life goals. Issues must be clarified with patient and family, taking into account the patient's position on the disease trajectory. Recommendations for symptom management will vary depending on individual goals of care which reflect the patient and family's stated values and what is meaningful to them**

   D. **The interdisciplinary team (IDT) is the framework for palliative care and hospice**

   E. **The patient and family are the unit of care in palliative care and hospice and are included in the assessment, planning, decision-making and evaluation of interventions**

      1. Options and expected or possible outcomes are discussed with patient and family to inform their decision-making; the IDT is responsible for giving them information regarding the benefits and the burdens of any treatment that is proposed

      2. Patients and families require time, opportunity for clarification and review in anticipation of making decisions

   F. **The end of life can be a time of growth, reconciliation, peace, joy and hope for patients and families; appropriate symptom management can facilitate this process by maximizing patient comfort**

   G. **Patients may experience a variety of symptoms. Those covered in this chapter are some of the most often experienced by individuals with life-threatening illness**

II. **Alteration in Skin and Mucous Membranes**

A. **Definition: disruption in the integrity of the skin or oral mucous membrane**

B. **Possible Etiologies**

1. Skin integrity

    a) Pressure ulcers

        i. Pressure to the skin, causing a decrease in blood flow and eventual cell death

        ii. Shearing forces, in which two surfaces slide in opposite but parallel directions (e.g., a patient slides down in bed and bone and skin are displaced from one another)

        iii. Friction, in which two surfaces move across one another (e.g., patient is dragged across bed sheets)

        iv. Moisture (especially feces and urine)

        v. Obesity

        vi. Malnutrition

        vii. Cachexia

        viii. Immobility

        ix. Impaired circulation due to peripheral vascular disease, diabetes or cancer infiltration through skin

    b) Fistulas

    c) Tumor necrosis

2. Alteration of oral mucous membranes

    a) Dry mouth (xerostomia)

        i. Drugs (anticholinergics, antihistamines, phenothiazines)

        ii. Radiation and chemotherapy

        iii. Dehydration

        iv. Mucositis

        v. Mouth breathing

        vi. Metabolic disorders (hypercalcemia, hyperglycemia)

    b) Candidiasis

        i. Radiation and chemotherapy

        ii. Drugs (antibiotics, corticosteroids)

        iii. Altered immune system with disease

    c) Herpes simplex virus

    d) Mucositis caused by radiation or chemotherapy

3. Pruritus: uncomfortable itching of the skin

    a) Dry, flaky skin

    b) Wet, macerated skin

    c) Contact dermatitis caused by ointments or creams

    d) Infestations caused by scabies, lice, fleas

    e) Drugs (antibiotics, morphine, phenothiazines)

    f) Systemic disease (renal failure, hepatobiliary disease, infiltration of tumors into subcutaneous tissue)

    g) Fungal infections

C. Assess for

1. Skin integrity

    a) Inspect skin each time patient changes position. If pressure ulcer, grade wound according to stage[1]

        i. Stage I: Non-blanchable erythema of intact skin, the heralding lesion of skin ulceration

            (a) In individuals with dark skin, discoloration of the skin, warmth, edema, induration or hardness also may be indicators

            (b) Skin changes may be difficult to discern in some persons of color and the patient's report of pain may be the only clue to closely examine at-risk areas; be mindful of baseline skin color and monitor skin frequently for skin color change

        ii. Stage II: Partial thickness skin loss involving epidermis, dermis or both. The ulcer is superficial and presents clinically as an abrasion, blister or shallow crater

        iii. Stage III: Full thickness skin loss involving damage to or necrosis of subcutaneous tissue that may extend down to, but not through, underlying fascia. The ulcer presents clinically as a deep crater with or without undermining of adjacent tissue

        iv. Stage IV: Full thickness skin loss with extensive destruction, tissue necrosis or damage to muscle, bone or supporting structures; undermining and sinus tracts also may be associated with Stage IV pressure ulcers

    b) Wound location

    c) Wound appearance/characteristics: Consider use of a comprehensive assessment tool such as Pressure Ulcer Scale for Healing (PUSH) or Pressure Sore Status Tool (PSST)

        i. Size, length, width, depth, undermining

        ii. Presence of drainage (serous, serosanguineous, sanguineous, purulent) and amount

        iii. Tissue type (i.e., granulating or eschar)

        iv. Appearance of surrounding skin (redness, maceration, etc.)

    d)   Is wound painful?

    e)   If wound is due to tumor necrosis, does the location present a potential for serious complications (i.e., potential for hemorrhage or obstruction of blood flow due to the tumor located next to blood vessels)?

    f)   Is the wound malodorous or fungating?

    g)   A nutritional assessment is important, as malnutrition can impede proper wound healing and also cause pressure ulcer formation

2.   Alteration in Oral Mucous Membranes

    a)   Patient history of mouth dryness or sore mouth

    b)   Review of medications which may cause oral membrane alterations (i.e., antibiotics, chemotherapy drugs such as IV 5-Fluouracil, anticholinergics)

    c)   Examination of internal and external oral mucosa

       i.   Dry, cracked lips

       ii.   Sores or white patches on buccal membranes oropharynx or tongue

       iii.   Bleeding of gums, lips or tongue

    d)   Patient's current oral hygiene regimen

    e)   Patient and family knowledge of etiology and management of altered oral mucous membranes

3.   Pruritus

    a)   History of itching (including when, how long, what is tolerable)

    b)   Assessment of skin

       i.   Location

       ii.   Presence or absence of rash or lesions

       iii.   Overall skin integrity

       iv.   Quality of symptoms

       v.   Aggravating/alleviating factors

    c)   Review plan of care for medications that may cause pruritus

    d)   Patient and family knowledge of etiology and management of pruritus including its relationship to disease state, medications or other environmental factors

D. Diagnoses

1.   Impaired skin integrity, oral, related to dry mouth, oral lesions, infection

2.   Impaired skin integrity related to immobility and pressure over bony prominences

3.   Impaired skin integrity related to tumor necrosis or fistula

4.   Pain related to altered skin or oral mucous membranes or pruritus

5.   Body image disturbance related to malodorous or unsightly wounds

6.   Patient/family knowledge deficit related to etiology and management of wounds, altered oral mucous membranes or pruritus

E. Planning and Intervention

1. Wound management

a) Relieve pressure

i. Turn at least every two hours

ii. Place patient on pressure relief and pressure reduction support surfaces, such as low air loss or air fluidized bed

b) Reduce friction and shearing forces

i. Teach family proper techniques for moving patient in bed; physical therapy referral may be indicated

ii. Use transparent dressings or elbow and knee protectors

c) Consult team dietitian for nutritional assessment and plan of care

d) Consult enterostomal therapy (ET) nurse for wound management plan, if appropriate

e) Consult Agency for Healthcare Research and Quality (AHRQ) (formerly AHCPR) guidelines for skin and wound care

f) Wounds should be cleansed and irrigated with normal saline prior to being dressed

i. Irrigation with low pressure (pouring directly from the bottle or using bulb or piston syringe) if wound has granulation tissue present and very little serous to serosanguineous exudate[2]

ii. Irrigation with high pressure (35 cc syringe with 19 gauge IV cannula attached) if wound has debris, eschar or moderate to large amount of exudate (especially purulent)[2]

iii. Dressing selection

(a) The following should be considered when selecting a dressing[1]

(i) Moist wound bed

(ii) Dry surrounding skin

(iii) Exudate control

(iv) Caregiver time

(b) If wounds are malodorous, special dressings are required to assist with odor control

(i) Metronidazole tablets crushed and sprinkled into the malodorous wound will help minimize infection and odor

(c) Table I lists different types of dressings and the types of wounds for which they are appropriate

iv. Assure adequate pain control prior to changing dressings; schedule pre-medication with short-acting systemic medications and/or utilize topical pain relievers as appropriate for ongoing pain (i.e., topical lidocaine, cold packs, morphine mixed into the wound care ointment)

2. Alteration in oral mucous membranes

    a) Xerostomia

        i. Stimulate salivation

            (a) Peppermint water

            (b) Gum, mints, hard candy (preferably sugar-free to prevent dental caries)

            (c) Avoid preparations or candies containing lemon as lemon contributes to dryness and irritation

            (d) Ice chips or frequent sips of water

            (e) Pilocarpine 2.5 mg PO TID, titrate to 10 mg PO TID; do not use in patients with severe COPD or bowel obstruction[3]

        ii. Utilize saliva substitutes

            (a) Ice chips or frequent sips of water

            (b) Artificial saliva

        iii. Treat dehydration

            (a) Ice chips or frequent sips of water

            (b) Offer fluids throughout the day, especially with meals

            (c) Humidify the room

            (d) Place spray bottle and moistened oral swabs close to patient (avoid lemon-glycerin swabs)

        iv. Review medications and alter regimen if appropriate

3. Sore mouth due to oral Candida, herpetic lesions, mucositis or stomatitis

    a) For Candida

        i. Nystatin swish and swallow—for optimal treatment 2 minutes of swishing is required, which may be difficult for some patients

        ii. Fluconazole 150 mg PO once is the first line treatment

    b) Around-the-clock mouth care at least every two to four hours with moistened oral swabs and saline mouth rinse, if patient is able; be sure to apply water-soluble lubricant to lips

    c) 1:4 hydrogen peroxide and water rinse for mucous or hard debris in mouth[4]

    d) Do not serve hot or overly spicy foods; serve softened and moist foods rather than dry

    e) Several oral medications and medicated mouthwash cocktails are available for mouth pain and lesions. Some examples are

        i. Topical morphine

        ii. Viscous lidocaine

        iii. Cocktail of Milk of Magnesia, diphenhydrAMINE and viscous lidocaine

        iv. Sucralfate slurry

f) PCA with IV Morphine may be used for severe oropharyngeal pain[5]

4. Pruritus Interventions

   a) Non-pharmacologic measures

      i. Avoid skin irritants that may cause dryness or additional moisture[4]

         (a) Alcohol

         (b) Tight or heavy clothing

         (c) Frequent bathing with harsh soaps and hot water. Avoid soaps with deodorants and those with additives that can be drying

      ii. Avoid heat, maintain cool room temperatures; keep the patient cool to avoid sweating and frequently cleanse the skin with neutral pH cleansers and tepid water

      iii. Cool starch baths (be observant for any signs of candidiasis in skin folds of groin, axilla, under breasts)

      iv. Cold compresses can decrease itching; make sure to assess skin frequently during application and do not apply if patient's peripheral vascular system is compromised

      v. Apply lubricating ointments or creams to skin (i.e., lanolin) to avoid excessive drying

      vi. Avoid alcohol, foods/drinks containing caffeine, theophylline

   b) Pharmacologic Measures

      i. Moisturizers—the mainstay of treatment is hydration

      ii. Antihistamines—hydroxyzine and diphenhydrAMINE

      iii. Topical corticosteroids can be used for acute localized itching, but should be avoided for chronic pruritis[6]

      iv. Ondansetron has been used in cholestatic, uremic and opioid-induced pruritis[6]

      v. Antifungal creams for pruritus related to Candida

      vi. Transcutaneous electrical nerve stimulation (TENS) units may be helpful in localized pruritis[4,6]

      vii. Systemic corticosteroids to relieve pruritus related to inflammatory condition and neoplasms

      viii. Anesthetics for relief of intractable pruritus

      ix. For end stage liver induced itching—bile acid sequestrants (cholestyramine) may be helpful

F. Patient/Family Education

1. Wounds

   a) Demonstrate and observe caregiver performing, correct positioning to maximize pressure relief. Explain importance of changing patient's position every two hours, when appropriate, even if the patient is sitting in a chair

b) Demonstrate and observe caregiver performing, proper technique in moving patient up in bed to reduce friction and shearing force

c) Demonstrate correct procedures for cleansing and dressing wounds

d) Explain possible complications with tumor necrotic wounds; prepare family for bleeding or airway concerns and management

e) Explain management of ostomy bags if fistula present

f) Address nutritional needs of patient within context of palliative care goals

g) Mobility: address degree of activity, based on palliative care goals

2. Altered oral mucous membranes

a) Demonstrate and observe caregiver performing, proper technique for oral care; explain importance of frequent oral care

b) Explain medication usage and potential side effects

c) Introduce non-pharmacologic methods for preventing and relieving dry and sore oral mucous membranes

d) Address nutritional concerns related to altered intake due to mouth pain; within the context of palliative care goals

3. Pruritus

a) Explain etiology of pruritus

b) Explain ways of preventing pruritus (keep skin clean and dry, avoid soaps, etc.)

c) Explain actions of medications and potential side effects

d) Introduce non-pharmacologic methods for preventing and relieving pruritus [see Section E, 4 a) above]

G. Evaluate

1. Wounds

a) Response of patient/family to teaching

b) Effectiveness of interventions (i.e., is wound healing?)

c) Need for change in plan (i.e., change in dressing, referral to ET nurse)

d) Patient/family understanding of treatment and prevention of further alteration of skin integrity

2. Altered oral mucous membranes and pruritus

a) Response to interventions and patient/family teaching

b) Effectiveness of interventions: are patient/family satisfied with outcome?

c) Medication effects and side effects

d) Patient/family understanding of treatment and prevention of further alteration

H. Revise plan according to findings from ongoing evaluations, changes in patient status or family needs

Table 1: Indications and Uses for Dressings

Type of Dressing	Indications and Uses
Semipermeable film	Protects very early damage from shear forces. Prevents bacterial contamination. Maintains humidity in shallow ulcers, producing ideal conditions for granulation and healing. Provides immediate pain relief. Best applied when there is no exudation from the wound.
Hydrocolloids	For low-exudate wounds. Maintains moist environment. Fluidizes to produce a gel useful for debridement. Provides environment for granulation. Available as a paste to fill wound cavities.
Alginates	For heavy exudates; controls secretion and bacterial contamination by absorption and formation of hydrophilic gel.
Hydrogels/xerogels	For debridement in the presence of slough and infection: rehydrates eschar and makes it easier to remove.
Enzymatic	For eschar and necrotic tissue; loosens necrotic tissue by liquefaction, thereby aiding in its removal (Protect edges of wound with zinc paste and apply to eschar under an occlusive dressing).
Polysaccharide dextranomer	For exudative, infected wounds; on contact with wound exudates the beads absorb fluid and swell, forming a gel; bacteria and dead cells are drawn away from the wound. Applied every 24 hours until wound is clean and granulation tissue is developing.
Charcoal	Malodorous infected pressure sores: adsorbs bacteria, cellular debris, toxins and odors.

Reprinted from *Handbook of Palliative Care in Cancer*, 2nd ed, Waller A, Caroline NL, p. 97, Copyright 2000, with permission from Elsevier.

III. **Altered Mental Status: Confusion, Delirium, Terminal Restlessness, Agitation**

A. **Confusion/Delirium/Agitation**

1. Definitions

a) Confusion

i. "Confusion" is not an accurate descriptive term. It can mean anything from delirium, dementia, psychosis, obtunded, etc. Patients need a focused assessment, including a mini-mental examination[7]

ii. Clouding of consciousness, memory impairment

iii. Change in cognition/impaired cognitive function, impaired perceptions and emotional disturbances

iv. May be accompanied by reduced level of consciousness, disorientation and misperceptions

b) Delirium (Note: "Terminal delirium/restlessness" is addressed later in this chapter)

    i. Hallmark of delirium is an acute change in cognitive function; sleep disturbance, mumbling speech, memory and perceptual disturbances

    ii. Exaggerated emotions or memories with aggression, paranoia or terror displayed

    iii. Disturbance develops over a short period of time (hours or days) and tends to fluctuate over the course of the day

    iv. Delirium can either be a hyperactive/agitated delirium or a hypoactive delirium

        (a) Symptoms of hyperactive/agitated delirium include constant movement, trying to get out of bed, removing clothing, IV lines and catheters; hyperactive delirium may be misdiagnosed as an anxiety state and the patient sedated while overlooking the underlying cause

        (b) In hypoactive delirium psychomotor activity is decreased and the patient may be misdiagnosed as depressed and/or the delirium overlooked

c) Agitation

    i. Can occur at any time during a disease process and is an objective result of confusion or delirium

    ii. A group of symptoms that may include physically and/or verbally aggressive behaviors, hiding or hoarding behaviors and physically non-aggressive behaviors, i.e., pacing, inappropriate dressing/undressing, repetitive actions[8]

2. Potential Etiologies

a) Medications: opioids, phenothiazines, benzodiazepines, anticholinergics, beta-blockers, diuretics, dopaminergics, steroids, atropine, phenytoin, H_2 antagonists, digoxin (at toxic levels)

b) Unrelieved pain, discomfort or other unrelieved symptoms, especially where pre-existing condition, such as dementia, may alter the person's ability to identify and express symptoms

c) A full bladder or bowel are major causes of delirium

d) Infection (UTI, lung, septicemia)

e) Brain tumor, primary or metastatic or CNS pathology

f) Cardiac or respiratory failure

g) Metabolic disturbance (calcium, urea nitrogen, glucose, sodium)

h) Nicotine, alcohol, drug withdrawal

i) Extreme, uncontrolled anxiety

j) Other: fever, heart failure, sleep disruption

3. Assess for

a) Confusion vs. delirium vs. depression using available tools such as those listed below[8]

    i. Memorial Delirium Assessment Scale (MDAS)

    ii. Delirium Rating Scale (DRS)

       iii.   Neecham Confusion Scale (NCS)

       iv.   Confusion Assessment Method (CAM)

       v.   Mini-Mental Status Examination (or Brief Mini-Mental Status Examination)

       vi.   Bedside Confusion Scale[9]

b) Differentiation between hyperalert-hyperactive and hypoalert-hypoactive variants of delirium

c) Patient's previous personality and emotional coping abilities

d) Alcohol, drug use history; recent nicotine, alcohol or drug use

e) Signs of infection

       i.   Fever, flushing, tachycardia, tachypnea, perspiration

       ii.   These symptoms of infection may not be present in persons with immunosuppression due to corticosteroids, chemotherapy, disease process or in the elderly

f) Abdominal examination: palpate for bladder or bowel, abdominal distention

g) Bowel history, noting time and character of last bowel movement; rectal examination for impaction

h) If diabetic history or currently on corticosteroids, capillary blood glucose

i) Lab studies including: BUN, creatinine, electrolytes, glucose, calcium

j) Consider midstream clean-catch urinalysis, culture and sensitivity

k) Neurologic status: dysphasia, weakness, bilateral strength, coordination, poor coordination

l) Patient safety

m) Patient and family coping with change in mental status and ways of managing patient

n) Determine if and to what degree cognitive dysfunction is distressing to the patient; determine same for the family

o) Differentiate between confused agitated delirium and anxiety

4. Potential diagnoses

a) Altered mental status changes potentially related to (etiology)

b) High safety risk for fall related to altered mental status

c) Impaired bowel function related to constipation from (etiology)

d) Impaired bladder function related to retention from (etiology)

e) Disturbed physiologic response to infection related to corticosteroid use, aging

f) Impaired physiologic response related to alcohol, drugs, medication

g) Risk for alcohol, drug withdrawal due to recent use

5. Planning and Intervention

a) Etiology of altered mental status will determine intervention plan

b) Effective pain control and control of other disabling symptoms

    c)   Assess patient's current medications for compliance, effects and iatrogenic effects (side effects) contributing to altered mental status

    d)   Review with physician; consider discontinuation or reduction of medications thought to be contributing to patient's confusion

    e)   Correct metabolic imbalance, if appropriate

    f)   Support alcohol, drug withdrawal chemically as indicated

    g)   Treat infection as appropriate

    h)   For impaction, disimpact; establish aggressive bowel regimen

    i)   For urine retention, straight or retention catheter to relieve

    j)   Support withdrawal from nicotine, alcohol or drugs if withdrawal is contributing to agitation

    k)   Reassure patient and family and provide constant, consistent reorientation of confused patient (assess the degree to which the patient tolerates this, especially if there is underlying dementia; orient only to the extent necessary to maintain care)

    l)   Provide for patient's safety; follow agency/institutional policy regarding the use of restraints, both chemical and physical

    m)   Avoid sedation if possible

    n)   Psychotropic drugs do not reverse confusion or altered mental status, but they may calm distressing agitation, paranoia or hallucinations

        i.   Neuroleptics are considered first line pharmacological agents in managing delirium. Haloperidol, chlorpromazine are first line

        ii.   The newer atypical neuroleptics, such as risperidone, are particularly helpful in managing agitation and hallucinations in the elderly

6.   Patient and family education

    a)   Since confusion is most distressing to patients and families, much education and support is required

    b)   Identify and explore family/caregiver expectations for behavior; educate to adjust expectations if necessary

    c)   Intermittent nature of most confusion

    d)   Expected therapeutic response to interventions

    e)   Expected medication effects and potential side effects

    f)   Safety needs of patient during periods of confusion, agitation

    g)   Importance of compliance with bowel regimen, bladder emptying

7.   Evaluate

    a)   Effectiveness of interventions

        i.   Medications

        ii.   Non-pharmacologic interventions

    b)   Family participation and coping

    c)   Reassess to determine additional needs

8.   Revise plan according to findings from ongoing evaluations, changes in patient status or family needs

B. Terminal Restlessness

1.   Definitions

    a)   Excessive restlessness, increased mental and physical activity[10]

    b)   Commonly seen features are frequent, non-purposeful motor activity, inability to concentrate or relax, disturbances in sleep or rest patterns, potential for progression to agitation[11]

2.   Potential etiologies include

    a)   Full bladder, constipation/impaction

    b)   Hypoxia, dyspnea

    c)   Left ventricular failure, decreased cardiac output

    d)   Uncontrolled pain

    e)   Denial, anxiety, unfinished emotional and/or spiritual issues

    f)   Also consider the possible etiologies listed above for confusion/delirium/agitation

3.   Assess for

    a)   Etiology of terminal restlessness

    b)   Emotional, spiritual history related to issues, personal peace, resolution

    c)   Shortness of breath or labored breathing; lung sounds

    d)   Bladder and bowel status

    e)   Hallucinations, muscle twitching or jerking

    f)   "Sundowning"

4.   Potential diagnoses

    a)   Disturbed mental status related to (etiology)

    b)   High risk for injury due to agitation and uncontrolled restlessness

    c)   Family coping impairment related to severe stress of uncontrolled agitation

5.   Plan and interventions

    a)   Terminal agitation often constitutes active crisis and calls for emergent control of symptoms with aggressive and committed management

    b)   Etiology of restlessness will determine intervention plan

    c)   Disimpaction, bladder relief if distended

    d)   Consult physician for pharmacologic management. Medications may include

        i.   Analgesics for pain and sedation; propofol is used in combination with opioids for palliative sedation, but mainly in an inpatient setting

    ii. Antipsychotics

      (a) Chlorpromazine *(ThoRAZiNE)*

      (b) Haloperidol

      (c) The newer atypical neuroleptics such as risperidone, olanzapine and quetiapine are particularly helpful in managing agitation and hallucinations in the elderly

    iii. Benzodiazepines

      (a) Lorazepam (if no delirium)

      (b) Diazepam

      (c) Midazolam

    iv. Barbiturates

      (a) Phenobarbital

e) Medications should be given by the least invasive route possible: oral, rectal, transdermal, subcutaneous or intravenous; intramuscular route should be used only if absolutely necessary

f) Regular assessment of medication effects

g) Pharmacologic control of muscle twitching, jerking

h) Pastoral and psychological support of patient and family for emotional and spiritual issues

i) Non-pharmacologic approaches including

    i. Subdued, quiet, calm environment

    ii. Consistent, familiar faces and staff

    iii. Calm and reassuring presence

    iv. Relaxation techniques

      (a) Visualization

      (b) Distraction

      (c) Massage

    v. Pet therapy, if appropriate

    vi. Music therapy, especially by a trained music thanatologist, can be particularly helpful

6. Family education

a) Calm environment, presence with minimal stimulation

b) Non-pharmacologic methods for cueing patient with relaxation, visualization, massage, music, distraction

c) Expected therapeutic response to medications and potential side effects

d) Prepare family for patient's sedation response to medications

e) Prepare family for patient's death; encourage speaking with/to patient and using "letting go" language and phrases if family able

7. Evaluate

   a) Effectiveness of interventions

      i. Medications

      ii. Non-pharmacologic interventions

   b) Family participation and coping

   c) Reassess to determine additional needs

8. Revise plan according to findings from ongoing evaluations, changes in patient status or family needs

IV. Anorexia and Cachexia

A. Definitions

1. Anorexia: loss of appetite or inability to take in nutrients

2. Cachexia: weight loss and wasting due to inadequate intake of nutrients

B. Possible Etiologies

1. Anorexia

   a) Pain

   b) Constipation

   c) Nausea and vomiting

   d) Alteration in oral mucous membranes (candidiasis, xerostomia, mucositis)

   e) Impaired gastric emptying

   f) Change of taste in foods (dysgeusia); change in smell of foods

   g) Dental pain and/or dentures not fitting properly

   h) Altered mental status (depression, dementia, confusion, anxiety)

   i) Fatigue

   j) Medications (opioids, antibiotics)

   k) Radiation or chemotherapy

   l) Natural progression of disease; part of body's mechanism of dying

2. Cachexia

   a) Increased nutritional losses related to etiologies associated with anorexia

   b) Increased nutritional losses associated with[4]

      i. Bleeding

      ii. Diarrhea

      iii. Malabsorption of nutrients (i.e., pancreatic cancer)

c) Metabolic Disorders

    i. Abnormal protein metabolism (negative nitrogen balance and decreased muscle mass)

    ii. Abnormal carbohydrate metabolism due to inefficient energy metabolism

    iii. Abnormal lipid metabolism (overall depletion of total body fat)

    iv. Change in fluid and electrolyte balance (increase in extracellular fluid and total body sodium and decrease in intracellular fluid and total body potassium)[4]

C. Assess for

1. History of loss of appetite, including reasons for loss (i.e., change in taste or smell, dysphagia, nausea and vomiting)

2. Patient food likes and dislikes

3. Oral mucosa for dryness, sores, candidiasis

4. Medications that may cause a decrease in appetite

5. Symptoms of malabsorption, such as diarrhea

6. Decrease in bowel sounds

7. Signs and symptoms of constipation or fecal impaction

8. Signs and symptoms of metabolic disorder, such as hypoglycemia, hypernatremia, hypokalemia, dehydration, hypercalcemia

9. Patient/family knowledge of etiology of anorexia and cachexia

D. Potential Diagnoses

1. Nutrition less than body requirements related to anorexia

2. Fatigue, related to decreased nutritional intake secondary to anorexia

3. Body image disturbance, related to cachexia

4. Anxiety related to inability to eat as desired

5. Patient/family knowledge deficit related to etiology and management of anorexia/cachexia

E. Plan/Interventions[4]

1. Encourage patient and family to prepare foods the patient likes and have those foods available whenever the patient requests them

2. Refer to interdisciplinary team dietitian

3. Give patient permission to eat less than before

4. Encourage small, frequent meals rather than three large meals

5. Avoid strong odors; allow food to cool before serving

6. Serve small portions with a pleasing appearance

7. In cases where anorexia is due to nausea/vomiting, altered oral mucous membranes, constipation or diarrhea. Refer to the sections in this chapter on treating these symptoms

8. Encourage nutritional supplements if tolerated

9. Enteral feedings may be appropriate in certain cases if patient's GI function is adequate for digestion/absorption

10. Parenteral nutrition support (total or peripheral parenteral nutrition, i.e., TPN or PPN) if indicated and desired by patient/family (rare in hospice setting)

11. Address emotional needs of family in providing food and fluids

12. Pharmacologic interventions (see Table 2)

    a) Mirtazapine to treat anorexia, insomnia and depression

F. Patient/Family Education

1. Encourage patient to eat as often as desired, but assure patient it is okay not to eat if it is uncomfortable

2. Explain dying process to patient/family, especially that anorexia is normal in last days of life

3. Encourage open communication regarding nutrition

G. Evaluate

1. Has patient's appetite and nutritional intake increased, if this was a goal?

2. Patient/family response to interventions. Are they satisfied with outcome?

3. Are symptoms contributing to anorexia/cachexia treated, if appropriate?

H. Revise plan according to findings from ongoing evaluations, changes in patient status or family needs

V. Ascites

A. Definition: the accumulation of excessive fluid in the peritoneal cavity

B. Possible Etiologies

1. Portal hypertension: obstruction of portal vessels, causing leakage into abdominal cavity. Usually due to

    a) Cirrhosis

    b) Cancer (ovarian, endometrial, breast, colon, pancreatic, gastric, lymphoma, liver)

    c) Cardiac dysfunction: congestive heart failure, constrictive pericarditis

2. Decreased plasma oncotic pressure: decrease in plasma albumin levels, causing fluid to leave plasma and accumulate in abdomen. Usually due to

    a) Cirrhosis

    b) Nephrotic syndrome

    c) Malnutrition

Table 2: Anorexia/Cachexia: Pharmacologic Interventions

Class of Drug	Example(s)	Comments
Gastrokinetic Agents	Metoclopramide 10 mg PO TID *Reglan*	Useful in patients complaining of nausea or early satiety.
Corticosteroids	Dexamethasone 4 mg PO q am, then taper gradually to the minimum effective dosage	Highly effective in improving appetite in the short term, with side effects at the dosage recommended; may lose efficacy after a few weeks.
Progesterone Analogs	Megestrol acetate 400–800 mg PO QD MedroxyPROGESTERone acetate100 mg PO TID	80% of patients will show improvement in appetite; significant decreases in nausea and vomiting occur in more than 50%; abnormalities of taste are often reduced and weight gain (of fat, fluid and lean body mass) is seen in nearly all patients except those in the most terminal stages. Treatment with recommended dosage costs $2/day (more expensive but has fewer side effects than steroids).
Cannabinoids	Dronabinol 2.5 mg PO BID 1 hour PC	An effective appetite stimulant in low doses, without the usual side effects of drowsiness and muddled thinking.
Alcohol	1 glass of beer or sherry before meals	May improve appetite and morale in patients who enjoyed a drink before dinner when they were well.
Vitamins	Multivitamins Vitamin C, 500 mg QID	Anecdotal evidence of improved appetite (may be due to placebo effect).

Reprinted from *Handbook for Palliative Care in Cancer,* 2nd ed, Waller A, Caroline NL, p. 152, Copyright 2000, with permission from Elsevier.

3. Lymphatic obstruction due to tumor infiltration in the abdomen, causing a buildup of fluid in the abdomen

4. Other not related to malignancy: pancreatitis, TB, bowel perforation

C. **Assess for**

1. History relating to etiology (i.e., liver damage, cancer, alcoholism)

2. Weight gain

3. Tachycardia, dyspnea, orthopnea

4. Discomfort related to pressure

5. Decrease in mobility: unable to bend or sit straight

6. Peripheral edema

7. Abdominal signs

    a) Measure abdominal girth every visit

    b) Fluid wave test

    c) Shifting dullness test

    d) Abdominal striae

    e) Distended abdominal wall veins

8. Dehydration

9. Anorexia/early satiety

D. Diagnoses

1. Pain, related to increasing abdominal girth

2. Immobility and fatigue secondary to ascites

3. Impaired gas exchange related to ascites

4. Activity intolerance related to ascites

5. Patient/family knowledge deficit related to etiology and treatment of ascites

E. Planning and Intervention

1. Treatment is determined by the extent of fluid accumulation

2. Analgesics (usually low-dose opioids) can be used for the pain and discomfort of abdominal distention

3. Fluid and sodium restriction: limit fluid to 500–1000 cc/day and sodium to 200–1000 mg/day; may not be successful in malignant ascites[12]

4. Diuretics may be added if fluid and sodium restriction has not been successful after four to five days; spironolactone is drug of choice, with furosemide added if spironolactone alone is not successful

5. Paracentesis may be indicated for palliation if the patient's comfort is extremely compromised

6. Palliative chemotherapy may reduce tumor size and invasion, which may be causing ascites

7. Close monitoring of intake and output may be needed, depending on where patient is on disease trajectory

F. Patient/Family Education

1. Discuss dietary measures (fluid and sodium restriction) to reduce ascites

2. Explain effects of medication and potential side effects (including dehydration for diuretics)

3. Explain skin problems associated with ascites and demonstrate proper measures for maintaining skin integrity

4. Discuss signs and symptoms of infection if paracentesis is part of the treatment plan

5. Discuss/review patient's goals for overall quality of life; ongoing assessment re: when risks and inconvenience of paracentesis outweigh benefits

G. Evaluate

1. Effectiveness of interventions and patient/family teaching (are patient/family satisfied with outcome?)

2. Medication effectiveness and presence of side effects

3. Skin integrity

H. Revise plan according to findings from ongoing evaluations, changes in patient status or family needs

VI. Aphasia

A. Definition: absence or impairment of ability to communicate through speech, writing or signs

B. Possible Etiologies

1. Left cerebral hemisphere lesion from infarct, hemorrhage, tumor, trauma or degeneration

2. Advanced dementia, cerebral vascular disease

C. Assess for

1. Type of aphasia

    a) Sensory (receptive) aphasia: inability to comprehend spoken or written words

    b) Motor (expressive) aphasia: comprehension but inability or impairment of speech

    c) Global (sensory and motor) aphasia: failure of all forms of communication

2. Impairment of patient's ability to communicate pain, comfort needs

3. Difficulty in assessment of patient orientation, knowledge, judgment, abstraction, calculation ability and emotional responses, which can impact patient education, safety management

4. Caregiver's abilities, willingness to interpret patient's needs

5. Patient and family frustration, anxiety about deficits in communication

D. Potential Diagnoses

1. Speech and communication impairment related to type of aphasia and probable etiology

2. Compromised patient/family coping, stress, tolerance related to onset of aphasia

3. Patient knowledge deficit related to adjustment to impairment, disease process, therapeutic regimen related to aphasia

E. **Planning and Intervention**

1. Model acceptance and patience in communication

2. Speech therapy clinician consultation for recommendations for improving communication

3. Writing or picture boards for expressive aphasia

4. Ongoing inquiry and monitoring of patient's non-verbal behaviors for anxiety, pain, discomfort

5. Consistency in communication with patient from family and interdisciplinary team members

F. **Patient/Family Education**

1. Instruct, support caregiver/family in learning patient's non-verbal cues and developing signs, signals for communicating patient's needs: e.g., pain relief, toileting, thirst, hunger, repositioning, emotional feelings

2. Instruct in reducing excessive stimuli in environment that can distract communication

G. **Evaluate for Effectiveness of Interventions, Specifically**

1. Development of alternate communication tools

2. Patient/family coping and adaptation

3. Patient comfort: symptom progression or relief (pain or other)

4. Patient needs being met

5. Interdisciplinary team consistency

H. **Revise plan according to findings from ongoing evaluations, changes in patient status or family needs**

VII. Bladder Spasms

A. **Definition: intermittent, painful contractions of the detrusor muscle, leading to suprapubic pain and urgency**

B. **Possible Etiologies**

1. Indwelling catheter and/or problems associated with indwelling catheters (obstruction, size of catheter or balloon too large)

2. Urinary tract infection

3. Encroachment on bladder or urethra by tumor or impacted feces

4. Radiation or chemotherapy cystitis

5. Urethral obstruction by tumors or blood clots

6. Neurologic disorders: stroke, spinal cord lesions, multiple sclerosis

C. **Assess for**

1. Possible etiologies as documented in the medical history (history of bladder or prostate cancer, neurologic disorders, recent radiation or chemotherapy)

2. Signs and symptoms of urinary tract infection

3. Indwelling catheter function, assess catheter and balloon size as possible source of spasm

4. Hematuria

5. Food and fluid intake: some foods aggravate symptoms; adequate fluid intake important for urinary tract health

6. Presence of fecal impaction

D. **Potential Diagnoses**

1. Pain related to bladder spasm secondary to obstruction/infection/disease process

2. Altered urinary elimination related to bladder spasm

3. Patient and family knowledge deficit related to disease process, management of indwelling catheter and treatment of bladder spasm

E. **Planning and Intervention: Etiology will guide treatment**

1. Presence of indwelling catheter

   a) Reassess the need for urinary catheter

   b) Change catheter to appropriate size

   c) Partially deflate balloon

   d) Gently irrigate with normal saline

   e) May need to initiate continuous saline irrigation if etiology is related to blood clots

2. Urinary tract infection

   a) Antibiotics

   b) Reassess the need for urinary catheter

   c) Change catheter if catheterized

   d) Increase oral fluid intake if feasible

3. Disimpact if etiology is fecal impaction

4. Non-pharmacologic measures: assisting the patient to void every 4 hours, sitting or standing to void, teach relaxation techniques

5. Pharmacologic measures: antispasmodic drugs such as oxybutynin; NSAIDs; Belladonna and Opium (B & O) suppositories

F. **Patient/Family Education**

1. Explain etiology of bladder spasm and measures to reduce symptoms

2. Demonstrate proper catheter care and explain signs and symptoms of catheter obstruction

3. Explain signs and symptoms of urinary tract infection

4. Teach expected medication effects and potential side effects

G. **Evaluate**

1. Effectiveness of interventions and/or medications in decreasing pain related to bladder spasm

2. Effectiveness of antibiotic therapy, if appropriate

3. Patient/family understanding of interventions and medication regimen and recognition of symptoms

H. **Revise plan according to findings from ongoing evaluations, changes in patient status or family needs**

VIII. Bowel Incontinence

A. **Definition: the inability to control bowel movements**

B. **Possible Etiologies**

1. Obstruction, including fecal impaction or tumor (overflow incontinence)

2. Diarrhea (see Section XI: Diarrhea)

3. Sphincter damage due to rectal carcinoma, recto-vaginal fistula or inflammatory bowel disease involving the rectum

4. Sensory or motor dysfunction of the rectosphincter due to spinal cord lesions or compression, multiple sclerosis, diabetes

5. Changes in sphincter tone related to age or spinal cord compression

6. Dementia or mobility related (unable to verbalize or recognize need or unable to reach the toilet)

C. **Assess for**

1. Rectal urgency and passage of loose or formed stool without patient control; incontinence of formed stool usually related to dementia,[13] fecal impaction

2. Functional status: is patient able to reach toilet?

3. Neurologic and sensory function

4. Skin integrity

D. **Potential Diagnoses**

1. Bowel incontinence related to obstruction, diarrhea, neurosensory dysfunction or impaired cognition

2. Risk for impaired skin integrity related to bowel incontinence

3. Patient/family knowledge deficit related to etiology and management of bowel incontinence

4. Patient/family anxiety related to bowel incontinence

E.   Planning and Intervention: Etiology will guide interventions

1.   Review bowel regimen and adjust laxative dose as needed if patient is taking opioids for pain

2.   Utilize opioids for constipating effect (codeine most effective)

3.   Disimpact if fecal impaction is causing incontinence; may need opioid or anxiolytic prior to disimpaction

4.   Modify dietary practices if appropriate and as tolerated

   a)   Decrease fiber intake to reduce bulk formation of stool

   b)   Increase fluid intake of lukewarm, room temperature or cool beverages (very cold or hot liquids can act as stimulants)

   c)   Avoid spicy, greasy, rich and fried foods; avoid caffeine and large amounts of milk products

   d)   Incorporate bananas, rice, applesauce into diet; eat several small frequent meals rather than large meals

5.   Alter environment to place patient closer to toileting facilities

6.   Initiate a bowel routine (i.e., taking patient to toilet after eating)

7.   Maintain skin integrity with adequate skin cleansing and liberal use of skin protectant ointment

8.   Utilize incontinence products

F.   Patient/Family Education

1.   Explain etiology of bowel incontinence and appropriate interventions relative to the etiology

2.   Explain effects of medication and potential side effects

3.   Demonstrate correct hygiene and skin care techniques to prevent skin breakdown

4.   Explain safety measures if altering environment for ease in toileting (i.e., have patient call for assistance, bowel routine, assuring clear path to bathroom)

G.   Evaluate

1.   Effectiveness of interventions and patient/family teaching (Are patient/family satisfied with outcome?)

2.   Medication effectiveness and presence of side effects

3.   Skin integrity

4.   Patient safety

H.   Revise plan according to findings from ongoing evaluations, changes in patient status or family needs

IX. Bowel Obstruction

A.   Definition: occlusion of the lumen of the intestine, delaying or preventing the normal passage of feces

B.   Possible Etiologies

1.   External compression of the lumen (i.e., tumor enlargement, metastases, adhesions, organomegaly)

2.   Internal occlusion of the lumen (i.e., tumor, intussusception)

3.   Ischemic or inflammatory processes (i.e., Crohn's disease, diverticulitis, peritonitis, pancreatitis, hernia)

4.   Fecal blockage (severe constipation can mimic obstruction)

5.   Adynamic ileus (i.e., pneumonia, metabolic/electrolyte problems)

6.   Metabolic disorders (i.e., Crohn's disease, hypokalemia)

7.   Drugs (i.e., diuretics can cause hypokalemia, which decreases peristalsis; opioids; chemotherapy)

8.   Often more than one etiology is present when a bowel obstruction develops

C.   Assess for

1.   History: predisposition to obstruction (most common in ovarian and pancreatic cancers, pancreatitis, etc.), history of bowel habits, medication usage, history of pain

2.   Pain

    a)   Crampy, colicky pain in the middle to upper abdomen relieved with vomiting suggests a small bowel obstruction

    b)   Crampy pain in the lower abdomen that increases over time suggests a large bowel obstruction

    c)   Severe, steady pain is a sign of bowel strangulation

3.   Abdominal distention: present and possibly severe in obstruction of the large intestine; visible peristalsis may be present; patient may complain of constipation and bloating

4.   Nausea and vomiting: moderate to severe in small bowel obstruction and can relieve pain. May develop later in obstruction of the large intestine

5.   Bowel sounds: hyperactive sounds and borborygmi; hypoactive or absent sounds with adynamic ileus

6.   Constipation and inability to pass flatus seen in complete obstruction

7.   Diarrhea due to overflow of feces related to fecal impaction

8.   Fever and chills could indicate bowel ischemia or strangulation

D.   Possible Diagnoses

1.   Pain related to bowel obstruction

2.   Potential for fluid and electrolyte imbalances related to vomiting secondary to bowel obstruction

3.   Anxiety related to pain and inability to defecate secondary to bowel obstruction

4.   Nausea and vomiting related to bowel obstruction

5.   Patient/family knowledge deficit related to etiology and treatment of bowel obstruction

E.   **Planning and Intervention**

1.   Goal of treatment is prevention whenever possible

2.   Disimpact if necessary, utilizing an opioid or anxiolytic if needed for patient comfort

3.   Surgery may be considered if

a)   This is patient's first obstruction

b)   The obstruction occurs in only one site

c)   The patient has a >2 months prognosis and good overall function[14]

d)   Surgery is not usually indicated for non-mechanical obstructions

4.   Medication for pain including antimuscarinic/anticholinergic drugs (loperamide or scopolamine, atropine, glycopyrrolate) and opioids

5.   Octreotide: lacks the adverse effects of the antimuscarinic agents. Can be administered as a SQ injection or a continuous IV infusion[15]

6.   Corticosteroids may be used to decrease inflammatory response and resultant edema, as well as relieve nausea

7.   Stimulant laxatives (senna, bisacodyl) and prokinetics (metoclopramide) should be discontinued if patient is experiencing colicky pain[13]

8.   Medication for nausea and vomiting (if symptoms are distressful for patient) including promethazine, prochlorperazine, haloperidol or lorazepam, if benzodiazepines not contraindicated

9.   Gastric decompression using NG suction may be necessary for relief of gastric distention and nausea; if symptoms persist, percutaneous gastrostomy placement can aid in venting

10. Oral fluids should be increased if tolerable and nausea and vomiting can be controlled; parenteral fluids may be considered if vomiting is not controlled and patient at risk for severe dehydration if consistent with patient goals

11. Treat constipation or diarrhea according to interventions outlined in Sections X and XI

F.   **Patient/Family Education**

1.   Explain etiology and treatment course of bowel obstruction

2.   Explain medication effects and possible side effects

3.   Demonstrate post-operative care of incisions/gastrostomy tube, if appropriate

4.   Explain importance of bowel regime and assist in initiating regime, if appropriate

5.   Support patient and family in review of goals and decision-making, including acceptance of this as an end stage event

[handwritten margin note: SANDOSTATIN]

G. **Evaluate**

1. Effectiveness of interventions and patient/family teaching

2. Effects and side effects of medications

3. Patient/family understanding of treatment and prevention of further obstruction

H. **Revise plan according to findings from ongoing evaluations, changes in patient status or family needs**

X. **Constipation**

A. **Definition: difficulty in passing stools or an incomplete or infrequent passage of hard stools**

B. **Possible Etiologies**

1. Intestinal obstruction: tumors in bowel wall, external compression of the bowel by pelvic or abdominal tumors

2. Medications: opioids, tricyclic antidepressants, phenothiazines, antacids, diuretics, iron, vincristine, antihypertensives, anticonvulsants, anticholinergics or drugs with anticholinergic effects, NSAIDs

3. Metabolic disorders: hypercalcemia, hypokalemia, hypothyroidism

4. Other disease processes or disorders: colitis, diverticular disease, diabetes

5. Dietary problems: low fiber intake, inadequate fluid intake, dehydration

6. Neurologic: confusion, depression, sedation

7. Weakness, inactivity and immobility

8. Pain associated with constipation, including anal fissures or hemorrhoids, straining at stool, etc.

9. Decrease in privacy or unfamiliar toilet facilities; patient reluctant to ask for help in toileting (embarrassment, loss of independence, do not want to be a burden, etc.)

C. **Assess for**

1. Bowel history

    a) Last bowel movement and bowel movement prior to last

    b) Amount, color, consistency

    c) Straining or pain during defecation

    d) Current bowel regimen: does patient need aids in defecation, such as laxatives, suppositories or digital removal

2. Food and fluid intake

3. Medications contributing to constipation

4. Mobility potential

5. Abdominal assessment: abdominal distension and/or tenderness; may report feeling of fullness or bloating; bowel sounds may be normal or hypoactive; percussion reveals dullness in otherwise tympanic areas; may be able to palpate stool in colon

6. Increase in flatus

7. Nausea, vomiting

8. Rectal examination: presence of hemorrhoids, anal fissures; digital examination might reveal hard stool or large amount of soft stool in rectum

9. Patient/family understanding of underlying cause of constipation, expected effects of medication or non-pharmacological remedies

D. Potential Diagnoses

1. Risk for constipation related to opioid or other constipating medication usage, immobility, decrease in food, fluid intake

2. Constipation related to opioid medication usage, immobility, decrease in food, fluid intake

3. Alteration in comfort related to constipation

4. Patient/family knowledge deficit related to appropriate bowel regimen

E. Planning and Intervention

1. Goal in control of opioid-induced constipation is prevention of constipation

2. Bowel obstruction should be ruled out and disimpaction considered if appropriate

    a) If digitally disimpacting, give an opioid or anxiolytic prior to intervention

    b) Digital disimpaction contraindicated in neutropenic or thrombocytopenic patients; may be contraindicated in end stage cardiac patients

3. Non-pharmacologic therapies

    a) Increase fluid intake: water and fruit juices are most effective (prune juice is especially helpful)

    b) Encourage high-fiber foods; examples include: whole grain breads and cereals, bran cereal, fresh, canned, frozen or dried fruits and vegetables

    c) Increase activity, including active or passive range of motion if possible

    d) Ask patient what has been effective in the past

4. Pharmacologic therapies

    a) If patient is at risk for constipation, prophylactic stool softener and stimulant laxatives should be started (example: senna with docusate sodium)[13]

    b) Patient may use own regimen, but regular use should be stressed, especially if using opioids

    c) Titrate bowel meds to changes in opioid dosing

    d) If no bowel movement in three days, regardless of intake, fluids should be increased and an osmotic laxative

        i. Lactulose can be used when there is liver involvement to treat constipation and elevated ammonia levels

   ii. Sorbitol less expensive than lactulose and can be used when there is no liver involvement

  e) For continuing constipation, a glycerin or bisacodyl suppository or sodium biphosphate enema may be added[13]

  f) Discontinue medications that may cause constipation if not medically necessary (i.e., iron or calcium supplements)

 5. Rectal pain or discomfort: consider hemorrhoid preparations or warm sitz baths (rule out herpes in the case of a patient with HIV disease)

F. Patient/Family Education

 1. Explain etiology of constipation and instruct in ways to manage

  a) Non-pharmacological interventions: increased food/fluid intake, increased activity

  b) Pharmacological interventions

 2. Continually reinforce necessity of bowel regime, even if patient is not constipated

 3. Explain medication effects and possible side effects

 4. Reinforce that bowel movement should occur at least every three days and further action should be taken if no bowel movement after this time

G. Evaluate

 1. Effectiveness of bowel regime

  a) How often is patient having bowel movement?

  b) Is patient having difficulty during passage of stool?

 2. Assess abdomen and rectum (externally and digitally, if appropriate)

 3. Patient/family understanding of bowel regime, including medications and non-pharmacologic measures to prevent constipation

H. Revise plan according to findings from ongoing evaluations, changes in patient status or family needs

XI. Diarrhea

A. Definition: the frequent passage of loose, unformed, liquid stool

B. Possible Etiologies

 1. Laxative therapy overuse or imbalance

 2. Side effect of other drugs (i.e., NSAIDs, antibiotics)

 3. Radiation and chemotherapy

 4. Food intolerances or tube feedings

 5. Malnutrition (cachexia related to cancer or AIDS)

Figure 1: Algorithm to Prevent and Manage Opioid-Induced Constipation

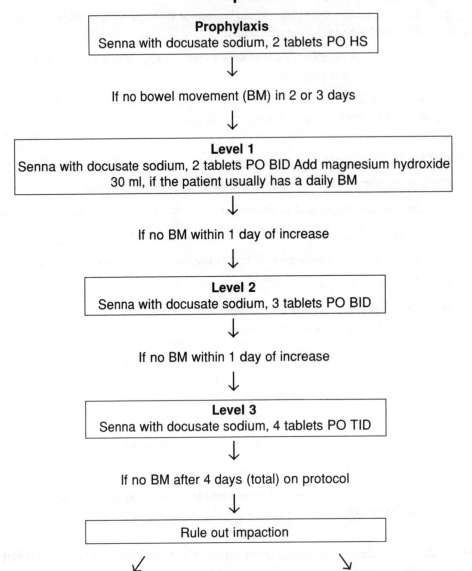

Prophylaxis
Senna with docusate sodium, 2 tablets PO HS

↓

If no bowel movement (BM) in 2 or 3 days

↓

Level 1
Senna with docusate sodium, 2 tablets PO BID Add magnesium hydroxide 30 ml, if the patient usually has a daily BM

↓

If no BM within 1 day of increase

↓

Level 2
Senna with docusate sodium, 3 tablets PO BID

↓

If no BM within 1 day of increase

↓

Level 3
Senna with docusate sodium, 4 tablets PO TID

↓

If no BM after 4 days (total) on protocol

↓

Rule out impaction

If impacted
• disimpact
• administer enemas until clear
• continue daily laxative protocol as outlined above

If no impaction, administer one of the following
• bisacodyl 2 to 3 tablets PO HS to TID
• sodium phosphate-sodium biphosphate enema
• sodium phosphate-sodium biphosphate oral solution (dilute 5 ml to 20 ml in 120 ml of fluid), followed by 240 ml of fluid
• lactulose 45 ml to 60 ml PO
• magnesium citrate 8 oz. PO

From: Plaisance L, Ellis JA. Opioid-induced constipation: management is necessary but prevention is better. *American Journal of Nursing.* 2002;102(3):72–73. Available at www.ajnonline.com. Accessed May 26, 2005. Used with Permission.

6. Surgical procedures: gastrectomy, ileal resection, colectomy

7. Fecal impaction

8. Infection (especially as seen in immunocompromised patients, such as those with AIDS and post-chemotherapy)

9. Partial intestinal obstruction

10. Tumors: gastrointestinal and carcinoid tumors, pancreatic islet cell tumors, small cell lung tumors

11. Gastrointestinal disorders: inflammatory bowel disease, pancreatic insufficiency, diverticulitis, ulcerative colitis, Crohn's disease

12. Other chronic disorders such as diabetes and hyperthyroidism

C. Assessment

1. History, including characteristic of stool, how often stool is occurring, medication usage, recent radiation or chemotherapy treatments or gastrointestinal surgery

2. Review diet, timing of movements in relation to ingestion of food or liquids and a description and quantity and quality of stool[16]

3. Physical exam

    a) Abdominal assessment: bowel sounds may be hyperactive (or hypoactive to absent if intestinal obstruction is present), patient reports of cramping or pain, palpable masses in abdomen may indicate partial obstruction

    b) Nature and consistency of stool (if available to assess): pancreatic insufficiency is indicated by steatorrhea (loose, pale, foul-smelling, greasy stool); fecal impaction may be indicated by small amounts of loose stool

4. Signs of dehydration

5. Skin integrity

D. Potential Diagnoses

1. Diarrhea related to infection, metabolic disorders, medications or therapies, partial obstruction, malnutrition or GI intolerance to food/feedings

2. Risk for impaired skin integrity related to diarrhea

3. Potential for fluid and electrolyte imbalance related to diarrhea

4. Patient/family knowledge deficit related to etiology and treatment of diarrhea

E. Planning and Intervention: Etiology will guide treatment options

1. Increase fluid intake, preferably with electrolyte replacement drinks

2. Clear liquid diet for first 24 hours, with light carbohydrates (rice, crackers, etc.), then advance as tolerated to diet high in protein and calories; avoid spicy, greasy, high-fiber foods and foods high in lactose or caffeine; small, frequent meals are usually better tolerated. Incorporate bananas, rice, applesauce into diet to help keep stool firm in consistency. Avoid milk and other lactose containing products

3. Disimpact if necessary, utilizing opioids or anxiolytics prior to intervention, if needed for patient comfort

4. Discontinue laxatives if certain etiology of diarrhea is not due to impaction

5. Antidiarrheals: loperamide; diphenoxylate HCl with atropine (absorbent and adsorbent agents do not work as fast, so are not indicated in advanced disease); opioids can also be considered if patient is not already taking

6. Pancreatic insufficiency: pancreatic enzymes with meals, with loperamide (slows peristalsis)

7. Maintain skin integrity with adequate skin cleansing and liberal use of skin protectant ointment

F. Patient/Family Education

1. Explain etiology of diarrhea and appropriate interventions relative to the etiology

2. Explain effects of medication and potential side effects

3. Demonstrate correct hygiene and skin care techniques to prevent skin breakdown

4. Explain signs, symptoms and treatment of dehydration

G. Evaluate

1. Effectiveness of interventions and patient/family teaching (are patient/family satisfied with outcome?)

2. Medication effectiveness and presence of side effects

3. Skin integrity

4. Fluid volume status

H. Revise plan according to findings from ongoing evaluations, changes in patient status or family needs

XII. Dysphagia/Odynophagia

A. Dysphagia: a subjective awareness of difficulty in swallowing

1. Possible etiologies

    a) Obstructive: cancer of esophagus and other cancers of the head and neck area, benign peptic stricture and lower esophageal ring (history of GERD [Gastroesophageal Reflux Disease]), compression of vessels or mediastinal nodes. This type of dysphagia is intermittent, usually occurring when eating or drinking; meat and bread are most difficult foods to swallow; some patients can tolerate only liquids[17]

    b) Motor: neuromuscular, esophageal dysfunction (stasis) related to smooth muscle hypertonia or dystonia: e.g., cardiospasm, esophageal aperistalsis, diffuse esophageal spasm (GERD), amyotrophic lateral sclerosis, scleroderma; this type of dysphagia is often for both solids and liquids[17]

Table 3: Pharmacologic Treatments for Diarrhea

Class of Drug	Examples	Mechanism of Action	Comments
Opioids	Diphenoxylate hydrochloride *lomotil*	Suppress forward peristalsis and increase sphincter tone.	5 mg PO QID
	Loperamide hydrochloride		Start at 4 mg PO, then 2 mg after each loose stool, not to exceed 16 mg a day
Bulk-Forming Agents	Psyllium *Metamucil*	Promote absorption of liquid and increase thickness of stool.	Give 1–3 times a day, many preparations available Patient must be able to drink at least 8 glasses of water daily; if they are unable to do so, this is not the appropriate choice of medication
Antibiotics	Metronidazole *Flagyl*	To eliminate infectious processes.	Antibiotic choice is based on etiology
Steroids	Dexamethasone	Decrease inflammation in the gut and provides some relief in partial bowel obstruction and ulcerative colitis.	
Somatostatin	Octreotide	Slows transit time by decreasing secretions.	Suppress diarrhea associated with carcinoid tumors and AIDS

American Association of Colleges of Nursing and the City of Hope National Medical Center. (2000). Pharmacologic treatments for diarrhea, In Module 3: Symptom Management module. *The End-of-Life Nursing Education Consortium (ELNEC)-Core Training Curriculum.* Duarte, CA: Authors. Used with permission.

B.   **Odynophagia: a report of painful swallowing**

    1.   Odynophagia possible etiologies

        a)   Inflammatory process: candidiasis, conditions favoring overgrowth of fungal *Candida albicans* e.g., broad spectrum antibiotics, diabetes mellitus, compromised cellular immunity (AIDS, leukemia, chemotherapy)

        b)   Dry mucous membranes due to xerostomia (decreased quantity or quality of saliva) from radiotherapy, anticholinergic or other medications

        c)   Corrosive esophagitis (ingestion of substance damaging to mucosa)

        d)   Bronchoesophageal fistula with chief complaint: "coughing after ingesting fluids"

C.   **Assess for**

    1.   Etiology of dysphagia or odynophagia, which will direct intervention plan

    2.   Common complaints of swallowing difficulty include choking on fluids, protracted meal times, nasal regurgitation of fluids, difficulty getting swallow started, dry mouth, solids caught in throat, regurgitation or emesis after swallowing, sour taste in mouth after eating and pain on swallowing[3]

3. If odynophagia only, treatment of underlying cause may relieve symptom

    a) Assess oral cavity including tongue, gingiva, mucosa, lips, presence and amount of saliva

    b) Note onset and duration of painful swallowing

    c) Assess voice quality, swallowing ability, oral hygiene

    d) Oral intake: review 24 hour quantity food/liquid

    e) Review history for AIDS, diabetes, chemotherapy, radiotherapy

    f) Review current medications for contributing agents (steroid inhalers, steroids, antibiotics, sulfa)

    g) Presence of creamy white curd-like patches in oropharynx, tongue; patches usually scrape off easily with 4X4 gauze; may cause bleeding

4. Current nutritional status related to disease process, goals of therapies, patient and family expectations

5. If dysphagia, odynophagia are accompanied by anorexia, evaluate patient for disease progression, current nutritional status; discuss management options with interdisciplinary team, patient and family

D. Potential Diagnoses

1. Swallowing impairment, nutritional impairment related to dysphagia × time or odynophagia × time

2. Oral mucous membranes impairment related to: candidiasis, mucositis, xerostomia

3. Patient/family knowledge deficit of: nutrition; types of food, liquids; safety in food selection, expected medication, therapy effects and side effects

E. Planning and Intervention

1. If candidiasis: antifungal swish and swallow QID × 7–10 days; antifungal PO × 5–7 days or fluconazole 150 mg once

2. If mucositis or esophagitis from radiotherapy: topical anesthetic, antihistamine, antacid combination e.g., lidocaine/diphenhydrAMINE/antacid in 1:1:1 ratio as swish and swallow IF patient has gag reflex

3. If obstruction from tumors/nodes: limited dose steroids may reduce inflammatory edema

4. If poor esophageal motility: prokinetic agents (e.g., metoclopramide)

5. If gastroesophageal reflux disease: anti-reflux agents (e.g., omeprazole, ranitidine)

6. If neuro-motor etiology: speech therapy consult may be helpful to evaluate swallow and make recommendation

7. If dry mucosa induced from medications or radiotherapy: artificial saliva, lip balm, exquisite oral care, increase hydration

8. Determine food consistency best tolerated by patient: liquids may have thickening agents added to facilitate swallowing

9. If medications are etiology of dysphagia or odynophagia, consider alternative medicines if appropriate

10. Artificial feeding may be considered for obstructive or fistula processes in some palliative care situations depending upon the patient's place on the disease trajectory, current nutritional and functional status and other factors

F. **Patient/Family Education**

1. Importance of excellent oral hygiene

2. Avoid nicotine, alcohol and caffeine, which increase esophageal and vasospasm and have mucosal drying effects

3. Cool, non-irritating foods and liquids generally better tolerated

4. Encourage patient to chew food well and to avoid large boluses of meat, bread; modify food consistency if necessary, e.g., ground or pureed meats

5. Anticipated medication effects and potential side effects

G. **Evaluate for Effectiveness of Interventions, Specifically**

1. Resolution of candidiasis

2. Improvement in mucosal lubrication

3. Oral hygiene

4. Nutritional status

5. Patient/family understanding of instructions, recommendations

H. **Revise plan according to findings from ongoing evaluations, changes in patient status or family needs**

XIII. Dyspnea/Cough

A. **Definitions**

1. Dyspnea: subjective sensation of shortness of breath

2. Cough: a natural defense of the body to prevent entry of foreign material into the respiratory tract[18]

B. **Possible Etiologies**

1. Dyspnea: lung tumor or metastases, pleural effusion, COPD, CHF, ascites, pneumothorax, pulmonary embolism, anemia, neurologic insult

2. Cough: infection, inflammation, cardiac (left ventricular failure), pulmonary disease (pleural effusion, bronchospasm, bronchogenic cancer), medications (ACE inhibitors), smoke, tobacco abuse or irritation from second-hand smoke, allergic conditions, GERD

C. **Assess for**

1. Dyspnea: etiology will direct intervention plan

   a) Look for simple answers—oxygen on, oxygen tubing kinked, fluid overload, anxiety, pain, constipation, etc.

       b)   Onset of dyspnea. Respiratory rate, depth, quality of respiration, lung sounds, accessory muscle use, stridor

       c)   Past interventions that have provided relief/comfort

       d)   Appropriate use and understanding of current medications for relief of dyspnea and accompanying anxiety

       e)   Whether patient is a carbon dioxide (CO_2) retainer; this will influence decisions regarding oxygen delivery rate, opioid and anxiolytic dosing

       f)   Patient/family anxiety, coping, understanding of dyspnea triggers and etiology and interventions to control dyspnea

   2.   Cough: etiology will direct intervention plan

       a)   History and physical to determine etiology and appropriate treatment

           i.   Productive vs. nonproductive cough

          ii.   If productive, sputum quantity, appearance, including color

         iii.   Diagnostic studies as appropriate

       b)   Effect of cough on patient/family's quality of life

       c)   Need for cough suppressant or cough expectorant based on etiology and patient need

       d)   Fever

D. Potential Diagnoses

   1.   Respiratory alteration related to: impairment of airway clearance, breathing pattern or gas exchange

   2.   Patient/family knowledge deficit of: etiology or triggers of dyspnea and/or cough, steps to relieve dyspnea or anxiety; medication use, effects or side effects

   3.   Patient discomfort related to inability to control cough and/or mobilize secretions

   4.   Patient/family anxiety related to perceived situational powerlessness, fear, breathing impairment

E. Planning and Intervention[18]

   1.   Review of medical history, progression of disease, current medications; etiology of dyspnea will direct intervention plan

   2.   Non-pharmacologic interventions

       a)   Dyspnea

           i.   Position patient in high Fowler's position as appropriate; COPD patients do better leaning forward with upper arms supported on a table

          ii.   Encourage pursed lip breathing in COPD patients

         iii.   Palliative thoracentesis or paracentesis may be considered in selected patients

         iv.   Model calm reassurance

          v.   Encourage intake of nutrient-dense beverages (e.g., commercial supplements) if oral intake is limited because of dyspnea; liquids take less eating effort

vi. Fan directly in front of patient; cool room environment

vii. Complementary therapies such as relaxation techniques, guided imagery, therapeutic touch

viii. Oxygen as appropriate: nasal cannula is better tolerated than a mask, especially in a terminal setting. Oxygen is not always helpful. Try a therapeutic trial, based on symptom relief, not pulse oximetry

b) Productive cough: chest physiotherapy (if able to tolerate), oxygen, humidity and, elevate head of bed, frequent sips of water, throat lozenges

 i. Suctioning rarely indicated unless secretions are accessible in throat or upper airway. Suctioning can worsen congestion by irritation of the mucous membranes

c) Pharmacologic interventions

d) Dyspnea and productive cough

 i. Opioids (PO, SL, SQ, IV or nebulized) for bronchodilatation

  (a) Start low and titrate dose slowly for opioid-naïve patients and patients with CO_2 retention

  (b) For opioid tolerant patients, the dose of opioid is at least equal to the dose used for breakthrough pain

  (c) Monitor respiratory rate and depth

 ii. High dose steroids for obstructive or inflammatory etiologies

 iii. Bronchodilators

 iv. Anticholinergic agents

 v. Expectorant such as guaifenesin

 vi. Antibiotics for infection if appropriate

 vii. Anxiolytic medications may help to reduce the anxiety that often accompanies dyspnea: use and titrate slowly in elderly and patients with CO_2 retention; monitor respiratory rate and depth

 viii. For uncontrolled dyspnea in hospice home-care setting, may consider short-term inpatient management

 ix. Sedation at end of life for refractory dyspnea is an option

 x. Ethical consideration: the fear of using opioids, due to the potential for respiratory depression, to ease terminal dyspnea often leads to inadequate symptom management. The use of these drugs to ease terminal dyspnea is often mistakenly equated with euthanasia or assisted suicide. NOTE: There is no justification for withholding symptomatic treatment to a dying patient out of fear of potential respiratory depression. Excellent communication with family and staff is required to avoid misunderstanding[19]

e) Nonproductive cough

 i. Non-opioid (dextromethorphan, benzonatate) or opioid antitussives

           ii.   Nebulized lidocaine 2% for 10 minutes q 2–6 hours

                (a)   NPO for 1 hour post treatment due to risk of aspiration from loss of gag reflex from anesthetic agent

      f)   Cough associated with CHF

           i.   Diuretic

           ii.   Beta blocker

          iii.   ACE inhibitor

F. Patient/Family Education

1. Reassurance and empowerment of patient/family by review, rehearsal of steps to take when patient's shortness of breath begins

2. Treatment options, medication effects, side effects

3. Demonstrate relaxation techniques when patient/family is not in crisis

4. Instruct others not to crowd dyspneic person and to remain calm, in control of emotions

5. Consistency in information with rehearsal, review by all members of the interdisciplinary team

G. Evaluate

1. Understanding, compliance and effectiveness of medications for dyspneic episodes

2. For patient/family coping; reduction of, improvement in management and control of dyspneic episodes

3. For progression of disease process related to uncontrolled dyspnea

H. Revise plan according to findings from ongoing evaluations, changes in patient status or family needs

XIV. Edema

A. Definition: presence of excessive fluid in the intercellular tissues especially in the subcutaneous tissues

B. Possible Etiologies

1. Protein deficiency

2. Obstruction of venous return: peritoneal tumors, DVT, CHF, superior vena cava syndrome (SVC)

3. Renal failure

4. Lymphedema: blockage of lymphatic return in the periphery or the abdomen from surgical procedures, pressure from tumor

5. Ascites of liver failure; peritoneal inflammation

Table 4: Pharmacologic Treatment of Dyspnea

Class of Drug	Examples	Mechanism of Action	Dosages/Comments
Opioids	Morphine	Exact mechanism for dyspnea is not completely understood	IV—1–4 mg q15 min—4 hrs SQ—1–4 mg q30 min—4 hrs PO—5–15 mg, capsule/tablet or liquid form q 1–4 hrs Rectal—5–15 mg q 1–4 hrs suppository. May need to be compounded.
	Fentanyl		IV—25–40 mcg q 15 min PRN SL—25–40 mcg q 15 min PRN Nebulizer—25 mcg (Coyne et al, 2000)
Bronchodilators (Used frequently in airway obstruction, COPD and asthma conditions)	Albuterol Ipratropium Metaproterenol Salmeterol	Relax smooth muscles of respiratory tract relieving bronchospasm Stimulates β2 agonist, adrenergic receptors of sympathetic nervous system. Relaxing smooth muscles of bronchial tree	Dosages are highly variable and dependent on patient's overall health status, smoking history, age and presence of co-morbid factors. May cause anxiety, cough while worsening dyspnea. Drugs are available in metered dose inhalers, nebulizers or orally
Diuretics (Used in heart failure, reduce fluid overload)	Furosemide	Inhibits reabsorption of electrolytes in ascending limb of the loop of Henle, enhancing excretion of sodium chloride, potassium, calcium and other electrolytes	PO—20–80 mg IV—20–40 mg Dosage varies widely and should be adjusted to patient's requirement and response
Benzodiaze-pines	Lorazepam (There are conflicting reports about the efficacy in the treatment of dyspnea. Therefore it should not be considered a first line treatment)	Appear to act on thalamic/hypothalamic areas of the CNS producing anxiolytic, sedative, hypnotic and skeletal muscle relaxation	IV—0.5–2 mg q8-q12 hrs PO—0.5–2 mg q8-q12 hrs IM—0.5–2 mg q 6-q 12 hrs All routes q8-q12hrs for anxiety. Dosages may vary significantly and should be adjusted to patient's requirements and responses
Non-benzodiaz-epine anxiolytic	BusPIRone	No effect on pulmonary function tests or arterial blood gases, but improves exercise tolerance and decrease sensation of breathlessness in patients with COPD	

(continued)

Class of Drug	Examples	Mechanism of Action	Dosages/Comments
Steroids (Used in asthma and COPD)	Dexamethasone	Mechanism not fully understood. Affects antibody systems. Appears to decrease inflammation (especially associated with vena cava syndrome) and suppresses immune response	Aerosol—0.25 mg–20 mg IV—0.25–20 mg PO—0.25–20 mg IM—0.25–20 mg
Antibiotics Antifungals (used to treat pulmonary infections)	Penicillin Fluconazole	Varies by agent Varies by agent	Varies according to antibiotic given Dose varies, typically 200 mg PO day one then 100 mg qd.
Anticoagulants	Heparin Warfarin	Prevents clot formation which may prevent future incidence of pulmonary emboli	Varies according to lab results

American Association of Colleges of Nursing and the City of Hope National Medical Center. (2000). Pharmacologic treatment of dyspnea, In Module 3: Symptom Management module. *The End-of-Life Nursing Education Consortium (ELNEC)-Core Training Curriculum.* Duarte, CA: Authors. Used with permission.

C. **Assess for**

1. Review of medical history and progression of disease process

2. Etiology of edema, which will direct intervention plan

3. New, increased or returning edema

4. Extremity edema, pitting, non-pitting, tissue perfusion, warmth, cold, presence or absence of leaking from tissues

5. Superior Vena Cava Syndrome (SVC)

    a) Upper body edema, i.e., papilledema, facial edema, distended neck veins, one or both arms depending on where the obstruction is located: note onset, tissues involved

    b) Other symptoms: dyspnea (most common), headache, chest pain, dry cough, visual or mental status changes, dizziness, vertigo

    c) SVC is considered an oncologic emergency and may be palliated with radiotherapy with or without steroids depending on the etiology

    d) Not responsive to diuretics

6. Ascites: abdomen size, tenderness, distention, fluid wave; if elevated diaphragm, may have dyspnea, pleural effusion

7. Patient/family understanding of disease process related to poor perfusion, expected medication effects and possible side effects

Table 5: Pharmacological Interventions for Cough

Class of Drug	Examples	Mechanism of Action	Dosages/Comments
Bronchodilators	Terbutaline	Relax smooth muscles and decrease cough in airway disease	Dosages vary widely
Cough Suppressants —Opiates —Local anesthetics	Morphine Sulfate Benzonatate (Tessalon Perles®)	Central CNS action, suppresses cough Suppresses cough stimulus (anecdotal reports) Inhibits cough by anesthetizing stretch receptors which mediate cough reflex	5 ml of 2% Lidocaine via nebulizer q 4 hrs prn 100 mg PO 3 times a day; may be administered q 4 hours up to 600 mg daily Should not be chewed or dissolved in mouth
Cough Expectorants	Guaifenesin	Increases bronchial secretion viscosity	
Antibiotics	Penicillin	To treat pneumonias or infections of the airway passages	Infrequently used in palliative care but may prove useful in an infectious process
Steroids	Dexamethasone	To decrease inflammation of airways or compression of an airway by tumor	
Anticholinergics	Atropine Hydroscine Ipratropium	Decrease secretion production; decrease cough	
Nebulized saline or humidifier		Used to thin secretions	

American Association of Colleges of Nursing and the City of Hope National Medical Center. (2000). Pharmacologic interventions for cough, In Module 3: Symptom Management module. *The End-of-Life Nursing Education Consortium (ELNEC)-Core Training Curriculum.* Duarte, CA: Authors. Used with Permission.

D.   Potential Diagnoses

1.   Tissue perfusion alteration related to: peripheral edema, ascites, upper body, head and neck edema

2.   Skin integrity impairment and risk related to poor perfusion, subcutaneous tissue edema, increased pressure points

3.   Respiratory alteration related to gas exchange impairment (for dyspnea related to ascites, SVC syndrome)

4.   Patient/family knowledge deficit of disease process, expected medication effects or possible side effects, non-pharmacologic measures

E.   Planning and Intervention

1.   Etiology of edema will direct intervention plan

2.   Symptomatic relief of ascites: spironolactone, paracentesis; diuretics are rarely successful in reducing ascites

3.   Symptomatic relief of peripheral edema: compression stockings; diuretics usually appropriate when there are also crackles heard in lungs; meticulous skin care; active or passive exercise to help venous return if patient can tolerate; limb elevation above level of heart

4.   Lymphedema

a)   Does not respond to diuretics unless there is a true peripheral edema component

b)   May not resolve despite elevation, compression stockings

c)   In the palliative care patient not actively dying, manual lymph drainage therapies may promote better quality of life

d)   Refer patients to therapists specially trained in lymphedema management

F.   Patient/Family Education

1.   Explain etiology of edema and instruct in ways to manage or reduce

2.   Expected medication effects and possible side effects

3.   Application of compression stockings prior to ambulation

4.   Post paracentesis care

5.   Counsel for prevention of lymphedema must be stressed at the beginning and throughout any treatments (surgery, radiation) that predispose to its development; lymphedema has an enormous, long-term impact on quality of life and there is little reversibility once it develops

G.   Evaluate

1.   Effectiveness of medication

2.   For level, return, extension of edema

3.   Patient/family understanding of disease process, medications, application and use of compression stockings and/or manual lymph drainage therapies; non-pharmacologic interventions

H.   Revise plan according to findings from ongoing evaluations, changes in patient status or family needs

XV.   Extrapyramidal Symptoms (EPS)

A.   Definition: involuntary movements, hyperkinetic (akathisia) or hypokinetic (dystonia); tardive dyskinesia is a late-effect, which may not respond to reversal therapies

B.   Possible Etiologies

1.   Iatrogenic drug-induced from

a)   Neuroleptics

b)   Phenothiazines: e.g., chlorpromazine

c)   Butyrophenones: e.g., haloperidol

d)   Clozapine

e)   Metoclopramide

f)   Opioids (myoclonus)

g)   Others

2.   Parkinson's disease, chorea

3.   Cerebral lesions

C.   Assess for

1.   Etiology of EPS from medical history, medication review which will direct intervention plan

2.   Possible iatrogenic response to a medical therapy used to treat a symptom

3.   Patient safety with ambulation, activities of daily living (ADLs)

4.   Patient/family anxiety relating to EPS, understanding of medication effects and side effects

D.   Diagnosis

1.   Impaired physical mobility related to neurologic impairment caused by etiology

2.   Self-care deficit related to immobility, hyperactivity, loss of coordination

3.   Patient/family knowledge deficit related to medication effects or side effects, safety needs

E.   Planning and Intervention

1.   For phenothiazine toxicity

a)   Stop phenothiazine

b)   Benztropine mesylate, trihexyphenidyl, diphenhydrAMINE

2.   For akathisia (inability to sit still, pacing, agitation, restless movements)

a)   Benzodiazepines (lorazepam, diazepam)

b)   Beta-blockers (propranolol)

3.   For dystonia, slow, retarded movements: physical or occupational therapy may be an adjunct if appropriate according to patient's place in the disease process, trajectory

4.   In elderly or others who may have sensitivity to anticholinergics: amantadine

5.   Review of symptoms being treated with medication that may cause EPS; if symptoms remain present, discussion with medical team regarding alternative medications to control

F. **Patient/Family Education**

1. Stopping medication that may be contributing to EPS

2. Expected medication effects and potential side effects

3. Monitoring patient activity; safety in ambulation

G. **Evaluate for Effectiveness of Interventions, Specifically**

1. Effect of medication change on EPS symptoms

2. Patient/family compliance, comfort with new medications

3. Control of symptoms

H. **Revise plan according to findings from ongoing evaluations, changes in patient status or family needs**

XVI. Hematologic Symptoms

A. **Definitions**

1. Hemorrhage: excessive bleeding

2. Clotting: systemic response to disease or medication that initiates coagulation cascade causing clotting

3. Cytopenia: reduction in bone marrow blood cell components, which can precipitate a systemic response

    a) Neutropenia: reduction in white blood cells; decreases patient's ability to respond to infection

    b) Thrombocytopenia: reduction in platelets; increases potential for frank, uncontrolled bleeding

    c) Anemias: reduction in production or maturation of red blood cells; low hemoglobin; decreased oxygen carrying cells; increased dyspnea, fatigue

    d) Pancytopenia: reduction in all blood cells

B. **Possible Etiologies**

1. Initiating coagulation cascade: deep vein thrombosis (DVT)

2. Immunologic processes (AIDS), drug-induced processes, prosthetic cardiac valves, veno-occlusive liver disease initiating coagulation cascade: hemorrhage, disseminated intravascular coagulopathy (DIC)

3. Chemotherapy, radiotherapy or disorders of spleen: thrombocytopenia, pancytopenia

4. Tumor erosion of blood vessels: hemorrhage

5. Pulmonary embolism (PE)

C.   Assess for

1.   Review medical history and current medications for potential hematology problems

2.   Review current medications, foods, herbals for interactions with anticoagulant therapy

3.   For DIC: petechiae, ecchymosis, oozing blood from mucous membranes, body orifices, puncture sites, signs of decreased perfusion to brain, kidneys, gastrointestinal, cardiovascular and peripheral vascular systems, lungs

4.   For DVT: possible peripheral phlebitis, noting vascular access devices, streaking, erythema, heat over vein

5.   For pulmonary embolism: sudden onset dyspnea, chest/back pain, hemoptysis

6.   For thrombocytopenia: periorbital petechiae, epistaxis, gingival bleeding, blood-streaked sputum, emesis, urine or stool; acute shortness of breath, inspiratory pain, vaginal bleeding, petechiae, ecchymosis, joint pain, change in mental status, paresthesias

7.   Patient/family understanding of and coping with changes in blood clotting response or pancytopenia; non-pharmacologic therapies, safety

D.   Potential Diagnoses

1.   Injury risk due to altered clotting patterns related to etiology

2.   Infection risk due to neutropenia and body's reduced ability to control or fight infection

3.   Patient/family knowledge deficit related to expected medication effects or side effects, safety needs, e.g., injury or infection

4.   Medication risk related to anticoagulant therapy and other medications, herbals, foods

E.   Plan and Intervention: treat underlying problem if appropriate

1.   For DVT: anticoagulant therapy; monitor for other medications, foods and herbals that may interfere with anticoagulant therapy; antiembolic stockings

2.   For PE: anticoagulant therapy; monitor other medications, food and herbals that may interfere with anticoagulant therapy; antiembolic stockings, treatment of dyspnea, pain

3.   For thrombocytopenia

     a)   If palliative care: bleeding precautions, platelet transfusion for platelets <10,000, if appropriate

     b)   If hospice: bleeding precautions, treat bleeding with compression, other non-pharmacologic interventions

4.   For DIC: replenish clotting factors, e.g., platelets, fresh frozen plasma, antithrombin factor in palliative care; patient should be in an acute care facility for ongoing monitoring during therapy

5.   For neutropenia: institute precautions against introduction of bacteria, infections to patient

6.   Patient/family support, instruction, reassurance during bleeding and in anticipation of bleed

F.   **Patient/Family Education**

1.   Bleeding precautions

   a)   Soft toothbrush and gentle motions for tooth brushing

   b)   Care when using eating utensils

   c)   Rinses for mouth

   d)   No suppositories

   e)   Safety in ambulation; prevent falls, injury

   f)   Use electric razor rather than straight razor

2.   For active bleed: long pressure for active bleed; use of dark towels; whom to call

3.   For PE: elevate head of bed for dyspnea; palliative oxygen if needed

4.   For DVT: use of antiembolic stockings applied before ambulation; expected anticoagulation medicine effects and side effects

5.   Medicines, food and herbals that can affect anticoagulation including vitamin E, theophylline, carbamazepine, phenytoin, vitamin K (especially high in dark green vegetables)

6.   For neutropenia: regular and frequent hand washing; plants, flowers not in direct proximity; support of family in encouraging visitors with colds, illness to visit when they are well

7.   Review, rehearse with patient and family the steps to take if bleeding begins

G.   **Evaluate**

1.   Effectiveness of medical therapies

2.   Patient compliance with anticoagulant therapy; for therapeutic PTT/PT (partial thromboplastin time/prothrombin time)

3.   Safety in ambulation

4.   Patient/family understanding regarding disease process, safety, expected medicine effects and potential side effects

H.   **Revise plan according to findings from ongoing evaluations, changes in patient status or family needs**

XVII. **Hiccoughs**

A.   **Definition: an involuntary contraction of the diaphragm, followed by rapid closure of the glottis**

B.   **Possible Etiologies**

1.   Gastric distention: impaired gastric motility, excessive gas

2.   Central nervous system: neoplasm, stroke, multiple sclerosis, ventriculoperitoneal shunts, atriovenous malformations, hydrocephalus, lesions from head trauma

3.   Peripheral nervous system: irritation of phrenic or vagus nerve

4.   Tumors of the neck, lung, mediastinum

5. Chest surgery or trauma

6. Respiratory disorders: pulmonary edema, pneumonia, bronchitis, asthma, COPD

7. Gastrointestinal disorders: esophagitis or esophageal obstruction, gastritis, peptic ulcer disease, gastric cancer, pancreatitis, pancreatic cancer, bowel obstruction, cholelithiasis/cholecystitis

8. Renal/hepatic disorders

9. Metabolic disorders: uremia, hypocalcemia, hyponatremia

10. Infectious disease: sepsis, influenza, herpes zoster, malaria, tuberculosis

11. Pharmacologic agents: general anesthesia, IV corticosteroids, barbiturates, benzodiazepines, diazepam, chlordiazepoxide

12. Psychogenic: stress, excitement, grief reactions, anorexia, personality disorders

C. Assess for

1. Include subjective review of how much distress the hiccoughs cause the patient

2. Etiology of hiccoughs related to medical/psychological history and/or medication usage

3. Associated signs and symptoms (underlying disease process, etc.)

4. Severity and duration of current episode and previous episodes

5. Relationship of hiccoughs to sleep: hiccoughs that stop during sleep suggest a psychogenic cause

6. Patient/family concerns and knowledge: are the hiccoughs troublesome? Does anything help to alleviate hiccoughs?

D. Diagnoses

1. Alteration in comfort related to hiccoughs

2. Risk for fluid/nutritional deficit related to dysphagia secondary to hiccoughs

3. Risk for sleep pattern disturbance related to hiccoughs

4. Patient/family knowledge deficit related to etiology and treatment of hiccoughs

E. Planning and Intervention: etiology of hiccoughs can guide intervention plan (i.e., possible reversal of metabolic disorders)

1. Non-pharmacologic interventions: before suggesting non-pharmacologic techniques, assure patient safety and do not suggest techniques that may be harmful, depending upon diagnosis

    a) Nasopharyngeal stimulation

        i. Swallowing one teaspoon of granulated sugar

        ii. Lifting uvula with a spoon or cotton-tip applicator

        iii. Gargling with water

        iv. Biting on a lemon

        v. Swallowing crushed ice

      b)   Interference with normal respiratory function

          i.   Induction of sneezing or coughing

          ii.   Re-breathing into paper bag

          iii. Breath holding or hyperventilation

      c)   Etiology related to gastric distention

          i.   Nasogastric suction

          ii.   Gastric lavage

      d)   Complementary therapies

          i.   Hypnosis and/or behavior modification

          ii.   Acupuncture

      e)   Distraction

2. Pharmacologic Techniques

      a)   If etiology is related to gastric distention

          i.   Simethicone before or after meals

          ii.   Metoclopramide alone or with simethicone before meals

      b)   Peppermint oil relaxes lower esophageal sphincter and is useful for hiccoughs related to esophageal disorders; has opposing action with metoclopramide

      c)   Baclofen if simethicone and metoclopramide fail

      d)   Calcium channel blockers, e.g., NIFEdipine

      e)   Chlorpromazine 25–50 mg tid effective for uremic etiology, but useful in other etiologies as well; postural hypotension a significant side effect, especially when used IV. This is the only FDA drug approved for hiccoughs

      f)   Anticonvulsants: carbamazepine, phenytoin and valproic acid. Reported effectiveness in patients with a CNS etiology of their hiccoughs[20]

      g)   Nebulized lidocaine (3 cm^3 of 4% topical lidocaine nebulized in a standard small-particle nebulizer)

3. Invasive Techniques

      a)   Phrenic nerve interruption with bupivacaine or surgery

      b)   Pacing electrodes for direct phrenic nerve or diaphragmatic stimulation

F.   Patient/Family Education

1. Explain etiology and instruct in ways to treat

2. Explain appropriate, safe non-pharmacological techniques that are realistic for individual patient

3. Expected medication effects and side effects

4. Post-surgical care, if indicated

G. Evaluate

    1. Effectiveness of non-pharmacological techniques and/or medication

    2. Control of hiccoughs

    3. Patient/family understanding of regimen

H. Revise plan according to findings from ongoing evaluations, changes in patient status or family needs

XVIII. Impaired Mobility, Fatigue, Lethargy, Weakness

A. Definitions

    1. Impaired Mobility: a loss or abnormality of function due to physiological, anatomical, psychological or fatigue factors

    2. Fatigue: an overwhelming sustained sense of exhaustion with decreased capacity for physical or mental activity[10]

    3. Lethargy: a condition of functional torpor or sluggishness; stupor[10]

    4. Weakness: a subjective term to indicate a lack of strength as compared to what patient feels is normal

B. Potential Etiologies

    1. Disease process

        a) Sudden onset of weakness or impaired mobility: consider neurologic deficit, e.g., spinal cord compression or other CNS tumor effects; sudden generalized weakness may be adrenal failure or septicemia

        b) Chronic disease: chronic obstructive pulmonary disease (COPD), congestive heart failure (CHF)

        c) Tumor infiltration of bone marrow

        d) Liver disease with coagulopathy

        e) Hypothyroidism: adrenal or hormonal insufficiencies (including chemical and hormonal response to tumor)

        f) Uremia: related to kidney failure, tumor or use of nephrotoxic drugs

        g) Metabolic: hypercalcemia from metastatic disease, parathyroid disease

    2. Uncontrolled pain or other symptoms, anemia, blood loss

    3. Some medications or therapies may contribute to lethargy, weakness: beta blockers, antihistamines, benzodiazepines, phenothiazines, zidovudine, myelosuppressive chemotherapy, radiation therapy

    4. Nutritional deficiencies

        a) Decreased iron, B-12, folate

        b) Anorexia, nausea, vomiting, weight loss

        c) GI malabsorption

5. Infectious processes

    a) AIDS-related infections

    b) Pneumonia

    c) Urinary tract infections

6. Emotional factors: depression, anxiety, sleep disturbance, psychological or spiritual distress, family distress

7. Environmental factors: multiple sensory stimuli (noise, lights, odors)

C. **Assess for Etiology, which will determine intervention plan**

1. Thorough history

    a) Onset, history of or change in functional status

    b) Patient's own description of fatigue, weakness: does it relate to activity? Is it constant? Intermittent? What makes it better or worse?

    c) Effect of lethargy, fatigue, weakness on quality of life scores[21]

    d) Patient's place on disease trajectory of end-stage or terminal illness

2. Symptom management: review adequacy of pain control and management of other debilitating symptoms (including nausea, vomiting, dyspnea, anxiety, depression)

3. Current medications for appropriate use and dose for patient's current weight

4. Psychosocial factors

    a) Sleep, rest disturbance

    b) Depression, anxiety component

    c) Unresolved psychological or spiritual issues or distress

5. Family, caregiver perceptions and impact of patient's fatigue; understanding of disease process

6. Infectious or disease process

7. Dyspnea if anemic

D. **Potential Diagnoses**

1. Activity alteration from fatigue due to (etiology)

2. Self-care deficit related to activity intolerance

3. Risk for altered nutritional, functional status due to activity disturbance

4. Patient/family knowledge deficit of non-pharmacologic interventions, expected medication effects, side effects

5. Impaired physical mobility related to (injury, potential for injury, pain)

6. Alteration in perceived quality of life from fatigue

7. Altered self-image and role disturbance related to change in functional abilities and endurance

E.   Planning and Interventions: etiology of fatigue, impaired mobility, lethargy and weakness will determine intervention plan

1.   Patient's place on disease trajectory for end-stage or terminal illness, wishes and advance directives will influence treatment decisions

2.   Treat specific underlying causes as appropriate

a)   If anemia: based on classification of anemia, consider treatment of cause

b)   If endocrine disorder: determine appropriate therapy

c)   If medication-induced (iatrogenic)

i.   Consider tapering or discontinuing medicine

ii.   If opioid induced, fatigue may resolve when patient develops tolerance (usually 48–72 hours after dose increase)

iii.   If opioid induced lethargy continues and other etiologies have been ruled out and lethargy is unacceptable to the patient/family, consider adding methylphenidate 5 mg PO in the A.M. and at noon to combat sedation and to improve appetite and mood.[22] Titrate if not effective

3.   For depression, anxiety: see Chapter 6

4.   Non-pharmacologic interventions

a)   Balance activities with rest

b)   Hospital bed and other equipment as needed to decrease fatigue from exertion

c)   Set realistic goals for ADLs and other activities

d)   Exercise, physical and occupational therapy as indicated, if tolerated

e)   Increase team services for personal care as needed

F.   Patient/Family Education

1.   Instruct regarding balancing activities and rest

2.   Set activity priorities: e.g., a bedside commode may help patient to conserve the energy used walking to the bathroom for other activities

3.   Expected medication effects and potential side effects especially as they may contribute to fatigue or sedation

4.   Educate family of hospice patient in terminal phase regarding end-stage disease process and encourage setting of realistic expectations

5.   For the palliative care patient who is not in terminal phase of disease process, discourage prolonged bedrest or excessive inactivity explaining possible adverse physical (deep vein thrombosis [DVT], pulmonary embolism [PE], pneumonia, increased weakness) and emotional (depression, decreased motivation, social isolation) effects

G.   Evaluate

1.   Effectiveness of interventions and ability of the caregivers to provide care

2.   Improvement in activity tolerance

3.   Patient for signs of disease progression

4. Patient/family understanding, coping with ongoing fatigue, balancing activities, prioritizing to accomplish essential or preferred activities

5. Further adjustments in team visit frequency to assist in personal care as needed

H. Revise plan according to findings from ongoing evaluations, changes in patient status or family needs

Table 6: Pharmacologic Treatments for Fatigue

Class of Drug	Examples	Mechanism of Action	Comments
Corticosteroids	Dexamethasone PrednisoLONE Methyl-prednisoLONE	Mechanism of action is unclear Duration and benefits limited to weeks	Insufficient data on optimal type and dosage. (Can improve appetite & elevate mood, thus improving a sense of well-being, but the duration of effect may be limited)
Stimulants	Methyl-phenidate	Stimulates CNS and respiratory centers, increases appetite & energy levels, improves mood, reduces sedation[23]	Starting dose 2.5–10 mg q AM and 12 Noon, titrate to effect
Anti-depressants		Reduces depressive symptoms associated with fatigue. Can improve sleep. Primary choice for treatment of depression in cancer patients	
Selective Serotonin Reuptake Inhibitors (SSRIs)	Paroxetine Fluoxetine	Inhibits Serotonin reuptake	Some SSRIs have long half-lives and should be used cautiously in the terminally ill.
Tricyclic Anti-depressants	Desipramine Nortriptyline	Block reuptake of various neurotransmitters at the neuronal membrane. Can improve sleep	Starting dose 10–25 mg q HS
Erythropoietin		Increases hemoglobin with effects on energy, activity & overall quality of life while decreasing transfusion requirements[24]	150 Units/kg SQ q 3 times a week

American Association of Colleges of Nursing and the City of Hope National Medical Center. (2000). Pharmacologic treatments for fatigue, In Module 3: Symptom Management module. *The End-of-Life Nursing Education Consortium (ELNEC)-Core Training Curriculum.* Duarte, CA: Authors. Used with Permission.

XIX. Increased Intracranial Pressure (ICP)

A.   **Definition: increase in the pressure within the cranial cavity due to increased volume of fluid or mass**

B.   **Possible Etiologies**

1.   Space occupying tumors, metastatic lesions with surrounding edema

2.   Intracranial hemorrhage

3.   Inflammatory process: abscess, encephalitis, meningitis

4.   Obstruction of CSF flow

C.   **Assess for**

1.   Sudden unanticipated changes in patient condition with signs of increased ICP: new headache, vomiting, changed respiratory pattern, decreased motor function, lethargy to altered mental status, increased restlessness, agitation, blurred vision

2.   Documentation of possible etiologies of increased ICP in past medical history

3.   Patient/family anxiety, ability to cope with changes in condition; knowledge and/or understanding of presenting changes, disease process, treatment options

D.   **Potential Diagnoses**

1.   Altered mental status due to increased ICP

2.   Cerebral alteration related to increased ICP

3.   Patient and family knowledge deficit related to: disease process, current symptom changes, coping strategies

E.   **Planning and Interventions**

1.   Treat underlying etiology if appropriate

2.   Steroids to reduce edema/inflammation

3.   Anticonvulsant if seizure activity

4.   Palliative radiotherapy when appropriate

5.   Analgesia for headache

a)   Keep in mind that opioids can mildly increase ICP due to vasodilatation effects and mild respiratory depression

b)   Tramadol should not be used in increased ICP as it may lower seizure threshold[25]

6.   Non-pharmacologic measures: head of bed 45–60 degrees, darkened room, reduce external stimuli in environment, calm presence

F.   **Patient/Family Education**

1.   Reassurance and instruction regarding possible cause for changes in patient condition

2.   Review goals of therapy to reduce intracranial pressure symptoms and increase patient comfort and safety

3. Preparation for changes that may indicate advancement of disease and decline of patient condition; support of family/caregiver goals, needs

4. Consider transfer of home hospice patient to inpatient hospice facility or palliative care facility bed if management is beyond physical, emotional capacity of family or caregiver

G. Evaluate

1. Effectiveness of medications, patient comfort and relief, reduction of increased ICP symptoms

2. Patient/family understanding, coping, anxiety related to current symptoms, plan

H. Revise plan according to findings from ongoing evaluations, changes in patient status or family needs

XX. Myoclonus

A. Definition: twitching or brief spasm of a muscle or muscle group

B. Possible Etiologies

1. High dose opioid therapy: related to increased levels of the 3-glucuronide opioid metabolites which are the most likely cause of the neuro-excitatory side effects. Co-morbid factors include renal failure, electrolyte disturbances and dehydration[26]

2. Metabolic derangement, e.g., uremia

3. Inflammatory or degenerative CNS diseases, e.g., Jakob-Creutzfeldt, subacute sclerosing panencephalitis, end-stage Alzheimer's disease

4. Hypercalcemia from osteoblastic activity of bone metastases

C. Assess for

1. Onset, duration of myoclonus and its impact on patient and patient functional status

2. Interruption of sleep, rest

3. Patient/family anxiety related to myoclonic jerking

4. Patient/family understanding of disease process, medication effects and side effects

5. Potential etiology which will direct intervention plan

   a) If opioid-induced, evaluate adjuvant use that would allow for pain to be managed using a reduced opioid dose or rotate opioids. Dose can often be decreased because of incomplete cross tolerance

   b) If hypercalcemia, evaluate patient's place on the disease trajectory

6. Patient safety if ambulatory or if bed bound due to uncontrolled muscular jerking movements

D. Potential Diagnoses

1. Alteration in metabolic status related to: uremia, hypercalcemia, etc.

2. Alteration in functional status due to impairment of neuro-musculoskeletal system

3. Disturbance of sleep and rest pattern due to myoclonus

4. Patient/family knowledge deficit regarding: medication effects, disease process, safety precautions

E. Planning and Intervention: Etiology of myoclonus will direct intervention plan

1. Non-pharmacologic adjunct therapies including local heat, gentle massage, relaxation

2. If hypercalcemia etiology

    a) In palliative care, may consider pamidronate q 3–4 weeks to decrease serum calcium

    b) In hospice, supplementary hydration (IV or PO) may decrease serum calcium and relieve symptoms

3. If opioid-induced, consider adjuvant medicines for the specific type of pain (neuropathic or bone) at the most appropriate dose that may allow reduction in opioid dose

4. Rotate opioids

5. If unable to treat underlying metabolic or degenerative disorder because of advanced stage of disease, patient/family wishes, treat symptoms with clonazepam, valproic acid

6. Occasionally muscle relaxants provide benefit

    a) Diazepam

    b) Baclofen

    c) Cyclobenzaprine

        i. Cyclobenzaprine should be used cautiously in elderly or debilitated patients

        ii. Increases side effects of other medications often taken by the elderly and has side effects that can contribute to conditions often already present such as CHF, glaucoma, etc.

    d) Lorazepam

7. If night cramps only, quinine sulfate at bedtime

8. If restless leg syndrome, gabapentin

F. Patient/Family Education

1. Discuss possible etiologies and recommended interventions

2. Expected medication effects and potential side effects

3. Non-pharmacologic methods of intervention: heat, gentle massage, relaxation to decrease anxiety

G. Evaluate for Effectiveness of Interventions, Specifically

1. Decrease in or resolution of myoclonus

2. Maintenance of effective pain control

3. Patient/family understanding of instructions, recommendations

4. Patient safety

H.   Revise plan according to findings from ongoing evaluations, changes in patient status or family needs

XXI. Nausea and Vomiting

A.   Definitions

1.   Nausea is a subjectively perceived, stomach discomfort ranging from stomach awareness to the conscious recognition of the need to vomit

2.   Vomiting is the expelling of stomach contents through the mouth

B.   Possible Etiologies[4,13,27]

1.   Fluid and electrolyte imbalances (hypercalcemia, hyponatremia, uremia, dehydration)

2.   Gastrointestinal disorders (pressure due to tumor, organomegaly; distention; ascites; esophageal, gastrointestinal and hepatic malignancies; constipation; bowel obstruction; GI stasis)

3.   Other physiologic disorders (oral thrush; cough; pain; high fever)

4.   Neurologic disorders (primary and metastatic CNS tumors, increased intracranial pressure)

5.   Renal failure

6.   Vestibular (tumors and bone metastases at skull base; motion sickness)

7.   Chemical (radiation, medications such as chemotherapy, antibiotics, aspirin, iron, steroids, digoxin, expectorants, NSAIDs, opioids, theophylline)

8.   Psychogenic (anxiety; anticipatory nausea and vomiting; fear)

9.   Adverse response to certain foods especially high fat content

10.   Adverse response to certain drugs e.g., increase in opioids

C.   Assess for

1.   History of the onset of nausea and vomiting and concomitant symptoms i.e., heartburn, constipation, excessive thirst and other symptoms that can indicate etiology

2.   Pattern of nausea: when does nausea occur? Are there contributing factors?

3.   If possible, assess vomitus for volume, color, odor, presence of blood (vomitus with fecal odor or fecal material indicates possible bowel obstruction; coffee ground emesis indicates old blood, whereas fresh blood indicates current hemorrhage)

4.   Abdominal assessment: pain or cramps, bowel sounds, distention

5.   Oropharynx for infection (thrush) or presence of tenacious sputum

6.   Neurologic signs of increased intracranial pressure

7.   Other factors that could trigger nausea response: malodorous wounds, pain, fear, anxiety

D.   Potential Diagnoses

1.   Nausea related to metabolic disorders, tumor pressure, therapies, neurosensory disorders or anxiety

2. Risk for fluid volume deficit related to nausea and vomiting

3. Risk for altered nutrition due to intake less than body requirements related to inability to eat or keep food down secondary to nausea and vomiting

4. Patient/family knowledge deficit related to etiology and treatment of nausea and vomiting

E. **Planning and Intervention: Etiology of nausea and vomiting may guide interventions**

1. Modify diet to decrease nausea

   a) Bland foods that patient enjoys, e.g., baked potatoes, soft fruits, yogurt, soft drinks, crackers or dry toast, clear liquids such as Popsicles®, Jell-O®, sports drinks, foods without aggressive odors, non-gas-forming foods

   b) Cold or room temperature foods are often better tolerated than warm foods due to less odor

   c) Serve small, frequent meals

   d) Avoid fatty, greasy, spicy or very sweet foods

2. Correct reversible causes of nausea, including cough, hypercalcemia, increased intracranial pressure

3. Keep the patient cool; place a fan in the room or open a window to circulate air

4. Keep patient's head elevated

5. Medication regimen (see Table 7) should be prescribed according to etiology of nausea[4,28]

   a) A prokinetic agent (metoclopramide) can be used for delayed gastric emptying (do not use in bowel obstruction)

   b) Butyrophenones, i.e., haloperidol or droperidol for opioid-induced nausea (nausea related to opioid initiation generally resolves within one week)

   c) An antihistamine (meclizine, dimenhyDRINATE) can be used for bowel obstruction or other visceral irritation (liver metastases, constipation, etc.), disturbances in the vestibular system (vertigo, motion sickness), pharyngeal stimulation (tenacious sputum, oral thrush) or increased intracranial pressure (which can also be treated with a glucocorticoid such as dexamethasone)

   d) Anticholinergics (scopolamine patches, hydroxyzine) are used primarily for increased intracranial pressure and vestibular disturbances

   e) Nausea related to disturbances in the chemoreceptor trigger zone (CTZ) (usually due to metabolic disorders, medications and toxins produced from GI tumors, infection, poisoning, etc.), can be treated by discontinuing offending medication if possible and utilizing drugs which act on the CTZ (haloperidol, metoclopramide, phenothiazines)

   f) Nausea related to emetogenic chemotherapy can be treated with $5\text{-}HT_3$ serotonin receptor antagonists (ondansetron, granisetron)

   g) Nausea related to anxiety and fear can be treated with antihistamines or anticholinergics

   h) Consider switching opioids

   i) Treat constipation if present

6. Oral hygiene before and after meals

F.   **Patient/Family Education**

1.   Explain etiology and treatment course of nausea and vomiting

2.   Explain effects of medication and possible side effects

3.   Explain non-pharmacologic measures to treat nausea and vomiting, including diet, oral hygiene, etc.

G.   **Evaluate**

1.   Effectiveness of interventions and patient/family teaching (are patient/family satisfied with outcome?)

2.   Medication effectiveness and presence of side effects

3.   Patient/family understanding of treatment measures

H.   **Revise plan according to findings from ongoing evaluations, changes in patient status or family needs**

XXII.   **Paresthesia and Neuropathy**

A.   **Definitions**

1.   Paresthesia: a sensation of numbness, prickling or tingling; heightened sensitivity

2.   Neuropathy: any disease of the nerves; may include sensory loss, muscle weakness and atrophy and decreased deep tendon reflexes

B.   **Possible Etiologies**

1.   Central and peripheral nerve lesions

2.   Direct damage to peripheral and autonomic nerves

3.   Metabolic and vascular changes of diabetes mellitus

4.   Chemical or drug-induced: e.g., chemotherapy, isoniazid, alcohol

5.   Amputation, AIDS, Vitamin B-12 deficiency

6.   Tumor invasion with pressure on nerves or plexuses

7.   Spinal cord compression (considered an oncologic emergency)

C.   **Assess for**

1.   Sudden loss of sensation, motor function of lower extremities with or without loss of bladder or bowel control; **MAY INDICATE SPINAL CORD COMPRESSION WHICH IS A MEDICAL EMERGENCY.** Most common signs of pending cord compression are escalating back pain with or without bladder changes and before lower extremity weakness, worse when lying down, improved when standing. Amount of neurological deficit patient presents with is usually amount left with following treatment, therefore early recognition is imperative

2.   Location and degree of numbness: patient's subjective descriptions of pain or sensation assist in determining etiology

Table 7: Management of Nausea/Vomiting

Syndrome Pathway(s)	Causes	Clinical Features	Antiemetic Management	Adjuvant
S Gastric stasis and gastric outflow obstruction **P** Vomiting center, GI tract	Anticholinergic drugs, autonomic failure, ascites, hepatomegaly, tumor infiltration, peptic ulcer, gastritis	Epigastric fullness and discomfort. Early satiety. Flatulence, hiccough, acid reflux and gastric regurgitation. Large volume emesis which may contain undigested food. Nausea often relieved by vomiting	Prokinetic Metoclopramide 10–20 mg TID PO 40–80 mg SQ infusion/24 hours	Dietary advice. Paracentesis for ascites. Simethicone for flatulence. Steroid therapy may be used to improve the dysfunction induced by tumor infiltration of nerve plexuses. For total obstruction a venting gastrostomy or surgical bypass may be considered. H_2 blocker or proton pump inhibitor. Review drug regimen
S Stretch/ irritation of visceral and GI serosa **P** Vomiting center, GI tract	Liver metastases, ureteric obstruction, tumor, constipation, bowel obstruction, lymph nodes	Pain is often a feature. Colic. Altered bowel habits. Nausea. Vomiting of fecal fluid in obstruction	Antihistamine <u>DiphenhydrAMINE</u> 25–50 mg TID or QID PO/IM/IV <u>Promethazine</u> 12.5–25 mg TID or QID PO/IM/IV/PR Hydroxyzine 25–100 mg TID or QID PO/IM	Relieve the cause, e.g., constipation with stimulant laxatives and enemas as required. Steroid therapy for the reduction of peri-tumor edema
S Raised intracranial pressure/ meningism **P** Vomiting center	Cerebral tumor, intracranial tumor, intracranial bleeding, infiltration of meninges by tumor, skull metastases, cerebral infection	Neurological signs, e.g., drowsiness, dizziness, headache, nausea and/or vomiting, vomiting may be projectile in nature	Antihistamine <u>DiphenhydrAMINE</u> 25–50 mg TID or QID PO/IM/IV <u>Promethazine</u> 12.5–25 mg TID or QID PO/IM/IV/PR Hydroxyzine 25–100 mg TID or QID PO/IM Anticholinergic Scopolamine Transdermal patch q 3 days	High dose steroids may reduce cerebral edema and/or tumor mass Bisphosphonates if hypercalcemia present

(continued)

Syndrome Pathway(s)	Causes	Clinical Features	Antiemetic Management	Adjuvant
S Pharyngeal stimulation **P** Vomiting center	Tenacious sputum not easily expectorated, infection (*Candida*)	Retching	Antihistamine <u>DiphenhydrAMINE</u> 25–50 mg TID or QID PO/IM/IV <u>Promethazine</u> 12.5–25 mg TID or QID PO/IM/IV/ PR Hydroxyzine 25–100 mg TID or QID PO/IM	Treat the cause. Saline nebulizers. Antibiotics. Antifungal therapy. If an inner ear problem, treat with meclizine
S Esophageal obstruction **P** Vomiting center	Tumor, odynophagia (painful swallowing), functional dysphagia, *Candida*	Regurgitation, dysphagia	Anticholinergic Will help to reduce saliva and secretions Scopolamine Transdermal patch q 3 days Octreotide	Radiotherapy, brachiotherapy, laser therapy, high dose steroids, self-expanding stent, Celestin or Atkinson tube, Surgery (not for patients with metastatic spread)
S Anxiety **P** Vomiting center	Psychological and emotional distress, anticipatory emesis associated with chemotherapy	Nausea, waves of nausea and vomiting, distraction may relieve symptoms	Antihistamine or Anticholinergics if required	Address the anxiety with psychological techniques. Relaxation. Benzodiazepines. Ensure adequate pain control

Adapted with permission from: Campbell T, Hately J. The management of nausea and vomiting in advanced cancer. *International Journal of Palliative Nursing.* 2000;6(1):18–20,22–25.
Editor's Note: **S** = Syndrome, **P** = Pathway(s)

3. Patient's course in the diseases process/trajectory for assistance in intervention planning

4. Patient safety in ambulation, ADLs

5. Patient/family understanding of cause of sudden change in sensation or motor function, need for safety in ambulation/ADLs, understanding of treatment options

D. **Potential Diagnoses**

1. Alteration in comfort related to peripheral sensory and neuropathic changes

2. Safety risk related to alteration in sensation

3. Patient/family knowledge deficit related to safety needs, medication effects, treatment options

4. Compromised patient/family coping related to uncontrolled pain

E. Planning and Intervention: determining patient's course in disease process, trajectory will facilitate planning in the event of spinal cord compression

1. If patient is in advanced stage of disease (weak, bed bound, poor nutritional status), symptom management may be appropriate option, i.e., steroids to decrease edema around cord; neuroleptic analgesia, opioids

2. If patient is ambulatory, active and able to participate in self-care, palliative radiotherapy and steroids may provide significant benefit for quality of life

3. Tricyclic antidepressants (TCAs) are appropriate adjuvant analgesics to opioids for neuropathic pain (see Chapter 4)

   a) Titrate dose every few days based upon the patient's response

   b) Therapeutic levels achieved in 3–7 days

4. Anticonvulsants can be considered for neuropathic pain

   a) If gabapentin: start low; dose can be titrated to 3600 mg daily maximum (in divided doses) for therapeutic effect

   b) If carbamazepine or phenytoin: monitor for effect and for drug interaction. Monitor CBC and for adverse drug reaction of pancytopenia

5. Appropriate bowel regimen if patient has decreased activity, is bed bound or has lost sensation in rectum

6. Foley catheter for urinary retention

7. Condom or indwelling catheter for urinary incontinence if this causes skin irritation, patient anxiety and if patient/caregiver agree

8. Increase assistance with ADLs in home as indicated for patient personal needs and safety

F. Patient/Family Education

1. Expected medication effects and possible side effects

   a) Continue TCAs regularly

      i. It takes 3–7 days to become therapeutic for neuropathic pain

      ii. Give at night, which might aid in sleeping and reduce daytime sedation

   b) Prepare patient/family to expect that gabapentin may cause sedation when initiated or dose increased

   c) Carbamazepine may cause dizziness, drowsiness, anorexia and nausea

   d) Phenytoin may cause ataxia, diplopia, dizziness, drowsiness

2. Safety needs when ambulating related to decreased sensation, motor ability and medication effects

G. Evaluate for Effectiveness of Interventions

1. Compliance with medication regimen

2. Effectiveness of medication and any side effects

3. Return of sensation, function

4. Safety needs/issues

H. Revise plan according to findings from ongoing evaluations, changes in patient status or family needs

XXIII. Seizures

A. Definitions: usually intermittent tonic, clonic movements; convulsions caused by a large number of neurons discharging abnormally[29]

1. Primary (generalized) involving large parts of the brain and including grand mal and petit mal types

2. Focal (partial) involving specific regions of the brain with symptoms reflecting the location of the disturbance

B. Possible Etiologies[29]

1. Brain infarct, primary brain tumor or brain metastases, cerebral abscess, brain infection in HIV and AIDS

2. Increased intracranial pressure (may be associated with SIADH in some cancer patients)

3. Pre-existing seizure disorder

4. Medications (metabolites from normeperidine and propoxyphene) and their preservatives (sodium bisulfite); medications that lower seizure threshold include phenothiazines, butyrophenones, tricyclic antidepressants, tramadol lowers seizure threshold

5. Infection, stroke, hemorrhage, oxygen deprivation, paraneoplastic syndromes

6. Metabolic instability (hyponatremia, hypercalcemia, hypomagnesemia, hypoxemia, hypoglycemia)

7. Drug toxicity, drug withdrawal

C. Assess for

1. Acutely seizing patient: intervene with first intervention below

2. Underlying etiology reviewing medical history, disease process, current medications, history of trauma or recent fall, differentiate from myoclonus

3. Question patient and/or family to determine onset and type of seizure, presence of aura, headache, nausea and projectile vomiting

4. Drug levels if previously taking anticonvulsants; EEG may be warranted

5. Patient/family coping with seizure activity, their understanding of patient protection/safety during seizure, medication effects and side effects

D. Potential Diagnoses

1. Safety precautions (e.g., risk for falls) for seizures from (etiology)

2. Potential risk for medication toxicity or withdrawal side effects

    a) Dexamethasone is commonly given to those with seizure disorder; interaction between this drug and phenytoin is problematic

        i. Phenytoin increases bioavailability of dexamethasone

        ii. Dexamethasone inhibits metabolism of phenytoin

    b) Steroids must not be suddenly stopped—seizures may occur

3. Metabolic impairment related to: hyponatremia, hypercalcemia, hypomagnesemia, hypoxia, hypoglycemia

4. Patient/family knowledge deficit related to: etiology, disease process, medication effects/side effects, safety

E. Planning and Intervention

1. For actively seizing patient

    a) Assess airway, breathing, circulation and ensure adequate airway

    b) Protect patient from harm and ensure safety

    c) Model calm demeanor

    d) Medical therapy may include

        i. IV or SL lorazepam

        ii. Diazepam enema, IV diazepam

        iii. Clonazepam

        iv. Initiation of phenytoin, carbamazepine, valproic acid or phenobarbital[29]

2. Determine potentially treatable etiologies

    a) Hypoglycemia: glucose PO/IV or glucagon SQ as indicated

    b) Hyponatremia: fluid restriction, IV NaCl, adjustment of diuretics

    c) Hypercalcemia: increase fluids PO/IV, pamidronate may be appropriate depending on disease trajectory

    d) Hypoxemia: supplemental O_2; further evaluation of this etiology

    e) Hypomagnesemia: supplemental magnesium

    f) Infectious process (cerebral abscess, encephalitis, meningitis): antibiotics as indicated and according to patient's place on disease trajectory and advance directives

    g) Substance abuse: support withdrawal, consult substance withdrawal specialist

F. Patient/Family Education

1. Anticipate potential for seizure activity and prepare family for patient safety, preemptive interventions, whom to call

2. Calmly rehearse, review caregiver interventions

3. Expected medication effects and potential side effects

G. Evaluate

1. Effectiveness of seizure management interventions

2. Family preparedness and coping

3. Patient safety

4. Medication effects and side effects

5. Blood draws to monitor levels of medications such as phenytoin

   a) Phenytoin has a narrow therapeutic range and drug interactions may lead to alterations in its plasma concentration

   b) This may result in either phenytoin intoxication or in decreased effectiveness of the drug[30]

   c) Assess free or unbound phenytoin levels, linked to hypoalbuminemia

H. Revise plan according to findings from ongoing evaluations, changes in patient status or family needs

XXIV. Urinary Incontinence/Retention

A. Definition: the inability to control urination

B. Possible Etiologies

1. Urge incontinence: urge to void sensed, but cannot control urine flow long enough to reach toilet

   a) Due to bladder irritation such as infection, tumor, radiation or chemotherapy

   b) Nervous system damage: spinal cord lesions (neurogenic bladder), stroke, multiple sclerosis, Parkinson's disease, Alzheimer's disease

   c) Decreased mobility or difficulty reaching the toilet in time

2. Stress incontinence: leakage of urine when intra-abdominal pressure is raised

   a) Damage or dysfunction of bladder sphincter due to

      i. Tumor infiltration in GU system or CNS or spinal cord lesions

      ii. Multiparity or post-menopausal changes in women

3. Overflow incontinence: bladder unable to empty normally

   a) Bladder outlet obstruction due to fecal mass, tumor, calculi, prostatic hypertrophy

   b) Detrusor muscle failure due to anticholinergic drugs, CNS lesions or debility and confusion

4. Functional incontinence: an involuntary or unpredictable passage of urine with no impairment of the GU tract

   a) Cognitive dysfunction: depression leading to self-neglect, confusion, excessive sedation

   b) Mobility or functional problems: immobility, unable to undress, inaccessible toilet facilities, final stage of illness

5. Many drugs can lead to any of the aforementioned urinary incontinence problems

   a) Diuretics increase volume and frequency

   b) Sedatives decrease awareness of need to void, as well as decrease bladder contraction and outlet resistance

   c) Anticholinergics decrease bladder contraction

   d) Antiparkinson drugs increase outlet resistance

6. Metabolic disorders: hypercalcemia

7. Atonic bladder: no awareness of bladder fullness or urgency

   a) Diabetic neuropathy

   b) Spinal cord lesions or cord compression

   c) Neurologic dysfunction

8. Fistula

C. Assess for

1. History, including nature and duration of symptoms, medications, recent treatments for cancer

2. Physical exam: bladder distention, perineal swelling, fecal impaction, simple neurologic exam (including sensation and sensorimotor deficits), signs of hypercalcemia, functional assessment (mobility, able to dress/undress self, presence of aphasia or dysphasia), skin assessment

3. Urge incontinence: nocturia, frequency with urination

4. Stress incontinence: leakage of urine upon laughing, coughing, sneezing, lifting or bending

5. Overflow incontinence: bladder distention, discomfort, urgency, continual dribbling and only voiding small amounts, large residual urine after voiding, fecal impaction

6. Functional incontinence: mobility, ability to perform ADLs, cognitive level, depression

D. Diagnoses

1. Altered urinary elimination related to anatomic dysfunction or obstruction, medications or metabolic disorder

2. Urinary incontinence, urge, related to bladder irritation, sensory-motor disorder or decreased mobility

3. Urinary incontinence, stress, related to decrease in bladder or sphincter support

4. Urinary incontinence, functional, related to cognitive dysfunction or mobility problems

5. Risk for impaired skin integrity related to urinary incontinence

6. Patient/family knowledge deficit related to etiology and management of urinary incontinence

7. Patient/family anxiety related to urinary incontinence

8. Risk for falls trying to get to the bathroom

E.   **Planning and Intervention**

1.   Review medications and discontinue those that may be causing incontinence (if appropriate)

2.   If appropriate, establish a regular voiding schedule (i.e., every 2 hours)

3.   Alter environment to make toileting easier (i.e., move patient closer to toilet or utilize a bedside commode, urinal or bedpan, assuring modesty and dignity is maintained)

4.   Decrease fluid intake at night and limit intake of food/fluids containing caffeine or alcohol

5.   If fecal impaction is present, disimpact and teach bowel regime to patient and family to avoid further problems

6.   Consider catheterizing, either indwelling or external

7.   Utilize incontinence supplies, such as pads, briefs, etc.

8.   Teach patient and family hygiene and skin care measures

9.   Urge incontinence: antibiotics for UTI, urinary tract analgesics such as phenazopyridine, imipramine for neurogenic bladder

10.   Stress incontinence: teach pelvic floor muscle exercises (PFME) and voiding schedule, pessary or penile clamp, imipramine at bedtime for anticholinergic effect

11.   Overflow incontinence: discontinue anticholinergic medications, if possible; disimpact if necessary; cholinergic drug such as bethanechol; indwelling catheterization if obstruction persists

12.   Functional incontinence: interventions rely on cause of incontinence; indwelling catheter may be only choice

13.   Incontinence related to fistulas is treated by establishing voiding schedules, catheterization and, if indicated, urinary diversion (if life expectancy is not short)

F.   **Patient/Family Education**

1.   Expected medication effects and potential side effects

2.   Demonstrate correct hygiene and skin care techniques to prevent skin breakdown

3.   Explain correct catheter care and signs of catheter malfunction

4.   Explain safety measures if altering environment for ease in toileting (i.e., have patient call for assistance, voiding schedules, assuring clear path to bathroom)

5.   Explain signs and symptoms of urinary tract infection (UTI)

G.   **Evaluate**

1.   Effectiveness of interventions (are patient/family satisfied with outcome?)

2.   Skin integrity

3.   Medication effects and side effects

4.   Patient safety

H.   **Revise plan according to findings from ongoing evaluations, changes in patient/family needs**

CITED REFERENCES

1. Bergstrom N, et al. *Pressure Ulcer Treatment: Clinical Practice Guideline. Quick Reference Guide for Clinicians, No. 15*. Rockville, MD; U.S. Department of Health and Human Services, Public Health Service, Agency for Health Care Policy and Research; 1994.

2. Barr JE. Principles of wound cleansing. *Ostomy/Wound Management*. 1995; 41(Supp 7A):15S–22S.

3. Dahlin CM, Goldsmith T. Dysphagia, dry mouth, & hiccups. In: Ferrell BR, Coyle N, eds. *Textbook of Palliative Nursing*. New York, NY: Oxford University Press; 2001:122–138.

4. Waller A, Caroline NL. *Handbook of palliative care in cancer*. 2nd ed. Boston, MA: Butterworth-Heinemann; 2000.

5. Coda BA, O'Sullivan B, Donaldson G, Bohl S, Chapman CR, Shen DD. Comparative efficacy of patient-controlled administration of morphine, hydromorphone, or sufentanil for the treatment of oral mucositis pain following bone marrow transplantation (Abstract). *Pain*. 1997;72(3):333–346. Retrieved October 9, 2001 from the Ovid Bibliographic Records database.

6. Rhiner M, Slatkin NE. Pruritus, fever and sweats. In: Ferrell BR, Coyle N, eds. *Textbook of Palliative Nursing*. New York, NY: Oxford University Press; 2001:245-261.

7. Weissman D. Fast Facts #1: Treating terminal delirium. End of Life Physician Education Resource Center. Available at www.eperc.mcw.edu/. Accessed May, 2000.

8. Kuebler KK, English N, Heidrich DE. Delirium, confusion, agitation and restlessness. In: Ferrell BR, Coyle N, eds. *Textbook of Palliative Nursing*. New York, NY: Oxford University Press; 2001:290–308.

9. Stillman MJ, Rybicki LA. The bedside confusion scale: development of a portable bedside test for confusion and its application to the palliative medicine population. *J Palliat Med* 2000;3(4):449–456.

10. Taber CW. *Taber's Cyclopedic Medical Dictionary*. 18th ed. Philadelphia, PA: A. Davis; 1997.

11. Kuebler KK. *Hospice and Palliative Care Clinical Practice Protocol: Terminal Restlessness*. Pittsburgh, PA: Hospice and Palliative Nurses Association; 1997.

12. Collins CA. Ascites. *Clinical Journal of Oncology Nursing*. 2001;5(1):43–44.

13. Kemp C. *Terminal Illness: A Guide to Nursing Care*. 2nd ed., Philadelphia, PA: Lippincott; 1999.

14. Baumrucker SJ. Current concepts in hospice care: Management of intestinal obstruction in hospice care. *The American Journal of Hospice and Palliative Care*. 1998;14(4):232–235.

15. von Gunten C, Muir C. Fast Facts #45: Medical management of bowel obstruction. End of Life Physician Education Resource Center. Available at www.eperc.mcw.edu/. Accessed July, 2001.

16. Alderman J. Fast Facts #96: Diarrhea in palliative care. End of Life Physician Education Resource Center. Available at www.eperc.mcw.edu/. Accessed August, 2003.

17. Preston FA, Cunningham RS. *Clinical Guidelines for Symptom Management in Oncology: A Handbook for Advanced Practice Nurses*. New York, NY: Clinical Insights Press; 1998.

18. Dudgeon D. Dyspnea, death rattle and cough. In: Ferrell BR, Coyle N, eds. *Textbook of Palliative Nursing*. New York, NY: Oxford University Press; 2001:164–174.

19. Weissman DE, Ambuel B, Hallenback J. Improving end-of-life care: a resource guide for physician education. Medical College of Wisconsin. 2000:50.

20. Farmer, C. Fast Facts #81: Management of hiccups. End of Life Physician Education Resource Center. Available at www.eperc.mcw.edu/. Accessed January 2003.

21. Grant M, Padilla GV, Ferrell BR, Rhiner M. Assessment of quality of life with a single instrument. *Seminars in Oncology Nursing*. 1990;6(4):260–270.

22. Chochinov HM, Breitbart W. *Handbook of Psychiatry and Palliative Care*. New York, NY: Oxford University Press; 2000.

23. Bruera E, Chadwick S, Brennis C. Methylphenidate associated with narcotic treatment of cancer pain. *Cancer Treatment Reports*. 1985;70:295–297.

24. Krammer L, Muir C, Gooding-Gellar N, Williams M., von Gunten, C. Palliative care and oncology: Opportunities for nursing. *Oncology Nursing Update*. 1999;6:1–12.

25. McCaffery M, Pasero C. *Pain: Clinical Manual*. St. Louis, MO: Mosby; 1999.

26. Wilson RK, Weissman D. Fast Facts #57: Neuroexcitatory effects of opioids: Patient assessment. End of Life Physician Education Resource Center. Available at www.eperc.mcw.edu/. Accessed December, 2001.

27. Rousseau P. Nonpain symptom management in terminal care. *Clinics in Geriatric Medicine*. 1996;12(2):313–327.

28. Campbell T, Hately J. The management of nausea and vomiting in advanced cancer. *International Journal of Palliative Nursing*. 2000;6(1):18–20, 22–25.

29. Paice JA. *Neurological disturbances*. In: Ferrell BR, Coyle N, eds. *Textbook of Palliative Nursing*. New York, NY: Oxford University Press; 2001:262–268.

30. Nation RL, Evans AM, Milne RW. Pharmacokinetic drug interactions with phenytoin (Part I). *Clinical Pharmacokinetics*. 1997;18(1):37–60.

ADDITIONAL REFERENCES AND RESOURCES

Ferrell BR, Coyle N, eds. *Textbook of Palliative Nursing*. New York, NY: Oxford University Press; 2001.

Ferris, F, and von Gunten, C. Fast Facts #40: Pressure ulcer management: Part 1 Prevention. End of Life Physician Education Resource Center. Available at www.eperc.mcw.edu/.

Herfindal ET, Gourley DR, eds. *Textbook of Therapeutics: Drug and Disease Management*. Baltimore, MD: Williams & Wilkins; 1996.

Kaye P. *Notes on Symptom Control in Hospice and Palliative Care*. rev. 1st ed. USA version. Essex, CT: Hospice Education Institute; 1990.

Quijada E, Billings JA. Fast Facts #60: Pharmacologic management of delirium: update on newer agents. End of Life Physician Education Resource Center. Available at www.eperc.mcw.edu/.

Sander R. Promoting urinary continence in residential care. *Nursing Standard* 2000;14(13):49–54.

Smith SA, ed. *Hospice and Palliative Care Clinical Practice Monograph: Treatment of End-stage Non-cancer Diagnoses*. Dubuque, IA: Kendall/Hunt Publishing Co.; 2001.

von Gunten C, Ferris F. Fast Facts #37: Pruritus. End of Life Physician Education Resource Center. Available at www.eperc.mcw.edu/.

Weissman DE. Fast Facts #27: Dyspnea at end of life. End of Life Physician Education Resource Center. Available at www.eperc.mcw.edu/.

Wrede-Seaman, L. *Symptom Management Algorithms for Palliative Care*. Yakima, WA: Intellicard; 1999.

CHAPTER VI

CARE OF THE PATIENT AND FAMILY

Terry Altilio, LMSW
Rose Anne Indelicato, MSN, APRN, BC-PCM, OCN

First Edition Authors
Judith B. Eighmy, RN, BSN, CHPN®, Elayne J. Nahman, MSW, LCSW

I. Introduction

    A. Hospice and palliative care provides

        1. A holistic approach which focuses on the patient and family as the unit of care

        2. Care which incorporates the expertise of several disciplines who collaborate to meet the needs of patient, family and caregiver and who, in addition to their own expertise, have knowledge about physical, psychosocial, spiritual and bereavement issues that enhance their ability to recognize the need for referral to team specialists

        3. Care that is based in recognition that assessment, planning and intervention are the ongoing responsibility of all team members and reflect attention to all dimensions of the patient/family situation[1]

        4. Care which respects the reality that patients and families form unique relationships with both past medical providers and with team members and that the perspectives and expertise of these individual clinicians can be invaluable in the identification of needs, in solving problems, clarifying conflicts and facilitating resolutions[2]

        5. Care which recognizes that the needs and perspectives of patients, family and caregivers are unique to them as individual and unique to their relationship to the patient and that each view the illness experience through their own experience, feelings and fears

II. Definitions

    A. Family can be defined as blood relatives, relationships established through an emotional commitment or a group of individuals with whom a person feels most connected[2]

        1. The family as a system

            a) A complex entity comprised of interrelated and interacting individuals functioning within a socio-economic, political, environment as well as a healthcare setting

        b)   The primary objective of this system is to maintain equilibrium in environment, which facilitates individual and family development

        c)   System seeks to maintain equilibrium through dynamic process of homeostasis

B.   Caregiver refers to anyone who provides and/or arranges for assistance to someone else who requires it.[2,3] Informal caregiver is a term used to refer to an unpaid individual such as family members and friends who provide care. Formal caregivers are volunteers or paid care providers associated with a service system[2]

III. Psychosocial Aspects of Care

A. Assessment

1.   Is an ongoing shared responsibility of the interdisciplinary team (IDT) and the specialty of social workers who are specifically prepared in this area

2.   Requires reassessment along the continuum as illness evolves and patient, family and caregiver adaptation is required, needs change and consequently plans may have to be altered

3.   Involves understanding the individual as well as the family as a unit; their history, current functioning, expectation and vision of the future

4.   Is shared and enhanced by the observations, input and clinical expertise of interdisciplinary team members as well as those medical providers who have provided care earlier in the illness trajectory

5.   Presupposes that the patient/family/caregiver perspectives and coping may differ, that they impact each other and that clinicians need to inquire, respect and intervene according to these unique views

6.   Involves verbal and non verbal behaviors and observations from patient, family, caregivers and interdisciplinary colleagues

7.   Is based in verbal, non verbal and symbolic communication impacted by

        a)   Literacy/numeracy levels

        b)   Language/cultural differences

            i.   Adopt an attitude of cultural respect, humility and inquiry

            ii.   Acquire knowledge about the predominant cultures in your community

            iii.   Make efforts to avoid using family as translators; use professional interpreters, colleagues, ATT language line

            iv.   Provide education material in the language of choice

        c)   Communication challenges

            i.   Physical—symptoms e.g., shortness of breath, pain, tracheostomy, mouth sores, cognitive impairment, visual/hearing impairment

            ii.   Environmental—noise, interruptions, lack of privacy

            iii.   Psychological—depression, anxiety, distress

      iv.   Accommodate assessment tools, environment and questions; when necessary, minimize need for patient to speak—ask questions that can be answered in few words or in a nonverbal response

8.   Involves specific areas of assessment which apply to patient/family/caregiver

    a)   Past and present patient/family (including children and adolescents)/caregiver functioning—physical, psychological, social, spiritual

    b)   Developmental tasks, sexual orientation, life cycle stage of family

    c)   Risk factors such as psychiatric illness, addiction, physical and or sexual abuse

    d)   Understanding of medical situation, history and impact of illness on roles, relationships, values and hopes

    e)   Individual/family coping styles, strengths and skills

      i.   Individual attitudes and beliefs about information and the need to know; how much, how little, specifics or generalities, who is to know and who is to tell

      ii.   Learning styles and decision making process of individuals to assist in customizing interventions

      iii.   Need for control; range of ability to delegate and maintain sense of self as valued and life as meaningful in the setting of progressing illness and the consequent emotional, social and physical impacts

      iv.   History of and experience in coping with the unknown, with healthcare systems, with change and with losses (physical, psychological, social, spiritual)

      v.   Values and attitudes that infuse individual/family coping and may be expressed by such phrases as "live one day at a time," "God only gives you what you can bear"

    f)   Patient, family and caregiver individual needs, distress and perspectives related to pain, symptoms, illness progression, caregiver tasks, prognosis, advance care planning, caregiver fatigue, unresolved issues, place of death

    g)   Needs of extended or geographically distant family

    h)   Ongoing evaluation of impact of illness to inform an evolving IDT care plan that might include respite care, alternate care settings and enhanced supports such as continuous home care, volunteer services and agency referrals

    i)   Community supports and resources including friends, neighbors, clergy and church community

    j)   Emotional and cognitive functioning of patient, family and caregivers (see Chapter 5 for Symptom Management). The following symptoms or behaviors can be very distressing to patients, family, caregivers and staff and require vigilant and expert assessment and interventions

      i.   Anger and hostility

        (a)   Possible etiologies—feelings of isolation, loneliness, infantilization, helplessness, frustration; actual or perceived loss of control or autonomy, perceived threats to feelings of competence, fears of abandonment, medical factors i.e., reaction to medication

ii.   Anxiety

(a)   Possible etiologies—fear, existential/spiritual distress, perceived loss of control, perceived threats of abandonment or physical injury; response to a new environment, new personnel in setting of serious illness and dependence; uncontrolled symptoms or fear of such; physical etiology, medication effect, impaired cognition, withdrawal symptom

iii. Confusion, delirium, agitation, terminal restlessness, near death awareness (dream, visions or communication with dead family/friends or with spiritual being). Many believe that this is a transitional experience prior to death. However it is important not to assume but rather to assess in relation to status of disease, goals of care and level of distress created by the behaviors

(a)   Possible etiologies—fear, existential/spiritual distress, perceived loss of control, perceived threats of abandonment or physical injury; response to a new environment, new personnel in setting of serious illness and dependence; uncontrolled symptoms or fear of such; physical etiology, metabolic disturbances, medication effect, impaired cognition, withdrawal symptom

iv.   Denial

(a)   Definition—an unconscious process designed to protect against an overwhelming reality as distinguished from avoidance which is a conscious process that protects individuals from bringing distressing aspects of their reality to the forefront. As an "unconscious" process, any decision to challenge denial requires thorough clinical evaluation

(b)   Possible etiologies—disbelief, fear, needing more time and experience with the distressing reality; uncertainty about ability to cope and in some situations what looks like denial is actually a reflection of the fact that appropriate, understandable and timely information has never been given

v.   Depression—emotional indicators such as guilt, hopelessness, helplessness, absence of pleasure and low self esteem are major indicators as the physical indicators such as disturbed sleep, anorexia, constipation, fatigue, reduced libido and emotional lability are often present consequent to serious illness, treatment and/or medications

(a)   Possible etiologies—existential/spiritual distress, despair, perceived loss of control, perceived threats of abandonment or physical injury; response to a new environment, new personnel in setting of serious illness and dependence; uncontrolled symptoms or fear of such; physical etiology, medication or treatment effect, impaired cognition, withdrawal symptom

vi.   Despair/loss of meaning

(a)   Possible etiologies—grief, pain and disability, spiritual/existential distress, loss of control, untreated depression, overload (emotional, medical, demands associated with uncontrolled symptoms), inability to find any meaning in the illness and/or caregiving experience

vii. Fear and worry

(a)   Possible etiologies—abandonment, uncontrolled pain and symptoms, inadequate resources (personal, healthcare, community, financial) dependency, fear of dying and death and future ability of survivors to manage

viii. Guilt

(a) Possible etiologies—unresolved issues, feelings of failure, troubled relationships, existential/spiritual turmoil, dependence on others

ix. Sleep disturbances

(a) Possible etiologies—physical such as side effect of medication, reaction to stimulants such as caffeine, alcohol, theophylline or theobromine containing fluid food; psychological including fear of nightmares, dying in one's sleep, nighttime quiet invites fears and worries such as unresolved relationship issues. Excessive sleep may be medication related, a symptom of depression or an expected part of the dying process

x. Suicidal/homicidal ideation/wish for hastened death

(a) Possible etiologies—may be transient or persistent; depression, psychiatric illness. despair, uncontrolled symptoms, need for control, hopelessness, perceived loss of dignity, sense of self as a "burden," delirium, misuse or abuse of medications

B. **Interventions—are the shared responsibility of the IDT and the individualized responsibility of the team clinician whose expertise and relationship establish their role as primary**

1. Are individualized and based in an ongoing assessment of the unique and potentially different needs of the patient, family and caregiver

2. Provided in collaboration and consultation with IDT who have a shared knowledge base as well as individual areas of expertise

3. Include medical management and education as well as advocacy, psychosocial, spiritual complementary techniques and expressive therapies which may be provided by nurse, MSW, physician or chaplain

4. Balance respect for patient, family and caregiver pace and adaptation with the teams need to provide information, educate and foster decision making

5. Reinforce aspects of experience that remain stable at the same time that patient, family, caregiver cope with change caused by illness progression and changing goals of care

6. Presuppose that psychosocial and spiritual suffering cannot be totally alleviated

7. May be delivered in person, via phone, email or internet

8. Include counseling and referral to interdisciplinary colleagues (social worker, chaplain, music/art therapist, holistic clinician) and involve modalities such as

a) Individual counseling

b) Supportive counseling

c) Group counseling

d) Family counseling

e) Family meetings which may focus on

i. Acceptance, ventilation and validation of a range of feelings, including coexisting seemingly incongruous awareness such as acceptance of poor prognosis while at the same time hoping for a miracle

    ii.   Acknowledging the ambivalent responses and feelings often associated with being ill, being a caregiver or family member

    iii.   Validating and reinforcing the efforts of family and caregiver

    iv.   Teaching and/or reinforcing skills especially during transitions between care settings that are often disruptive of prior learning

    v.   Teaching caregiver techniques for patient care along the continuum of illness and through the dying process, when culturally and clinically appropriate

    vi.   Reinforcing the commitment of the clinical team to non abandonment, competent proactive symptom management and continuity of care

    vii.   Encouraging techniques such as life review, reminiscence, storytelling, memory making, journaling which have the potential to enhance quality of life, explore and expand the patient/family/caregiver experience beyond illness to the whole of one's life/family experience

    viii.   Ongoing clinical review of decisions and changing goals of care with team and/or patient, family and caregivers

    ix.   Educating and providing information titrated to patient, family and caregiver need and adapted to learning styles, cultural values, language and communication needs

    x.   Enhancing patients' control in setting of evolving illness and physical decline

    xi.   Proactive inquiry regarding advanced care planning, caregiver emotional and physical wellbeing

    xii.   Reframing hope beyond cure of illness to expanded areas of meaning

    xiii.   Promoting and teaching family, caregiver self care

    xiv.   Ongoing advocacy with team to access resources, supports, maximize insurance benefits and opportunities for respite

IV. Spiritual Aspects of Care

A. Assessment: patients and families may choose to discuss spiritual issues with any IDT member. Spirituality as with psychosocial aspects of care is an ongoing shared responsibility of the IDT and the specialty of chaplains and clergy who are specifically trained in this area

    1.   Spirituality can be described as

        a)   The search for ultimate meaning and purpose of life which may involve connection to a higher power

        b)   The capacity to persevere with hope in the face of challenges to quality of life

        c)   A way of describing the organizing center in a person's life

    2.   Definitions related to spirituality

        a)   Religion: organized, codified and often institutionalized beliefs and practices that express one's spirituality. Can be described as the formal expression on one's spirituality[1]

b)   Faith: the acceptance, without objective proof, of something, e.g., God[1]

3.   Common concerns which can cause spiritual distress

a)   Alienation from the religious or spiritual community

b)   Lack of access to religious or spiritual rituals or contact with faith of choice

c)   Existential distress, despair, anxiety related to the struggle to find meaning in the experience of illness, suffering, death and dying

d)   Need to reconcile with God, others and self

e)   Spiritual beliefs opposed by family, peers and/or healthcare professionals

4.   Assessment and interventions

a)   Loss of hope or meaning

   i.   Possible causes: grief, overwhelming pain or disability, spiritual distress, emotional overload, fear of death, depression

   ii.   Interventions

     (a)   Effective symptom management to ensure maximal comfort

     (b)   Explore and acknowledge feelings

     (c)   Enhance sense of meaning and value to include respect for the full life experience of the individual and family

     (d)   Consider referral to spiritual and/or social work counselor, if appropriate

     (e)   Evaluate for depression/consider antidepressants and multidimensional interventions such as counseling, cognitive behavioral interventions

     (f)   Explore priorities and achievable goals to broaden the scope of hope and hope-related activities beyond cure of illness as the only acceptable and meaningful outcome

     (g)   Encourage life review

     (h)   Explore the value of rituals

     (i)   Enhance patient sense of control by offering options and choices

b)   Spiritual distress or unresolved spiritual issues

   i.   Possible causes: guilt, regrets, lack of meaning, loss of sense of self, problematic relationships, fear of unknown, wish or need for forgiveness

   ii.   Interventions

     (a)   Acknowledge spiritual suffering

     (b)   Encourage verbalization and elicit patient, family and caregiver values, relationships, fears, hopes and unfinished business

     (c)   Work with chaplains and spiritual counselors to provide requested prayers, readings, hymns, pastoral visits

     (d)   Work with IDT to consider most appropriate way to assist with issues of forgiveness, fractured relationships

     (e)   Respect individual belief systems

V.   **Cultural Aspects of Care**

    A.   **Assessment—requires consideration of the reality that cultural beliefs, values and practices infuse professional caregiver experience as well as the experience of the patient, family and caregiver. Professionals have the responsibility to**

        1.   Develop a knowledge base about the major cultures served in the programs in which they work

        2.   Adapt and accommodate assessment and interventions to respect cultural and spiritual variation

        3.   Understand that it is the clinician and team's responsibility to work through challenges and misunderstandings that can evolve when the culture of the healthcare professional differ from the culture of the family

        4.   Avoid using family as translators as family translate through the filter of their own emotional and cognitive reactions and clinicians cannot know what is being said or understood

        5.   Avoid stereotyping—do not assume all people from a certain country, region or nationality hold the same beliefs

        6.   Explore how assimilation, acculturation and generational differences influence family member's customs, language, beliefs and attitudes. Persons who have been in the United States for several generations may no longer follow the same customs as those who have recently arrived

        7.   Know that American healthcare is based on Western values such as individualism, open disclosure, desire for control and a future orientation which may be incongruous with the beliefs and values of the family

        8.   Know the areas of healthcare that can be impacted by cultural and/or religious beliefs and values including

            a)   Time orientation: emphasis on past versus present or future

            b)   Decision making style: self-determination/autonomy versus family, community decision making

            c)   Ideas about the causation of illness

            d)   Preferences and comfort with concept of "advance care planning"

            e)   Appropriateness of clothing, food preferences, traditional remedies

            f)   Issues related to privacy, gender, eye contact, personal space

            g)   Communication styles and preferences; truth telling, direct, non-verbal, respect for silence

            h)   Taboos, rituals and healing practices

            i)   Treatment decisions such as nutrition/hydration, discontinuing treatments, organ donation

            j)   Customs and belief systems related to death, transitions, after life etc.

            k)   Expectations and perceptions of healthcare relationships i.e., egalitarian, hierarchical, informal or paternalistic

            l)   Practices and behaviors related to illness, pain, treatments, suffering and end of life

Case Example: A 33-year-old Muslim woman from Mali is diagnosed with ovarian cancer. She and her husband have been in America for 5 years having come to work and sent money home to Africa to support family. She does not speak English and through the use of AT&T interpreters, staff is informed that she wishes to delegate all decisions to her husband. The AT&T interpreter is asked to explore the patient's understanding of her illness. The interpreter reports that in her culture it is not appropriate to ask or to tell a person that they are seriously ill and might die of their disease. Both patient and husband expect expert input and treatment from the doctor rather than being engaged in collaborative decision-making and husband is incredulous that in America this disease cannot be contained or cured. The husband cannot talk openly about the potential that his wife may die as acknowledging this is considered a challenge to the will of Allah. No one knows who will live and who will die. Staff insures that the patient is facing east toward Mecca and understands the importance of the prayers and verses from the Qur'an that are valued ritual at the time of death. There can be no planning for a funeral until, after the death and at that time, only family or Muslim staff can care for the body. Husband and friends from the mosque will wash and dress the body in an unsewn white cloth. The Imam from the community Mosque assists the staff to understand and provide respectful care and provides ongoing support to the husband after the death.

VI. Education

A.   **Definition: the knowledge or skill obtained or developed by a learning process; an instructive or enlightening experience**

   1.   Assess caregiver strengths and limitations as well as emotional (depression, anxiety, etc.), cognitive (fears, worries), cultural and physical (fatigue, insomnia, symptoms, etc.) factors to determine appropriateness, ability and readiness to integrate and carry out specific tasks

   2.   Teach primary caregivers specific techniques for patient care, e.g., medication administration, dressing changes, tube feedings

   3.   Language and cultural variations may require adaptation of teaching tool and approaches

   4.   Identify and consider individualizing factors that impact ability, style or environment of learning

      a)   Personal factors, e.g., patient or caregiver illiteracy, learning disabilities, impairments of vision or hearing, preferred learning style

      b)   Environmental challenges, e.g., noise, frequent interruptions, general chaos

      c)   Family dynamics and/or cultural factors which impact appropriateness of asking family members to provide care e.g., in some cultures it is not "proper" for a daughter to provide personal care for her father

      d)   Language differences and communication challenges, i.e., inability to speak, read and/or write English; no available bilingual professionals, no teaching materials in preferred language

   5.   Six steps to effective teaching[4]

      a)   State the purpose/goal/objective of the learning experience

      b)   Determine the needs of the learner, to match content and presentation to learner's needs

         i.   Assess language and cultural differences, readiness and motivation of learner

         ii.   Assess literacy, numeracy level, if appropriate

    c)   Devise a plan or a method of presenting the material to the learner; include members of the IDT in the planning and as instructors

    d)   Provide time for the learner to clarify content

        i.   Discuss using their own words

        ii.   Questions

        iii.   Observe

        iv.   Demonstrate

        v.   Example

    e)   Schedule time for the learner to practice the newly acquired knowledge or skills

        i.   Joint visits

        ii.   Patient/caregiver practice

        iii.   Observation

        iv.   Journal results

    f)   Schedule time for the learner's new skills to be evaluated. Involve other IDT if doing so enhances the comfort of the learner

        i.   Review

        ii.   Observation/return demonstration

        iii.   Verbal recall

        iv.   "What if" sharing

    g)   Utilize principles of adult learning[4]

        i.   Collaborating

        ii.   Critically reflective thinking

        iii.   Learning for action

        iv.   Learning in a participative environment

        v.   Empowering learners

        vi.   Dialoguing in the learning process

        vii.   Self-directed learning

6.   Monitor primary caregivers ability to provide care

    a)   Verbalization of understanding of instructions and willingness to provide care

    b)   Return demonstration of technique(s) taught

    c)   Observe, support and positively reinforce actual care during patient contact, i.e., visits to home, palliative care unit, acute care setting

    d)   Conduct on-going proactive assessment of caregiver physical and emotional status as over time caregiver's fatigue, mood and physical abilities change (a reality that may go unrecognized or unarticulated by the caregiver)

7. Instruct patient, family and caregiver on

   a) End Stage disease processes (see Chapter 3)

   b) Pain and Symptom management (see Chapters 4 and 5)

      i. Teach complementary, non-pharmacological modalities as well as pharmacological interventions e.g., cutaneous therapies (heat, cold, vibration), focused breathing, relaxation techniques, distraction, humor, massage, aromatherapy, etc.

8. Signs and symptoms of impending death (see Chapter 9)

VII. Advocacy

A. **Definition: the act of pleading or arguing in favor of something, such as a cause, idea or policy; also see active support**

B. **Monitor needs for changes in levels of palliative/hospice care and/or IDT services**

   1. Assess patient, family and caregiver needs at each contact

   2. Encourage family and caregiver to report changes in patient status as well as changes in their own physical and emotional state when they occur

   3. Encourage all team members who have patient/family contact to assess needs and report changes in patient condition and in the physical and emotional state of the caregiver and family

   4. Facilitate effective communication between patient, family and care providers; sit down, minimize personal distractions, take a couple of deep breaths to focus self

   5. Observe expressions, body language, etc. Pay special attention when they do not reflect what is being said

   6. Communicate in terms the listener understands, verbal and nonverbal

   7. Be sure you understand what the speaker intended to communicate, e.g., solicit feedback

C. **Assess and compensate, when possible, for barriers to communication**

   1. Language challenges

   2. Unwillingness or inability to concentrate on what is being said

   3. Lack of interest

   4. Environmental challenges, e.g., noise, interruptions, physical distance

   5. Physical barriers, e.g., visual or hearing impairment

D. **Encourage and support patient and family in sharing their individual decision-making style regarding illness related decisions and treatment options, i.e., empower patient and family; inquire about cultural dimensions**

E.   In collaboration with the primary physician and other members of the IDT and with consideration of individual and cultural differences, inform patient/family of treatment options available to them

1.   Assist the patient/family in clarifying their goals vs. focusing on specific treatments and/or interventions

2.   Discuss with patient/family each option with consideration of both physical and psychological benefits and burdens for patient, caregiver and family members

3.   Answer questions truthfully and as completely as possible

    a)   Utilize available resources as needed

    b)   Seek input from primary physician and other IDT members

4.   Support the patient/family in the decision making process

    a)   Acknowledge their right and ability to make the decision

    b)   Reassess decisions as medical and/or psychosocial situation changes

    c)   Be *non-judgmental*

    d)   Insure that needs of children, adolescents and extended family are met all along the continuum of illness and that expert clinical help is provided to assist family member of all generations. Refer to social worker who is specifically trained in this area (see Chapter 8)

F.   Make referrals for IDT consults

1.   Therapy services, e.g., physical therapy, speech therapy, occupational therapy

2.   Counseling services, e.g., spiritual, dietary, bereavement

3.   Medical social worker for counseling, crises intervention, family meetings and/or counseling, group intervention, resources

4.   Complementary and alternative modalities, e.g., massage therapy, music and other expressive therapies

G.   Participate in the shared process of advance care planning, e.g., advance directives, life support, DNR status, wills

1.   Inform patient of the teams' desire to understand and respect their preferences (right of self-determination) recognizing that cultural and individual beliefs may be based in different value system

    a)   Be sure to identify the decision maker and or healthcare agent selected by the patient

    b)   In some cultures the decision maker designated by legal statute may not be the decision maker designated by family or culture

2.   Assess decision-making preferences of patient and family

    a)   Information and education may be helpful for some and not for others

    b)   In some family settings the presence and participation of elders, clergy, healers, etc. are essential

3. Provide information and education to assist the patient/family in the decision-making process; individualize according to cultural and family belief systems that may be incongruous with advanced care planning concepts

4. Answer questions as needed and/or refer patient/family to appropriate resources

5. Assure patient/family that they will receive good care and treatment regardless of resuscitation status

6. Assure patient/family of continued care in the most appropriate setting as long as they meet admission criteria and desire care by the agency

VIII. The Environment of Care

A. **Assessment—implicit in an assessment of the environment of care is the acknowledgement and respect for the clinician responsibility that accompanies any invitation to enter the home or living space of a patient whether that be a mansion, a hut, a hospital or nursing home room**

1. Assess patient/family/caregiver ability to respond to emergencies, including fire, power failure, weather and other natural disasters

2. Assess family/caregiver physical and psychological ability to provide assistance with patient's activities of daily living

3. Recognize that one's home has psychological significance and changes or additions such as medical equipment has the potential to change a home into a medical setting

   a) Evaluate need for durable medical equipment and assistive devices

4. Perform a systematic safety assessment with an emphasis on prevention of falls, infection control, fire prevention, proper storage of medications, use and storage of oxygen

   a) Assess adequacy of electricity, heat, indoor plumbing, smoke alarms

5. Recognize need to modify or supplement plan of care to accommodate psychological/ socioeconomic factors

   a) Based on assessment, collaborate with the interdisciplinary team and refer to social worker if appropriate

6. Education and monitoring

   a) Inform patient/family/caregiver how and when to access hospice/palliative care services 24 hours a day by providing appropriate contact phone numbers (agency and/or healthcare provider)

   b) Instruct patient/family/caregiver on the procedure to obtain medications, equipment and supplies from agency or healthcare provider

   c) Educate about current and potential symptoms creating a proactive care plan with the goal of avoiding crises and unnecessary distress for patient/family/caregiver and staff

   d) Monitor disposal of supplies/equipment, e.g., needles/syringes

      i. Instruct patient/family/caregiver on proper use, storage and disposal of supplies/ equipment

       ii.   Refer to the agency's policies/procedures related to delivery and/or pick up of biohazardous medical waste

      iii.   Needles and syringes require puncture proof containers

      iv.   Soiled dressings should be discarded using a double bagging technique

  e)   Enhancing patient/family/caregiver comfort in handling medication

  f)   Medication administration

      i.   Instruct patient/family/caregiver on the agency's policies and procedures related to medications (including over the counter, prescription and controlled substances)

      ii.   Provide patient/family/caregiver instruction regarding appropriate medication use (medication name, dosage, schedule, indications and side effect profile) and document in the patient medical record

      iii.   Suggest the use of assistive devices, e.g., pill boxes, counting and/or measuring devices to assure patient is following medication orders correctly

      iv.   Evaluate instances of problematic over or under use of medication which may be due to

        (a) Misunderstanding of directions

        (b) Patients' self medicating in an effort to manage under treated pain or other symptoms

        (c) Medications being withheld due to fears of side effects, worry about addiction or hastening death

        (d) Substance abuse

          (i)   Do a risk assessment which includes: history, home environment, IDT observations, patterns of medication management and comprehensive symptom assessment

          (ii) Distinguish from pseudoaddiction (relief seeking that mimics drug-seeking behavior but emanates from unrelieved symptoms)

          (iii) Ongoing observation, consultation and assessment with IDT and patient, family and caregiver to work toward the goal of altering the care plan to safely and effectively treat symptoms and addictive disease if diagnosed

          (iv) Consult with a substance abuse specialist, if appropriate

          (v) Follow the agency/institutional protocol if substance abuse is suspected

  g)   Handling of medications at time of death

      i.   Inform family/caregiver of legal requirement regarding disposition of Schedule II controlled substances and inform supervisor if family and caregiver refuse disposal as per policy

      ii.   Destroy drugs in the presence of a witness

      iii.   Document outcomes as per agency policy

h) Monitor care for neglect and abuse (of patient, family and caregiver) in collaboration with members of the IDT, especially the social worker. The presence of any of these indicators does not necessarily mean the individual is abused; it should alert the nurse to the need for ongoing assessment and discussion with the other members of the IDT

   i.   Potential physical indicators include

      (a)   Unexplained or neglected injuries and/or those incompatible with history

      (b)   Evidence of inadequate care, e.g., gross pressure ulcers, soiled clothing or bed

      (c)   Evidence of inadequate or inappropriate administration of medication

      (d)   Dehydration and/or malnourishment without illness-related cause

      (e)   Lack of bandages on injuries or stitches when indicated or evidence of unset bones

      (f)   Cuts, lacerations, puncture wounds, burns

      (g)   Bruises, welts, discoloration, e.g., bilateral on upper arms, morphologically similar to an object, clustered in one general area

   ii.   Potential behavioral indicators in patient, family or caregiver include

      (a)   Fear, withdrawal, helplessness, hesitation to talk openly, implausible stories, ambivalence/contradictory statements not due to mental dysfunction, resignation, non-responsiveness

      (b)   Aggressive behavior toward patient or aggressive behavior toward caregiver that may emanate from anger, frustration at being sick, feeling dependent or trapped or a reflection of prior abuse history

      (c)   Patient/family/caregiver disclosure of abuse or observation of physical, emotional abuse or neglect

   iii.   Potential behavioral indicators on part of family/caregiver

      (a)   Patient/client not given the opportunity to speak for self or to be alone with team members

      (b)   Family declines visits from members of the IDT

      (c)   Absence of necessary, available assistance, attitudes of indifference or anger toward patient

      (d)   Family and caregiver blames patient for their illness or incapacitation

   iv.   Interventions

      (a)   Confer with members of the IDT especially the social worker. Signs of neglect and abuse have multilevel etiologies such as

         (i)   Caregiver fatigue and depression

         (ii)   Patient anger, rage, helplessness or prior history of abuse in family

         (iii)   Patient's inability or unwillingness to cooperate with family/caregivers

(iv) Inadequate symptom management e.g., pain, delirium

(v) Increased stress, financial, physical, emotional

(vi) Psychiatric illness, alcoholism, drug abuse, cognitive impairment

(b) Report according to applicable state law

(i) If possible, inform patient/caregiver that a report is being made

IX. The Death Event

A. Provide expertise and support to family/caregiver at time of impending death, in consult with IDT, as the experience of the death itself has the potential to profoundly impact the surviving family member's/caregiver's perceptions and memories

1. Management of acute physical symptoms

2. Consult members of IDT to determine who is most appropriate or able to provide support

3. Enhance dignity for the patient both in the physical care provided and in verbal communication to and around the patient

4. Visit at time of death whether at home, in hospital or long-term care facility

5. If the death is at home activities might include pronouncement, notification and arranging transportation of the body

6. Attendance at the death provides support for the patient/family/caregiver and is often helpful to clinicians as well

7. Notify healthcare professionals who have been important caregivers over the history of the illness

X. Grief and Loss

A. Theory and concepts of grief and loss

1. Definitions of key concepts[5]

a) Bereavement is the period after a loss which may result from death, divorce, loss of employment etc.

b) Grief is the emotional response associated with loss

c) Mourning is the process of adaptation, including the cultural and social rituals prescribed as accompaniments

d) Anticipatory grief: precedes the death and results from the expectation of the death event

e) Complicated grief represents a pathological outcome involving psychological, social or physical morbidity (see Table 1)

f) Disenfranchised grief: represents the hidden sorrow of the marginalized where there is less social permission to express many dimensions of loss (e.g., death of a homosexual partner)

g) Grief counseling assists in facilitating uncomplicated or normal grief to a healthy completion of the task of grieving

h) Grief therapy includes specialized techniques which are used to help people with abnormal or complicated grief reactions (see Table 1)

2. Risk factors for complicated grief[5]

a) Nature of the death

i. Untimely within the life cycle (e.g., death of a child)

ii. Sudden and unexpected

iii. Traumatic

iv. Stigmatized (e.g., AIDS or suicide)

b) Strengths and vulnerabilities of the caregiver/bereaved

i. Past history of psychiatric disorder

ii. Personality and coping style (e.g., intense worrier, low-self esteem)

iii. Cumulative experience of losses

c) Nature of the relationship with the deceased

i. Overly dependent (e.g., clinging, symbiotic)

ii. Ambivalent (e.g., anger related to abuse, infidelity)

d) Family and support network

i. Problematic, distressed family (e.g., poor cohesiveness and communication, high conflict)

ii. Isolated (e.g., new migrant, new residential move)

iii. Alienated (e.g., perception of poor support)

3. Assess family/caregiver for risk of complicated grief and refer for appropriate bereavement interventions

4. Interventions

a) Support family/caregiver to facilitate and promote healthy grieving following the death of the patient

b) Ensure adequate symptom management along the continuum of illness

c) Support and encourage life review

d) Use audio visual tools (e.g., photographs, memorabilia, music)

e) Demonstrate sensitivity to cultural and/or religious bereavement customs

f) Notify bereavement coordinator according to agency/institutional policy for follow up

g) Facilitate transition into bereavement services

h) Participate in formal closure activity (e.g., visit, call, sympathy card)

i. Condolence call to be made by appropriate member(s) of the IDT

ii. Participate in signing of sympathy card for family/caregiver

iii. Attend patient's funeral/memorial service if appropriate

      iv. Seek, accept or create an individual ritual or process to assist in your own integration of the loss, either as individual or with IDT

      v. Attend agency/institutional memorial service if appropriate

i) Counsel or provide emotional support regarding grief and loss for family and caregiver as a natural extension of the relationship established with clinicians over time[6]

      i. Help the survivor explore the significance of the loss

      ii. Help the survivor to identify and express feelings, lingering questions and reminiscences

      iii. Assist in practical aspects of living without the deceased

      iv. Encourage time to grieve

      v. Interpret and affirm "normal" grief behavior

      vi. Encourage acceptance of individual differences in family members grief behaviors and emotions

      vii. Provide continuing support

      viii. Refer those who need further intervention to appropriate professionals/resources

Table 1: Differences between Grief and Trauma[7]

Grief	Trauma
Sadness	**Terror**
• Often does *not* contain trauma	• *Trauma reactions generally include grief Especially in children, are hidden and unknown*
• Can talk about what happened	
• **Pain** is acknowledgement of the loss	• ***Pain*** *triggers terror, powerlessness and a loss of safety*
• **Anger** is generally non-assaultive	
Identity: does not generally distort nor disfigure identity	• Anger **often becomes destructive and assaultive**

• **Guilt**
  —If only . . .
  —I wish I would have/not have
	Identity: Attacks, distorts, disfigures identity ("I wasn't myself")

• **Dreams: focus is on the loss**	• **Guilt:**
	  —It was my fault
	  —I could have prevented it
	  —It should have been me

	• **Dreams: focus on self as potential/ perennial victim**

Schneider, John (2000) The Overdiagnosis of Depression, Seasons Press, Traverse City, MI. www.seasonspress.com.

Table 2: Comparing Grieving With Depression[7]

Issue	Grieving	Depression
Is there a loss?	Yes	Maybe/maybe not
What do you think about?	At times, you may be obsessed with the loss. At other times, you can think of other things.	Often obsessed with yourself and how this loss is unfair or a punishment.
What are your dreams & fantasies?	Vivid, clear dreams, sometimes of the loss, which can sometimes be comforting.	Flashbacks, nightmares, same disturbing dreams over and over
What is the physical effect?	Gain or lose some weight; Exercise a lot or stops entirely. Have trouble getting to sleep. Feel tired a lot.	Weight change is extreme. Exercise is also at extremes. Have trouble getting up; awaken with disturbing dreams. Always restless *or* always sleeping or tired.
What is the spiritual effect?	A connection is felt to something beyond the self, e.g., a belief in God and that this is happening for a reason. Able to challenge, revise, or maintain previously held beliefs.	Especially a year or more past a loss, a persistent failure to find meaning and a continued focus on "why me," on the unfairness & meaninglessness of the loss. Resist any "pat" answers when you question beliefs. Tends to discard previously held beliefs.
How do you feel?	Moody: Shifts in mood from anger to sadness to more positive feelings in the same day.	Can be hard to "read" emotionally, or you can be at an extreme, either crying all the time *or* not at all, angry all the time *or* not at all. Rarely feel "good."
How do you respond to others?	Generally respond to warmth, pressure, and reassurance. You appreciate being left alone but not ignored.	Either can't stand people at all or can't be without them. You respond to promises and urging *or* you remain unresponsive. Often feel abandoned and unloved when alone.
What happens to having pleasurable experiences?	As long as the pleasure isn't something that only came from the loss (e.g. sex after losing partner), it can be okay	Either extreme—you eat, drink, and are merry *or* you experience no pleasure at all. Pain as the absence of pleasure.
How do you attach and relate to others?	Likes to have close friends or someone who will listen to your story. Misses being loved or able to love others.	Feel unloved and incapable of loving. Often go about proving it!

Schneider, John (2000) The Overdiagnosis of Depression, Seasons Press, Traverse City, MI. www.seasonspress.com.

CITED REFERENCES

1. Ferrell B, Coyle N, eds. *Textbook of Palliative Nursing*. New York, NY: Oxford University Press; 2001.

2. Matzo M, Sherman D, eds. *Palliative Care Nursing: Quality Care to the End of Life*. New York, NY: Springer Publishing Company; 2001.

3. Levine C, ed. *Always on Call: When Illness Turns Families into Caregivers*. New York, NY: United Hospital Fund; 2004.

4. Leonard DJ. Workplace education: adult education in a hospital staff development department. *Journal of Nursing Staff Development*. 1993;No 9:68–73.

5. Doyle D, Hanks G, Cherny N, Calman K, eds. *Oxford Textbook of Palliative Medicine*. 3rd ed. New York, NY: Oxford University Press; 2004.

6. Worden JW. *Grief Counseling and Grief Therapy*. 2nd ed. New York, NY: Springer; 1991.

7. Schneider J. The Overdiangosis of Depression. Traverse City, MI: Seasons Press; 2000. (www.seasonspress.com).

ADDITIONAL REFERENCES AND RESOURSES

Berzoff J, Silverman P, eds. Living with Dying: A Comprehensive Resource for Healthcare Practitioners. New York, NY: Columbia University Press; 2004.

Bhungalia S, Kemp C. (Asian) Indian health beliefs and practices related to the end of life. *Journal of Hospice and Palliative Nursing*. 2002:4(1):54–58.

Blackhall LJ, Frank G, Murphy ST, Michel V, Palmer JM, Azen SP. Ethnicity and attitudes towards life sustaining technology. *Social Science & Medicine*. 1999;48(12):1779–1789.

Borneman T, Stahl C, Ferrell B, Smith D. The concept of hope in family caregivers of cancer patients and home. *Journal of Hospice and Palliative Nursing*. 2002:4(1):21–33.

Bowman K. Communication, negotiation and mediation: dealing with conflict in end-of-life decisions. *Journal of Palliative Care*. 2000;16:S17–S24.

Chochinov HM. Dignity-conserving care—a new model for palliative care: helping the patient feel valued. *JAMA*. 2002;287(17);2253–2260.

Daaleman TP, VandeCreek L. Placing religion and spirituality in end-of-life care. *JAMA*. 2000;284(19):2514–2517.

Doorenbos AZ. Hospice access for Asian Indian immigrants. *Journal of Hospice and Palliative Nursing*. 2002:5(1):27–33.

Doug H, Kemp C. Culture and the end of life: Nigerians. *Journal of Hospice and Palliative Nursing*. 2002:4(2):111-115.

Ellis RR. Multicultural grief counseling. In: Doka KJ, Davidson JD, eds. *Living with grief: Who we are; how we grieve*. Washington, DC: Hospice Foundation of America; 1998:248–260.

Irish DP, Lundquist KF, Nelsen VJ, eds. *Ethnic Variations in Dying, Death and Grief: Diversity in Universality*. Washington, DC: Taylor & Francis; 1993.

Kagawa-Singer M. The cultural context of death rituals and mourning practices. *Oncology Nursing Forum*. 1998;25(10):1752–1756.

Kagawa-Singer M, Blackhall LJ. Negotiating cross-cultural issues at the end of life: "You got to go where he lives." *JAMA*. 2001;286(23):2993–3001.

Kemp C, Chang BJ. Culture and the end of life: Chinese. *Journal of Hospice and Palliative Nursing*. 2002:4(3):173–178.

Koenig B, Gates-Williams J. Understanding cultural differences in caring for dying patients. *Caring for Patients at the End of Life (Special Issue) Western Journal of Medicine*, 1997;163:244–249.

Lipson JG, Dibble SL, Minarik PA, eds. *Culture & Nursing Care: A Pocket Guide*. San Francisco, CA: UCSF Nursing Press; 2000.

McCaffery M, Pasero C. *Pain: Clinical Manual* 2nd ed. New York, NY: Mosby; 1999.

Nicoll LH. Sandy Chen Stokes: breaking down barriers to better end-of-life care for Chinese Americans. *Journal of Hospice and Palliative Nursing*. 2002:4(3):178–179.

Otis-Green S, Rutland C. Marginalization at the end of life. In: Berzoff J, Silverman P, eds. *Living with Dying: A comprehensive Resource for Healthcare Practitioners*. New York, NY: Columbia University Press; 2004.

Parker-Oliver D. Redefining hope for the terminally ill. *American Journal of Hospice and Palliative Care*. 2002;19(2):115-120.

Romesberg TL. Understanding grief: a component of neonatal palliative care. *Journal of Hospice and Palliative Nursing*. 2002:6(3):161–170.

Stephenson PL, Draucker C, Martsolf DS. The experience of spirituality in the lives of hospice patients. *Journal of Hospice and Palliative Nursing*. 2002:5(1):51–58.

Scannell-Desch E. Prebereavement and postbereavement struggles and triumphs of midlife widows. *Journal of Hospice and Palliative Nursing*. 2002:7(1):15–22.

Teno JM, Casey VA, Welch, LC, Edgman-Levitan S. Patient-focused, family-centered end-of-life medical care: views of the guidelines and bereaved family members. *Journal of Pain and Symptom Management*. 2001;22(3):738–751.

Vachon MLS. Burnout and symptoms of stress in staff working in palliative care. In: Chochinov HM, Breitbart W, eds. *Handbook of Psychiatry in Palliative Medicine*. New York, NY: Oxford University Press; 2000:303–319.

WEB SITE/INTERNET RESOURCES ON CULTURE, ETHNICITY AND RELIGION

Office of Minority Health Information Center
http://www.omhrc.gov/clas
Assuring Cultural Competence in Health Care: Recommendations for National Standards and Outcomes

Cross-Cultural Health Care Program
http://www.xculture.org/
National program providing training on healthcare that is linguistically and culturally appropriate

CultureMed
http://www.sunyit.edu/library/html/culturedmed/

Diversity Rx
http://www.diversityrx.org/
Clearinghouse of information on how to meet the language and cultural needs of minorities, immigrants, refugees and other diverse populations seeking healthcare

http://www.Beliefnet.com
Educational information about different religions and their views concerning death and grieving; also useful for finding congregations all over the country

EthnoMed: Ethnic Medicine Information center from Harborview Medical Center
http://ethnomed.org/

HHS Office of Minority Health
http://www.omhrc.gov/omh/programs/2pgprograms/cultural4.htm

National Center for Cultural Competence
http://gucchd.georgetown.edu/nccc/

WEB SITE/INTERNET RESOURCES FOR INTERPRETERS

Certified Language International
www.clilang.com; 800-237-8434

Language Line Services
www.languageline.com; 800-752-0093

Tele-Interpreters
www.teleinterpreters.com

Online Interpreters
www.onlineinterpreters.com; 888-922-3582

CHAPTER VII

THE DYING PERSON IN VARIOUS CARE SETTINGS

Marianne L. Matzo, Ph.D., APRN, FAAN

First Edition Authors
Marianne L. Matzo, Ph.D., APRN, FAAN, Joanne E. Sheldon, RN, MEd, CHPN®, CIC

I. **The Challenge for Nurses to Provide Quality End-of-Life Care**

    A. **There are opportunities for nursing leadership in providing quality end-of-life care in settings other than the traditional "hospice environment"**

    B. **Attention to the unique needs of patients and families at this time reflects a commitment to nursing excellence**

    C. **Mandates to integrate palliative care principles across illness trajectories and care settings stem from the increased awareness of inadequacies of care of the dying patients and their families**

        1. As the population ages and the incidence of chronic, progressive illness continues to increase there will be increased demands from patients and families as well as healthcare providers to have established standards of care for the dying and their families

        2. To respond to the demands, the nursing profession must ensure that core competencies in end-of-life (EOL) care serve as a foundation to guide professional nurses in expert care of the dying

    D. **Nursing is in the unique position to institute change/improvement within the system since the nurse is the conduit for assessing the needs of the patient and implementing the goals of a team care plan/treatment**

    E. **The following content is applicable when providing end-of-life nursing care in any setting**

II. **The Need for Improved Care at the End of Life**

    A. **Death and Dying in America: Changes over the Last Century**

        1. Late 1800s

            a) Healthcare professionals had little to offer the sick beyond the easing of symptoms associated with disease

169

    b)   Most deaths occurred at home with extended family members caring for the dying person[1,2]

    c)   Most died within days of onset of illness

2.   Early to middle 1900s (growth of science and industry brought about broad, sweeping changes)

    a)   Improvements in living and working conditions, sanitation and an emphasis on disease prevention

    b)   Life-saving and life-prolonging treatments such as antibiotics, cardiopulmonary resuscitation and advances in anesthesia[3]

    c)   The focus of healthcare shifted from easing suffering to curing disease

    d)   Society's expectations changed regarding treatments and interventions for curable as well as incurable illnesses[4]

        i.   Patients whose disease failed to respond to treatments were given less priority

        ii.   Death itself became equated with medical failure[2]

3.   Recent demographics and social trends

    a)   Decreased age-adjusted death rate

    b)   Increased life expectancy; as death rates declined, life expectancy rose sharply and has been primarily linked to the reduction in infant and child mortality[1]

    c)   Racial and ethnic differences

        i.   Significant variations exist among racial, ethnic, age, sex and economic status sub-groups

        ii.   Variations often highlight serious gaps in access to healthcare and adequate EOL care

        iii.   In most cases, socially disadvantaged individuals experience higher mortality rates and death at a younger age[1,5,6]

    d)   Aging of the population

        i.   Those > 65 years represent a progressively larger number and proportion of the population due to changing mortality patterns

        ii.   By the year 2030, as the baby boom generation reaches the age of 65, there will be approximately 70 million older persons, more than double the number in 1997[7]

        iii.   The number of people over age 85 will double to 9 million by the year 2030[7]

4.   Site of death

    a)   Institutions have replaced the home as the most common place where death occurs

    b)   Care is more likely to be given by strangers/healthcare professionals than family members[1]

5. Disease and dying trajectories illustrate differences in the dying experience by examining the duration of the dying process and the course of the disease or injury[1,3,8]

   a) Sudden, unexpected death

   b) Steady decline, short terminal phase

   c) Slow decline, periodic crises and death

6. Impact

   a) Americans are living longer

   b) The period of time of living with progressive and eventually fatal illness is generally prolonged and often marked by functional dependency on others

   c) There is a trend toward the separation of family members by great distances

   d) An individual may not experience the death of a significant other until well into his/her adult years

      i. Isolation from the death experience increases discomfort with death and the dying process; this also applies to healthcare professionals

      ii. These individuals are at risk of an increased, profound emotional response to the death of a relative, friend or other significant person[1,3,9]

   e) Scientific and technological advances have led to the medicalization of care at the end of life; efforts toward cure and eliminating physiological dysfunction often overshadow the obligation to provide appropriate treatment and compassionate care[10]

   f) The shift to a curative focus may actually bring about hope for cure of disease; the fact that some diseases have been cured leads to therapeutic optimism

   g) Health professionals have become increasingly uncomfortable in addressing end-of-life concerns with patients and families

7. SUPPORT Study

   a) The *Study* to *Understand Prognosis* and *Preferences* for *Outcomes* and *Risks* of *Treatment*

   b) Substantial shortcomings exist in care for seriously ill, hospitalized adults

   c) To improve the experience of seriously ill and dying patients, greater individual and societal commitment and more proactive and forceful measures may be needed[11]

   d) SUPPORT: Phase I Results

      i. 46% of DNR orders were written within 2 days of death

      ii. Of patients preferring DNR, <50% of their physicians were aware of their wishes

      iii. 38% of those who died spent >10 days in ICU

      iv. Half of patients had moderate-severe pain >50% of last 3 days of life

B. Disparity between the Way People Die and the Way They Want to Die

1. Patient/family perspective

   a) Most adults prefer to be cared for at home if terminally ill and the majority would be interested in a comprehensive program of EOL care, such as hospice[12]

b) The majority of adults (62% of those surveyed) believe it would take a year or more to adjust to the death of a loved one[12]

c) The two greatest fears associated with death are being a burden to family and being in pain[12]

d) Many have come to fear the prospect of prolonged death characterized by over-treatment and the use of life-sustaining technology and invasive, debilitating treatments

e) Patients and families worry that when "nothing more can be done," their healthcare providers will abandon them

f) Past experiences with the death of others may influence fears about unrelieved symptoms and increased dependence on others

g) Families may be uncertain about how to provide physical care and adjust to role changes[13]

h) Many families drain life savings in order to cover costs of care for terminally ill family members[14]

2. Barriers to quality care at the end of life

a) The realities of life-limiting diseases

i. Failure to acknowledge the limits of medicine may lead to futile care

ii. Inappropriate use of aggressive curative treatments can prolong the dying process and contribute to physical and emotional distress

b) Lack of adequate training of professionals

i. Professionals often receive little training regarding the safe and effective means of controlling pain and other symptoms, as well as strategies to address the physical, psychological, social and spiritual aspects of care

ii. Many health professionals are uncomfortable communicating bad news and prognosis

iii. Nurses cannot practice what they do not know; educational efforts must incorporate the preparation of students for a professional role that includes providing quality nursing care to those approaching death[15]

c) Delayed access to hospice and palliative care services

i. Services not well understood

ii. Lack of understanding of what comprehensive EOL programs offer leads to confusion over when it is appropriate to consult or transfer care to these services

iii. More timely referrals are necessary in order for patients and families to reap the full benefit of hospice and palliative care services

iv. Surveys indicate that patients prefer to die at home, yet only 29% of terminally ill patients enroll in hospice programs[1,16]; the numbers are higher (approximately 50%) for cancer patients[17]

v. Increased approval and development of new anti-cancer drugs and other medications may give the message that there is always "one more treatment we can try," and in some cases, delay referral to hospice and/or palliative care

d)   Rules and regulations

i.   Institutional regulations that impede good EOL care include restrictive visiting hours and inadequate policies for pain and symptom management

ii.   Regulation of controlled substances has led to fear of prosecution for prescribing and administering medications to relieve pain and other symptoms

iii.   Issues regarding access to care, insurance coverage and the potential need to hire a caregiver from outside the family contribute to financial barriers to care

C.   Costs of End-of-Life Care

1.   Managed care

a)   Today patients admitted to hospitals are more critically ill, length of stay has decreased and there is an increase in the use of ambulatory services

i.   Patients discharged to the home and long-term care facilities are more seriously ill

ii.   There is a trend towards increased utilization of home care services[18]

b)   The healthcare system is straining under the effects of rapid change, making the implementation of comprehensive EOL care more difficult

c)   Certain managed care plan restrictions particularly affect people with advanced illness[1] such as

i.   Limiting the scope of benefits to reduce costs

ii.   Financial incentives for practitioners and providers to provide less care

iii.   Patient services that require pre-authorization

iv.   Coverage for services provided only by designated physicians and healthcare providers

2.   Expenses for care at the end of life

a)   Spending for end-of-life in a particular year may not reflect the cumulative cost of care for an illness with a long disease/dying trajectory compared with costs of intensive treatment for an illness with a short trajectory

b)   Increased costs and healthcare spending for end-of-life care are influenced by factors such as the population growth, general inflation in the economy and medical inflation[1]

c)   Evaluation of outcomes and costs of care is necessary to validate palliative care services; continued development and utilization of outcome indicators should provide an objective evaluation of care and the development of standards to guide program development[19]

3.   Payment for care at the end of life

a)   Public funding

i.   Efforts to control costs and reduce spending are placing increased pressure on Medicare, Medicaid and Social Security programs[1]

ii.   Medicare: covers 83% of those who die each year who are age 65 or older; and younger persons with disabilities and certain illnesses

iii. The 63% of Medicare patients with 2 or more chronic conditions account for 95% of Medicare spending[7]

iv. Medicaid pays for a smaller portion of healthcare costs and larger portion of long-term care

b) Hospice Medicare Benefit

i. Created early 1980s, as both cost containment and improving the quality care of the dying

ii. For persons with "expected six month survival," but never defined that term

iii. Medicare Hospice Benefit developed to care for the *dying:* regulations require 6 month prognosis and decision to forego coverage for life prolonging care

c) Other

i. Private insurance

ii. Programs servicing veterans

iii. Out of pocket payments by patient/family

D. Access to End-of-Life Care

1. Current trends that limit access include

a) Restrictive rules regarding eligibility

b) The tendency to discourage new enrollment or to continue enrollment of sicker individuals in certain health plans

c) Poor access for populations at risk: the elderly, pediatric patients, the homeless and the uninsured

d) Delayed referral to hospice and palliative services

e) Reluctance of physician to refer—not wanting to look like this is "giving up on the patient"

f) Family may not request referral or may be reluctant to accept referral when offered

g) Cultural barriers

E. Resource Allocation for End-of-Life Care

1. Determining the benefit of treatments or therapies

a) Does a treatment or therapy match the patient/family goals for care?

b) Do the benefits outweigh the risks?

2. Allocation questions are shadowed by questions of cost; everything that can be done to ensure comfort and quality life closure should be pursued

3. Nurses must be conscious of financial costs as well as the burden of treatments and therapies on the patient/family

F.   Optimum Use of Community Resources for End-of-Life Care

1.   Interdisciplinary teamwork extends to community resources

2.   Early access of needed resources can significantly decrease stressors and the perception of burden especially for patients/families that do not have extended family to assist the primary caregiver

G.   Denial of Death

1.   Reluctance to take away "hope" may delay accessing needed services and may be one of the biggest barriers[8]

2.   Poor communication about patient and family preferences can impede timely referrals to comprehensive end-of-life services

H.   Patient/family Perspective of End-of-Life Care

1.   Caring for a dying patient can exhaust a family's financial resources[1] because of missed work and out of pocket medical costs

2.   1996 United States estimates: 25 million caregivers deliver care at home to a seriously ill relative

3.   Mean hours caregiving per week: 18. Cost equivalent of uncompensated care: 194 billion dollars (assume $8/hr)[20]

4.   An increasing amount of payment for care has shifted to the patient/family; for persons on limited budgets this may mean they would not be able to stay at home due to the expense of hiring assistive personnel[14]

5.   The inability to access services that allow patients to remain at home which forces them, instead, to turn to nursing homes or other institutional care that actually increases costs of care covered by private and public sources; custodial care in institutions is not covered by Medicare and thus, there is a greater financial burden to the family[21]

I.   Outcomes of End-of-Life Care

1.   American society does not view any death (even an expected one) as a desired outcome, but improved EOL care as evaluated by measuring outcomes that reflect quality end-of-life closure can help the public at large to see the dying process as a more positive part of life

2.   Attention to realistic outcomes of care, better understanding and utilization of advanced directives, discussions regarding and increased use of hospice and palliative care services are strategies that can reduce costs at the end of life[1]

III.   The Role of the Nurse

A.   Nurses as the Constant across all Settings

1.   Nurses are the healthcare providers who spend more time with the patients and their families than any other member of the healthcare team

2.   Extending palliative care principles across settings to improve end-of-life care

3. Integrating palliative care principles across settings

   a) Nurses enter into intense, intimate relationships with patients and families

   b) They are therefore in a key position to impact patients' and families' ability to accomplish life completion goals by incorporating the principles of hospice and palliative care across all healthcare settings

4. The American Nurses Association's *Code for Nurses*[22] emphasizes that "nursing care extends to anyone requiring the services of the nurse for the promotion of health, the prevention of illness, the restoration of health, the alleviation of suffering and the provision of supportive care of the dying"

5. In any setting, the application of knowledge and skills that reflect the principles of palliative care allow the nurse to recognize subtle shifts in the patient's condition that often affect patient and family care preferences; this allows for timely reevaluation and resetting of goals

6. Nurses can impact quality end-of-life closure by identifying persons with any life-threatening illness or condition

   a) Early identification means that palliative care can be started sooner, allowing patients and families to set and achieve goals[4]

   b) One very useful technique is to ask, "Is the patient now sick enough that it would not be a surprise if he/she died in the next 3-12 months?" This may identify patients who would otherwise not be recognized to be in need of palliative care[17]

B. Expanding the Concept of Healing

1. Ensuring quality EOL closure

   a) At the end of life, nursing care shifts from a focus of wellness/recovery to an understanding of "healing"[23]

   b) Because of their unique relationship to patients and families, nurses are in a position to promote comfort care for the dying as an active, desirable and important skill and an integral component of nursing care

2. Healing

   a) Comes from attention to the multiple dimensions that influence a person's quality of life[14]

   b) Healing requires the recognition of the human face of each person and the communication that both the healer and the healed share a bond that ties them to each other through their humanity and their mortality[24]

C. The Importance of "Presence"

1. Some things cannot be "fixed"

   a) Care at the end of life can frustrate health professionals, family and friends when attempts to decrease suffering are either not possible or interventions are not successful[9]

  b) Some things that cannot be fixed[9,25]

    i. We cannot change the inevitability of death

    ii. We cannot erase the anguish felt when someone we love dies

    iii. We all must face the fact that we too will die

    iv. No matter how hard we try, the perfect words or gestures to relieve patient and family distress rarely, if ever, exist

    v. It is often enough to just be with the person

 2. The use of "Presence" as a way of expressing compassionate caring

  a) To be present with dying patients and their families is to allow oneself to enter into another's world and to respond with compassion[26]

  b) The nurse can use therapeutic presence as a means of communicating care for the patient struggling with the emotional and spiritual elements of suffering associated with multiple losses

  c) "Presence may in fact be our greatest gift to these patients and their families"[27]

D. Maintaining a Realistic Perspective

 1. There is no right way to die, no cookbook approach

 2. Crises and difficulties arise along with unexpected and profound joys

 3. A flexible approach is essential to meet the changing needs of the patient and family

 4. Recognition that quality of life (QOL) is determined by the unique needs of the patient and family assists the nurse in remaining focused on goals of care

IV. The Nurse's Role in Improving Care Systems[28]

A. Reasons to Participate in and Lead Reform

 1. Current services and reliability are woefully inadequate

 2. The best of current practices would not yield a competent, reliable care system for those "sick enough to die"

 3. The special trust that society gives to healthcare professionals includes an obligation to ensure high quality, reliability and pursuit of excellence

 4. When the care system has especially serious shortcomings in serving its' community, professionals have similarly strong obligations to correct those shortcomings

 5. Specific skills, attitudes and behaviors are helpful in this work and they can (and should) be learned and taught

 6. The history of reform in end-of-life care has been dominated by nursing—from establishing hospice programs through quality improvement projects; nurse leaders and managers have the opportunity and track record to make improvements happen

 7. No one knows exactly how to put together trustworthy, reliable, effective and efficient care systems; the pace of useful change depends on the pace of learning, which largely depends on innovation, evaluation and communication

B. What would reform aim to do?

1. At the most general level, provide a care system that can promise to a person who has a life-limiting progressive illness

   a) Good medical treatment

   b) Competent symptom management

   c) Continuity, coordination and comprehensiveness

   d) Inclusion in the care-planning process

   e) Individualized care reflecting patient and family preferences

2. It helps to think of "the population of people who _____", rather than just the separate individual, i.e., not just how to help Mr. Smith, but also how to reliably and effectively serve patients like Mr. Smith

3. Nurses might conceive of improvement activities at various "levels": personal, service team, provider organization, region, state and federal policy

   a) Service Teams

      i. The strongest vehicle for improvement seems to be rapid cycle quality improvement. Many variations are possible, but fundamental elements include[17]

         (a) An aim—stated in demonstrable terms relevant to patients and "owned" by the team

         (b) A team that wants to achieve the aim and is willing to work to do so

         (c) A measure that will show whether the team is achieving the goal

         (d) A set of changes that might achieve the aim

         (e) Serial implementation of changes, with evaluation and learning, by the team, from each Plan-Do-Study-Act Cycle (PDSA cycle)

         (f) The expansion and implementation of effective changes, which sustains reform and builds on success

      ii. One of the most difficult arenas for change is "noticing" or "attending to" deficits in care; nurses must become uncomfortable with routine shortcomings in order to develop motivation and commitment to change

      iii. Changes that might be seen as shortening a patient's life require careful attention; be sure that many people are involved and that good intentions and thoughtful considerations are well evidenced

   b) Provider organizations

      i. Rapid cycle quality improvement (under various names) is central to improving organizational performance

         (a) The process is the same

         (b) Organizational leadership is often very important to sustained improvement

      ii. There is a strong track record of nurse-led success in improving end-of-life care when the team aims for improving performance in an arena that they "own"

c) Regional healthcare systems

    i. Most patients need the services of multiple organizations; promises need to be "durable" across time and organizations

    ii. Very little work has addressed continuity of people, care plans, advance directives or anything else across time and settings; yet, this is essential

        (a) Nurses can encourage, contribute to and collaborate with efforts to make transfers less frequent, less disruptive and better supported

        (b) Likewise, standardization of protocols and measures of success for populations are useful and worthwhile

    iii. At the least, nurses should be familiar with the settings that their patients utilize at the end of life, including their personnel, practices and potentials (i.e., the nursing home nurse needs to sit-in on a hospice team, visit the hospital discharge nurse, etc.)

d) State and federal policies

    i. The United States society built a healthcare system around acute illness—aiming mainly for prevention and rescue. The demographics are now different. Most people face many months of living with slowly progressive disabling disease—which will eventually be fatal

    ii. Eventually, all reform runs into dysfunctional coverage, reimbursement and regulation. Professionals have an obligation to act to correct these problems

    iii. Some resources for policy reform

        (a) Americans for Better Care of the Dying, http://www.abcd-caring.org

        (b) National Hospice and Palliative Care Organization (NHPCO), http://www.nhpco.org

V. Death and Dying in the Hospital Setting

A. Death in the hospital: What do we know about it?

1. Physical suffering

2. Poor to non-existent communication about the goals of medical care

3. Lack of concordance of care with patient and family preferences

4. Huge financial, physical and emotional burdens on family caregivers

5. Suffering in professional caregivers

6. Fiscal impact on hospitals

7. Poor inclusion of family in care of the dying

B. All staff trained to provide aggressive care to save life

1. CPR expected to be performed unless a specific order says otherwise

2. Goals are rigorous care, resuscitation and recovery

3. Hard to prepare the patient and family for death when intensive efforts are ongoing to save the life

4. Death in acute care settings seen as resulting from ineffective care

C. Standard hospital policies and procedures typically inconsistent with palliative and hospice care approaches

D. 98% of Medicare decedents spent *at least some time* in a hospital in the year before death[29]

1. Nurses are in the best position to help reform these policies because they are the core of the healthcare delivery system in the hospital

2. Whichever changes nursing addresses, they should include principles and domains of hospice and palliative care, specifically

   a) Interdisciplinary approach

   b) Patient centered reports and rankings of quality of care

   c) Family support

   d) Functional status

   e) Continuity of care

   f) Spirituality

   g) Advance care planning

   h) Projected survival time and decisions regarding the aggressiveness of care

   i) Physical and emotional symptom management

   j) Grief and bereavement

   k) Communication among caregivers, patients and families

E. Facilitating a Good Death in the Hospital

1. Palliative Care Pathways and Standard Orders should be in place

2. Symptom relief protocols and standing orders for the palliative care patient

3. Palliative Care consultation teams should include

   a) Nursing leadership

   b) Interdisciplinary team members

   c) Referral mechanisms

   d) Case management to maintain continuity across all settings

   e) Around the clock accessibility

4. Palliative care Units

   a) Provide a familiar environment for patient and family; allow family members to be present with patient as the patient and family desire

   b) All staff have training to care for the palliative care patient

    c)   May have some drawbacks

        i.   Members of the healthcare team on other units may not feel they "need" to learn palliative care principles

        ii.   Continuity of care may be compromised when patients transferred between units

5.   Bereavement Programs and Services

    a)   The death of the patient does not signal an end to the care provided which is typical in the acute-care setting

    b)   Family are also included in the unit of care, these services can meet a currently unmet need in hospital-based deaths

    c)   As an institution bereavement services can also include sending a sympathy note, providing bereavement resources and the timing of mailing the hospital bill[30]

F.   Ongoing education for medical and nursing staff: Developing standardized protocols to help staff respond to commonly occurring events (e.g., advance care planning, pronouncement of death)

G.   The intensive care unit (ICU) presents its own challenges

1.   Shift in the focus of care can be as short as minutes, giving little time for nursing staff to prepare the patient and the family for death

2.   15–55% of decedents had *at least one stay* in an ICU in the 6 months before death[29]

3.   ICU physically not set up for many visitors for long periods of time

    a)   This presents a challenge for the nurse but an issue that deserves close attention

    b)   Patients should have the opportunity to be with their loved ones while they are dying if that is their wish

4.   Communication with family members

    a)   Fast pace of the ICU makes this difficult and inconsistent

    b)   Multidisciplinary teams to work with the family so that their needs are met

    c)   Involve the family in providing care, to the extent possible

5.   Medical decision making challenges

    a)   What are patient wishes when not documented

    b)   Withholding and withdrawing life support

H.   Bereavement Follow up Programs

1.   Family contact by phone or mail monthly until the one-year anniversary of the death

2.   Also found to be useful for the healthcare providers to cope with their loss[31]

VI. The End-of-life in the Long-Term Care Setting

A. Epidemiology of Long-Term Care Residents

1. On a given day, 1.5 million Americans are in a nursing home

2. Half of Americans who live to 65 years of age by 2030 will enter a nursing home before they die

3. Nearly one in two persons who lives to his/her 80s will spend time in a nursing home prior to death

4. Federal policy in the 1980s has resulted in shorter hospital stays and increased use of nursing homes

5. 2/3 of persons who consider a nursing home their usual place of residence will remain in the nursing home until death

6. According to the two most recent years of the National Mortality Follow-back Survey, the probability that a nursing home will be the site of death increased from 18.7% in 1986 to 20.0% by 1993

7. By 2020, it has been estimated that 40% of Americans will die in nursing homes[32]

8. Already, some states have nearly 40% of Americans dying in nursing homes

9. Current healthcare trends are likely to promote the use of nursing homes as a site for terminal care

10. Nursing home hospice population expanded from 7.7% of all Medicare hospice beneficiaries in 1989 to 17% in 1995

11. Only 1% of the nursing home population enrolls in hospice care

12. 70% of nursing homes have no hospice patients[33]

B. Pain Management in Long-Term Care

1. As many as 83% of nursing home residents experience pain that impairs mobility, may cause depression and diminishes quality of life

2. Recent research has found that pain is often unrecognized and not treated by healthcare providers

3. A 1998 JAMA study found that 40% of cancer patients discharged to a nursing home had daily pain[34]

4. Of those in pain, one in four did not have any analgesic prescribed . . . NOT EVEN acetaminophen

5. This study found that 41.2% of persons who had pain at their first assessment (within 60 days of April, 1999) also had either moderate daily pain or an excruciating level of pain at their next assessment (completed 60-180 days later)[34]

    a) Of those persons with two MDS assessments, ONE in SEVEN were in persistent severe pain

    b) The rate of persistent pain recorded in states varied from 37.7% to 49.5%. Yet, the majority of states were near 40%

C.   Hospice and Palliative Care in Long-Term Care Facilities

1.   A long-term care facility is the home of the patient

2.   Staff members of a long-term care facility are caregivers to patients and as such, are recipients of hospice and palliative care

    a)   Showing and sharing respect and care

    b)   Giving appropriate and necessary information

    c)   Assisting in decision-making of patients/residents

    d)   Encouraging family members to participate in care of resident

3.   Long-term care facility staff also are professional members of interdisciplinary team. A challenge for all to

    a)   Balance needs of patient with family and staff

    b)   Recognize the needs of patient foremost rather than those of family or staff

D.   Goal of Hospice/Palliative Care in a Long-Term Care Facility

1.   Provide optimal end-of-life care

2.   Identify residents who have been diagnosed with a life-limiting, progressive illness and meet their needs

3.   Potential patients might include (not an all inclusive listing)

    a)   Advanced cancer patients

    b)   End-stage diabetic patients

    c)   End-stage pulmonary disease patients

    d)   End-stage cardiac/CHF patients

    e)   End-stage Alzheimer's patients

    f)   End-stage renal patients

4.   For eligibility requirements for admission to Medicare hospice benefits refer to Chapter 10

5.   Delivering end-of-life care may be provided within the dual regulations of the long-term care facility and the hospice, if the care plan reflects hospice philosophy and is based on an assessment of the patient's needs and specific living arrangement in the long-term care facility

6.   Preauthorization of individualized plan of care by hospice is required for each long-term care facility

    a)   The primary physician remains in charge and he works cooperatively with the interdisciplinary team

    b)   The primary physician generally continues medical care

    c)   The hospice Medicare benefit requires bereavement services to family

    d)   Medicare skilled nursing facility reimbursement often forces a choice after hospitalization between coverage for 30 days of long-term care or hospice

E.   Agreements with Long-Term Care Facilities

1.   Formal, legal agreements

   a)   Written contracts required by Medicare

   b)   Contracts required may vary from state-to-state

   c)   Negotiated by administrators

2.   Informal agreements

   a)   Administrative support needed

   b)   Need excellent, ongoing communication among all members of team

   c)   Maintaining up-to-date information for all on a long-term care facility patient and his status to both parties[35]

   d)   Ensure comfort care at the end of life

   e)   Hospice/palliative care team augment nursing facility services available to the terminally ill patient

F.   Educational Needs for Long-Term Care Facility and Staff

1.   Needs Assessment

   a)   Who needs to learn what

   b)   What are the best learning tools for each particular individual/group?

      i.   Didactic

      ii.   Role-playing/simulation

      iii.   Interactive discussions

      iv.   One-to-one teaching

      v.   Self-study

2.   Suggested topics for teaching

   a)   Hospice and palliative care concepts and philosophy

   b)   Facilitation of an interdisciplinary team

   c)   Collaboration with the hospice/palliative care team

      i.   Interdisciplinary Team

         (a)   Members

         (b)   Role of each

      ii.   Blending of roles

      iii.   Conflict resolution

   d)   Involvement of family as part of unit of care—becoming "Partners in Caring"

      i.   Building and maintaining relationships

      ii.   Support of family (teach coping skills, etc.)

   e)   Decision-making process

f) Pain and symptom management and other physical care issues

g) Spiritual and/or religious needs of the dying patient

h) Ethical issues of the dying

i) Cultural and ethnic effects and impact on dying patient

j) Grief, loss, mourning and bereavement for the resident, family and staff

k) Psychosocial Issues of the dying resident

 i. Loss of everything, especially independence and control

 ii. Transition from chronic status to terminally ill status

 iii. Feelings of relief/burden/"ready to go"

 iv. End-of-life decision making

 v. Signs of denial, bargaining, anger and acceptance

 vi. Signs of anxiety, depression and fear

 vii. Family signs of guilt, remorse, anger, resentment

 viii. Family members who suddenly appear on the scene

 ix. Need and use of counseling for family when needed

 x. Bereavement for family/caregiver

 xi. Communication issues among

  (a) Healthcare providers

  (b) Patient

  (c) Families/caregivers

  (d) Types of Communication

   (i) Verbal

   (ii) Non-verbal

 xii. Need to be truthful with the terminally ill patient, at his level of understanding and need

G. Documentation of Hospice Care in a Long-Term Care Facility

1. Must meet regulations for both agencies

2. Must indicate a coordination of the plan of care

3. Goals of hospice and the long-term care facility must agree

4. Hospice must manage the plan of care

H. Clinical care of the dying patient in a long-term care facility should model clinical care provided in a private residence

1. Comprehensive assessment of the patient

2. Continual evaluation

3. Appropriate pain and symptom management

4. Appropriate hydration/nutrition

5. Frequent and good oral care

6. Prevention of infection

7. Skin integrity

8. Bowel and bladder care

9. Preparation of patient and family for approaching death

10. Maintenance of dignity of each patient

I. **Collaborative Approach of Hospice/Palliative Care Team and Long-Term Care Facility Staff**

1. Shared expertise

2. Care for patient and family

3. Mutual support

4. Mutual learning

5. Shared resources for both organizations and patient/family

J. **Symptoms That May Indicate Resident Needs for Further Screening for Hospice/Palliative Care**

1. Decreasing appetite

2. Decreased mobility

3. Increased sleepiness and decreased alertness

4. Loss of interest in life

5. Expressed desire to die

6. Worsening symptoms of disease process or development of new symptoms

K. **Advantages of Partnership between Long-Term Care Facility and Hospice/Palliative Care**

1. For the resident/family

    a) Access to end-of-life care in their place of residence

    b) Access to those in need of end-of-life care

    c) Access to hospice Medicare benefit

    d) Medications for symptoms related to the terminal illness

    e) Durable medical equipment

    f) Aggressive pain and symptom management

    g) Bereavement follow-up

    h) Staff trained in end-of-life care

2.   For the long-term care facility

   a)   Mentoring resource

   b)   Training and education source

   c)   Decision making

   d)   Support of staff

   e)   Assistance with advance care planning

   f)   Reduction in utilization of acute care facility

   g)   Increase bond with the community

3.   For the hospice/palliative care team

   a)   Meet primary objective to increase quality of life provided for all persons receiving end-of-life care

   b)   Support primary caregiver's needs

   c)   Continued relationship with community

L.   Hospice Nurse Role in the Long-Term Care Facility

1.   Develop a trusting, honest relationship with long-term care facility staff and residents

2.   Maintain good communication with the staff at all times

3.   Be a teacher/mentor in a non-threatening manner

4.   Be a resource person

5.   Assist in maintaining care plans for both institutions so that they are in agreement with each other

6.   Attend team meetings of both institutions

7.   Maintain good communication with primary physicians

8.   Note any new physician orders and add to the hospice orders

9.   Keep long-term care facility up-to-date on patient-related issues

10. Frequently reevaluate patient's condition to monitor disease progression

M.   Future Challenges for Hospice and Long-Term Care Facilities

1.   Increase of co-morbid diseases leading to greater severity of illness within long-term care facilities

2.   Increase in number of terminally ill dementia patients in long-term care facilities

3.   Maintaining hospice services within the long-term care environment

4.   Recognizing that more than one hospice may have patients in the same facility, therefore efforts should be taken to avoid confusion in delivery of care

5.   Accessing appropriate level of care that is financially reasonable and avoids conflict of skill

6. Necessity of ongoing continuing education of long-term care staff about hospice philosophy and practices

7. Challenge of turnover of long-term care staff; often preventing consistency of care to be maintained

8. Decisions needing to be made

   a) Establishing a specific hospice unit within facility

   b) Utilizing beds as available throughout the facility

9. Continual evaluation of end-of-life care provided in a long-term care facility[36]

10. Challenge of conducting research in the long-term care environment

11. Coordinate plan of care with all individuals and agencies providing care

VII. The End-of-Life in the Assisted Living Setting

A. **The fastest growing senior residence option, numbering between 30,000 and 40,000 facilities and housing over an estimated 800,000 persons[37,38]**

B. **With the philosophy of "aging in place" central to the mission of many assisted living facilities (ALFs) and the desire of many older adults to remain in the ALF rather than relocate to a nursing home, they have also become a place for terminal care and death[39,40]**

C. **Regulations vary by state; however, most day-to-day care performed by nursing assistants with nursing oversight**

D. **Staff members of an ALF are caregivers to patients and as such, are recipients of hospice and palliative care**

E. **An emerging area for hospice and palliative nursing**

VIII. Summary

A. **Unprecedented gains in life expectancy: exponential rise in number and needs of the sickest older adults**

B. **Cause of death shifted from acute sudden illness to chronic episodic disease**

C. **Untreated physical symptoms**

D. **Unmet patient/family needs**

E. **Future doctors and nurses untrained**

F. **Fragmentation, poor coordination and an unresponsive healthcare and payment system despite enormous expenditure**

IX. Conclusion

A. **Quality EOL care encompasses physical, psychological, social and spiritual aspects and includes the patient and the family as the unit of care**

   1. These not only are defining features of the nursing role, but also support the philosophy and principles of hospice and palliative care as well as reflect the dimensions of quality of life

2. Because nurses cannot practice what they do not know; increased knowledge is essential to improved patient care

B. Palliative nursing is not only "doing for," but is also largely "being with" patients and families

C. Hospice and palliative care is best provided by nurses functioning as part of an interdisciplinary team and is not defined by location, but rather by the care needs of the dying patient and family

Cited References

1. Field MJ, Cassel CK. *Approaching death: improving care at the end of life*. Washington, DC: Institute of Medicine Task Force; 1997.

2. Saunders C. Forward. In: Doyle D, Hanks G, MacDonald N, eds. *Oxford Textbook of Palliative Care*. New York, NY: Oxford University Press; 1993.

3. Corr CA. *Death in modern society*. In: Doyle D, Hanks G, MacDonald N, eds. *Oxford Textbook of Palliative Care*. New York, NY: Oxford University Press; 1993;31–40.

4. Super A. *The context of palliative care within progressive illness*. In: Ferrell B, Coyle N, eds. *Textbook of Palliative Nursing*. New York, NY: Oxford University Press: 2001:27–36.

5. Rosenberg HM, Ventura SJ, Maurer JD. *Births and deaths United States, 1995*. Monthly Vital Statistics Report, Preliminary Data from the Centers for Disease Control and Prevention, National Center for Health Statistics; 1996.

6. Ventura SJ, et al., *Births and deaths: Preliminary data for 1997*. Hyattsville: National Center for Health Statistics; 1998.

7. Administration on Aging. *Older population by age: 1900 to 2050*. Administration on Aging; 2000.

8. Emanuel L, von Gunten C, Ferris F. *The education for physicians on end of life care (EPEC) curriculum*. Washington, DC: American Medical Association; 1999.

9. Rando TA. *Grief, Dying and Death: Clinical Interventions for Caregivers*. Champaign, IL: Research Press; 1984.

10. Scanlon C. Defining standards for end-of-life care. *American Journal of Nursing*, 1997;97(11):58–60.

11. SUPPORT, S.P.I. A controlled trial to improve care for seriously ill hospitalized patients: A study to understand prognoses and preferences for outcomes and risks of treatments (SUPPORT). *Journal of the American Medical Association*, 1995;274:1591–1598.

12. National Hospice and Palliative Care Organization. *Press release: New findings address escalating end-of-life debate*. Alexandria, VA: National Hospice and Palliative Care Organization; 1996.

13. Egan K, Labyak MJ. *Hospice care: A model for quality end-of-life care*. In: Ferrell B, Coyle N, eds. *Textbook of Palliative Nursing*. New York, NY: Oxford University Press: 2001:7–26.

14. Byock IR. *Dying Well: The Prospects for Growth at the End of Life*. New York, NY: Riverhead Books; 1997.

15. Ferrell BR, Virani R, Grant M. Analysis of end-of-life content in nursing textbooks. *Oncology Nursing Forum*. 1999;26(5):869–876.

16. National Hospice and Palliative Care Organization. *Hospice fact sheet*. Alexandria, VA: National Hospice and Palliative Care Organization; 2000.

17. Lynn J, Schuster JL, Kabcenell A. *Improving Care for the End of Life: A Sourcebook for Health Care Managers and Clinicians*. New York, NY: Oxford University Press; 2000.

18. Ferrell BR, Juarez G, Borneman T. Outcomes of pain education in community home care. *Journal of Hospice and Palliative Nursing*. 1999;1(4):141–150.

19. Teno J, Byock IR, Field MJ. Research agenda for developing measures to examine quality of care and quality of life of patients diagnosed with life limiting illness. *Journal of Pain and Symptom Management*. 1999;17(2):75–82.

20. Levine C. Loneliness of the long-term caregiver. *N Engl J Med* 1999;340:1587–90.

21. Lagnado L. Rules are rules: Hospice's patients beat the odds, so Medicare decides to crack down. *The Wall Street Journal*. New York, NY. 2000:p. A1, A18.

22. American Nurses Association. *Code for nurses with interpretive statements*. Kansas City, MO: American Nurses Association; 1985.

23. Coyle N. Introduction to palliative nursing. In: Ferrell B, Coyle N, eds. *Textbook of Palliative Nursing*. New York, NY: Oxford University Press: 2001:3–6.

24. Sulmasy DP. *The Healer's Calling*. New York, NY/Mahway: Paulist Press; 1997.

25. Yates P, Stetz KM. Families' awareness of and response to dying. *Oncology Nursing Forum.* 1999;26(1):113–120.

26. O'Connor P. Clinical paradigm for exploring spiritual concerns. In Doka KJ, Morgan J, eds. *Death and Spirituality*, New York, NY: Baywood Publishing Company; 1993.

27. Borneman T, Brown-Saltzman K. Meaning in illness. In: Ferrell B, Coyle N, eds. *Textbook of Palliative Nursing*. New York, NY: Oxford University Press: 2001:415–424.

28. Bednash G, Ferrell B. *End-of-Life Nursing Education Consortium (ELNEC)*. Washington, DC: Association of Colleges of Nursing; 2000.

29. The Dartmouth Atlas of Health Care. 1999. Available at http://www.dartmouthatlas.org/atlaslinks/ 99atlas.php. Accessed April 18, 2005.

30. Whedon MB. Hospital care. In: Ferrell B, Coyle N, eds. *Textbook of Palliative Nursing*. New York, NY: Oxford University Press: 2001:584–608.

31. Puntillo K, Stannard D. The intensive care unit. In: Ferrell B, Coyle N, eds. *Textbook of Palliative Nursing*. New York, NY: Oxford University Press: 2001:609–621.

32. Brock DB, Foley DJ. Demography and epidemiology of dying in the U.S. with emphasis on deaths of older persons. Hosp J. 1998;13:49–60.

33. Zerzan J, Stearns S, Hanson L. Access to palliative care and hospice in nursing homes. *Journal of the American Medical Association*. 2000;284(10):2489–2493.

34. Teno JM, Weitzen S, Wetle T, Mor V. *Persistent Pain in Nursing Home Residents. JAMA.* 2001;285:2081.

35. Jones DH. Caring for hospice patients in a long term care facility. *Caring Magazine*. 1993:228–230.

36. Keay TJ, Schonwetter RS. Hospice care in the long-term care facility. *American Family Physician.* 1998;56:491–494.

37. Allen JE. *Assisted Living Administration: The Knowledge Base*. New York, NY: Springer; 1999.

38. National Center for Assisted Living (NCAL). Assisted living resident profile. 2001. Available at http: //www.ncal.org/about/resident.htm. Accessed June 19, 2004.

39. Cartwright J, Kayser-Jones J. End-of-life care in assisted living facilities: perceptions of residents, families and staffs. *Journal of Hospice and Palliative Nursing.* 2003;5(3):143–151.

40. Chapin R, Dobbs-Kepper D. Aging in place in assisted living: philosophy versus policy. *The Gerontologist.* 2001;41(1):43–50.

ADDITIONAL REFERENCES AND RESOURCES

American Association of Colleges of Nurses. *A Peaceful Death*. Report from the Robert Wood Johnson End-of-Life Care Roundtable. Washington, DC: Author; 1997.

Byock I. The nature of suffering and the nature of opportunity at the end of life. *Clinics in geriatric medicine.* 1996;12(2):237–251.

Cassel E. The nature of suffering and the goals of medicine. *New England Journal of Medicine.* 1982;306(11):639–645.

Curtis JR, Rubenfeld GD. *Managing Death in the ICU: The Transition from Cure to Comfort*. Seattle, WA: University of Washington; 2000.

Doyle D, Hanks GWC, MacDonald N, eds. *Oxford Textbook of Palliative Care* 2nd ed. New York, NY: Oxford University Press; 1998.

Ferrell BR, Coyle N, eds. *Textbook of Palliative Nursing*. New York, NY: Oxford University Press: 2001.

Ferrell BR, ed. *Suffering* Sudbury, MA: Jones and Bartlett Publishers; 1996.

Frankl VE. *Man's search for meaning*. New York, NY: Washington Square Press; 1984.

Highfield MEF. Providing spiritual care to patients with cancer. *Clinical Journal of Oncology Nursing*, 2000;4(3):115–120.

Kane RA. Ethical themes in long term care. In: Katz RJ, Kane RL, Mezey MD, eds. *Quality Care in Geriatric Settings* New York, NY: Springer; 1995:130–148.

Kane RL. The evolution of the American nursing home. In: Tinstock RH, Cluff LE, VonMering O, eds. *The Future of Long Term Care: Social and Policy Issues* Baltimore, MD: Johns Hopkins University Press; 1996:145–168.

Lair GS. *Counseling the Terminally Ill: Sharing the Journey*. Washington, DC: Taylor & Francis; 1996.

Last Acts Task Force. *Precepts of Palliative Care*. Princeton, NJ: Robert Wood Johnson Foundation; 1997.

Matzo ML, Sherman DW, eds. *Palliative Care Nursing: Quality Care to the End of Life*. New York, NY: Springer Publishing Company; 2001.

Oncolink. *Hospice in the long-term care facility*. University of Pennsylvania Cancer Center; 1999, August 27. Available at http://www.oncolink.upenn.edu/resources/hospitals/wissahickon/services/nursing.html.

Rhymes JA. Hospice care in the long-term care facility. *Long Term Care Facility Medicine*. 1993;1(6):14–24.

Smith SA. *Hospice Concepts: A Guide to Palliative Care in Terminal Illness*. Chicago, IL: Research Press; 2000.

Waller A, Caroline NL. *Handbook of Palliative Care in Cancer*. Boston, MA: Butterworth-Heinemann; 1996.

World Health Organization. Cancer pain relief and palliative care. *Technical Report Series 804*. Geneva, Switzerland: World Health Organization; 1990.

Younger JB. The alienation of the sufferer. *Advances in Nursing Science*. 1995;17(4):53–72.

CHAPTER VIII

END-OF-LIFE CARE FOR THE CHILD AND FAMILY

Lizabeth H. Sumner, RN, BSN

I. Introduction

A. This section is intended to provide hospice and palliative care nurses with a brief practical reference and some symptom management guidelines for adapting practice to the care of infants, children and adolescents with life-limiting, progressive illnesses

B. It is assumed that the general practice of hospice or palliative nursing is adhered to based on the other sections in this curriculum

C. Adaptations will be based on the individual child's age, developmental level, diagnosis and family specific circumstances

D. Because the range of diagnoses for these infants and children is so varied, some important, generalized approaches will be offered that may cross many diagnoses

II. Common Pediatric Diagnoses Seen in Hospice/Palliative Services

A. Cancer[1]

    1. These diagnoses continue to be the #2 cause of death overall for children 0–14 yrs of age

        a) Leukemia is most common form of childhood cancer

            i. 80% are acute lymphocytic leukemia (ALL), then acute myelocytic leukemia (AML) is next highest in incidence of leukemia

            ii. History

                (a) Fever, bleeding, pain and symptoms of anemia (fatigue/weakness/lassitude, pallor, dyspnea)

                (b) Symptoms of thrombocytopenia (petechiae, purpura and bruising with minimal trauma)

                (c) GI symptoms (anorexia, abdominal pain and weight loss)

                (d) Symptoms of leukostasis/WBC clumping (headache, blurred vision and respiratory problems due to leukemic infiltration of CNS and lungs)

(e) Infections

(f) Generalized achiness

iii. Management: depending on the goals of child and family the following approaches may be considered. Follow CBCs, serum electrolytes (hyperkalemia, hypocalcemia, hyperuricemia and hyperphosphatemia associated with grossly elevated WBC count and/or massive organ infiltration by leukemic cells); fever, bleeding patterns, infection patterns, neurological status changes, GI changes, pulmonary changes, GU changes (painless gonadal swelling may indicate gonadal infiltrate), all pain and anxiety patterns, impact on quality of life and activities

iv. Discuss with patient/family and physician the goals of treatments, desires regarding transfusing and other treatment interventions as a palliative goal for comfort or to prevent acute bleeds, increase energy. Personal goals should be elicited

v. Anticipate side effects and symptoms that may be distressing to child and family; create a plan to respond to these both at home and in the hospital. Support discussions when transitioning goals of care. Utilize pertinent team members for holistic approach to child's needs and goals

vi. Educate child and family what to expect at home or inpatient, as disease progresses and how to interpret child's changes physically and emotionally. (Note: These are applicable to all disease conditions)

b) Osteosarcoma—most common bone tumor in children

i. History

(a) Original painful lesion in long bone (may or may not have been associated with soft tissue mass and/or local edema)

(b) History of lung metastases and respiratory dysfunction (most common metastatic site)

(c) History related to other potential metastatic sites: bone, pleura, kidney, adrenal gland, brain and pericardium

(d) History of malaise, fatigue, fever, anorexia, weight loss and pain

ii. Management: follow systems noted above; follow changes in weight, changes in pain patterns and fevers. Utilize a combined approach (combination of medications and non-pharmacological interventions) to pain for bone and tissue pain to insure continued mobility and ADLs

c) Rhabdomyosarcoma most common soft tissue cancer in children

i. History

(a) Varies with anatomic location of tumor and the presence/extent of metastases

(b) Metastatic spread is via the blood and lymphatic systems and frequent sites of spread are lung, bone, bone marrow, brain, spinal cord, lymph nodes, liver, heart and breast

(c) Early spread within the muscle of origin and to adjacent tissue is common

ii. If orbital in origin: history of orbital invasion, ptosis, exophthalmos, cranial nerve involvement (especially nerves II, III, IV and/or VI)

iii. If origin is non-orbital parameningeal sites: history of nasal obstructions, sinusitis, epistaxis, local pain, hypernasal speech, serous otitis media with facial palsy and conduction hearing loss; affected ear may have mucopurulent or sanguineous drainage; extension into meninges is common, with history of symptom of increased ICP. If ICP present child may have increased seizure activity and headaches, that needs to be treated accordingly and proactively

d) Wilms' tumor: nephroblastoma—malignant embryonal neoplasm of kidney, typically effects younger children

   i. History

   (a) Original abdominal mass and history of pain, fever, malaise, hematuria, possible hypertension due to cyclo-oxygenase-2 activity

   (b) Symptoms related to potential metastatic sites: lung, liver, brain, bone and contralateral kidney

   ii. Management: follow systems and issues noted above; in addition, watch for symptoms related to compression of inferior vena cava; changes in fever and pain patterns. Educate on variety of comfort measures for fever and discomfort

e) Neuroblastoma

   i. History

   (a) Original mass (usually abdominal, in adrenal gland or paraspinal ganglia)

   (b) May occur in neck, paraspinal area of thorax or pelvis

   (c) Symptoms related to metastases

   (d) In order of occurrence, these are bone marrow, bone, lymph nodes, liver, intracranial lesions from direct extension of bony sites in skull, skin and testes

   (e) Pain (especially bone pain, with high risk of pathologic fractures), abdominal masses—retroperitoneal lymph nodes

   (f) If thoracic masses, history of Superior Vena Cava (SVC) Syndrome or Horner's Syndrome (miosis, ptosis, exophthalmos, anhidrosis)

   (g) If any paraspinal involvement-spinal cord compression

   ii. Management: follow systems and concerns noted above; also follow weight; watch for intractable diarrhea and/or hypertension (both rare); follow neuro status for acute cerebellar encephalopathy (also rare); monitor CBCs, serum electrolytes to influence decisions regarding treatment goals and observe for changes in pain patterns. Discuss decreasing frequency and/or purpose and meaning of labs as condition progresses

f) Brain tumors

   i. Early signs/symptoms in child: irritability, lethargy, vomiting, anorexia, headache, papilledema, behavioral changes, bulging fontanels in infant

   ii. Late signs/symptoms in child: increased intracranial pressure causing headache, vomiting, papilledema, increased irritability, decreased level of consciousness, changes in vital signs, including widening of pulse pressure, bradycardia, (slowed, irregular pulse), displacement of brain structures (herniation), seizures, personality changes, loss of sensation, disturbances in coordination, malnutrition and dehydration. Side effects of anticonvulsant therapy may lead to gum hypertrophy, bleeding, gingivitis and changes in self esteem due to change in appearance, i.e., cushingoid syndrome

    iii.   Unique issues: prognosis has not changed in last 10 years; many symptoms drastically affect normal functioning

    iv.   Identify strategies to foster increased self-esteem, minimize and treat above side effects and impact of physical limitations and changes in appearance, physical and emotional changes

2.   Spectrum of cancer in children differs markedly from that in adults

    a)   Childhood cancer: usually involves hematopoietic system, nervous system and connective tissue

    b)   Neuroblastoma, Wilms' tumor retinoblastoma, hepatoma rarely occur in adults[2]

B. Non-Cancer Diagnoses[1]

1.   Congenital anomalies

    a)   Half of all childhood deaths occur in the first year of life

    b)   Congenital anomalies as a group, account for the third highest cause of death in children 0–14 and create the largest group of children who could benefit from a hospice or palliative care program and include

        i.   Trisomy 13 and 18

        ii.   Osteogenesis Imperfecta Type II

        iii.   Werdnig Hoffmann, Walker-Warburg Syndrome

        iv.   Anencephaly

        v.   Holoprosencephaly

        vi.   Severe hydrocephaly

        vii.   Cardiac anomalies not compatible with life or determined to be inoperable/surgery not elected

        viii.   Rare anomalies that are known/expected to have poor prognosis. Incurable from the start by their very nature of causality

    c)   Pathophysiology

        i.   Two major types

            (a)   Malformations, arising during embryogenesis (e.g., anencephaly)

            (b)   Deformations, late changes in previously normal structures due to pathologic processes or intrauterine forces (e.g., hydrocephalus)

        ii.   1/3 are "inherited" anomalies (spontaneous gene or chromosomal mutations)

        iii.   1/3 are multifactoral (including toxic/environmental factors)

        iv.   1/3 are of unknown causes

2. Muscular diseases include Muscular Dystrophy or Spinal Muscular Atrophy; metabolic disorders; late stage Cerebral Palsy has significant muscular involvement

3. Children who have been profoundly injured or had a sudden acute illness event and may not/will not have life support continued for prolonged period should be identified for hospice consultation and support

4. Other relevant conditions include metabolic/mitochondrial disorders, Tay Sachs, Cystic Fibrosis, "near drowning accident" victim; intrauterine or birth related trauma/events, i.e., Hypoxic Ischemic Encephalopathy (HIE)

5. Repeated admissions for chronic progressive conditions may be a trigger for a palliative care consult to review goals of interventions and desired intensity of care

6. A significant decline or change in child's condition—(regardless of diagnosis); failed response to treatments or interventions are also triggers for palliative care consult

C. Perinatal Hospice

1. A prenatal diagnosis of a potentially lethal condition can be the catalyst for a hospice referral to support the expectant parents and other family throughout the pregnancy, labor and delivery

2. Referral may come from genetic counselor; OB; perinatologist; social worker, parental-referral

3. "Traditional" hospice support and care for the baby if he/she survives the immediate time of delivery, especially if parents have a goal of taking baby home

4. Emotional and spiritual support is offered/provided in preparation and anticipation of the birth of their baby as well as the possibility of death

5. Provision of information, resources on condition, range of outcomes and planning needed, anticipated needs of each family member, identify keepsakes to plan for, things to consider at time of delivery; rituals religious needs desired at birth and beyond

6. Bereavement support to be made available for the family if/when the baby dies and afterwards

7. Includes the same preventative approach to minimize physical, emotional and spiritual suffering during pregnancy and after birth and to avoid the initiation of unintended, undesired or futile interventions; emphasis is on *quality of life* and creating opportunities for a personalized, family centered experience, regardless of the duration of the baby's life. Preserving hope while balancing realities of condition

8. The Born Alive Infant Protection Act of 2002 (Pub. L. 107–207) defines any child born-alive to be a person, human being, child and individual. The act includes the criteria to be considered "born-alive"

III. Differences between Pediatric and Adult Hospice Care

A. Pediatric Issues[3]

1. Not legally able to make decisions regarding treatment; yet want to participate in decisions; assent versus consent

2. The child's needs and goals may be perceived differently by parents than by the sick child or staff thus affecting provision of care and communication

3. May not have verbal skills to adequately express feelings and needs or describe symptoms

4. Have varied conceptions of and reactions to illness and death based on the following factors: age, developmental level; family/religious/cultural norms; cognitive, intellectual and emotional maturity

5. Has not achieved a "full and complete life"

6. Desire a sense of "normalcy" and typically prefer to be at home versus hospital and maintain routine activities

B. Family Issues[3]

1. Financial stressors: one or both parents may need to keep working, resulting in an inadequate and fragmented support system

2. Respite often needed and rarely available (nor paid for) from being around-the-clock caregivers

3. Parents and staff must deal with sibling's feelings, which may include: acting out, anger, regressive behavior, anticipatory grief, fear and/or problems at school

4. Fear of being alone and/or feelings of helplessness and burdened with responsibility of caring for their dying child at home

5. Adults often feel the need to protect the sick child and/or siblings by withholding information regarding diagnosis, treatment and/or prognosis

6. Parental belief and hope that "there must be something more that can be done" along with perception of children's hospitals as "The Miracle Maker"

C. Community/Agency Issues[3]

1. Must provide ongoing staff support and continuing education regarding staff's own grief and personal issues is essential

2. Lack of referrals from physicians hesitant to stop "curative" treatment, who may believe they have "failed the child and family." Black and white view of "all or nothing" can be done related to treatment options

3. Reimbursement for pediatric hospice care may be difficult to obtain and can be more costly than adult care

4. Assessment of hospice "eligibility" requiring prognosis of 6 months or less is often difficult to determine and commit to in infants and children. Variable trajectories for the range of conditions, the resiliency of children also contributes to this factor

5. Need ongoing commitment of agency or institution to sustain a pediatric program in spite of "small" pediatric hospice/palliative care population

D. Staff Issues[3]

1. Must be knowledgeable regarding physical assessment, pain and symptom management for infants and children and pediatric disease processes and younger family systems and family centered care approach

2. Staff may project fears for own children onto pediatric patient and family, i.e., "If it were my child . . ." "They should . . ." and parentify their relationship, even interfere with role of parents as primary caregivers

3.   Must be able to recognize developmental level of child regarding cognitive understanding about illness, death and dying as well as ability to describe, communicate about symptoms

4.   Need education on the real needs of dying children i.e., children feel pain, want honest information and worry about their condition and its effects on others; be able to focus on "the living" yet to be done within the context of the child's limitations

IV.   General Issues Related to Admission of Pediatric Patients

A.   Family centered approach to care

1.   Requires an interdisciplinary, collaborative team approach that focuses first and foremost on the needs of the *whole* FAMILY as a unit, to enable them to optimally thrive and cope within the context of the child's condition as it changes over time

2.   Creates an inclusive model that optimally benefits the family and child, as the team works together to meet *their* goals for care and for *living*

3.   Typically requires a broader scope of individuals and providers, beyond the "patient/ caregiver" model for adult hospice care

a)   *Whole* family care involves support and intervention for all of the family as the needs arise. May include the child's school as indicated or that of the sibling(s)

b)   May include Child Life Specialist, multiple medical specialists and community pediatrician; ancillary staff such as PT, OT, play therapy, music or art therapy etc.; other providers in the home, infusion provider, durable medical equipment and special equipment provider, outpatient as well as inpatient staff/team

4.   Sets a standard of involving the siblings in ongoing discussions and supports helping them understand the child's condition and clarify their perceptions of cause and expression of fears and concerns

a)   Siblings need to be included in the circle of care and their individual emotional, developmental and basic needs met throughout the sibling's illness and into bereavement

b)   Feeling validated and supported during the sibling's illness and offering ways for the child to participate in the experience may assist him/her in adaptation during the illness and after child's death

B.   Identify existing supports

1.   Determine what is available and also what is needed for the ill child's and/or sibling's school community as the child enrolls in hospice/palliative care and as condition progresses, through the child's death

2.   Collaborate with the social worker to maintain contact with child's school, mechanism for classmate contact (counselor, teacher, school nurse etc.)

3.   Identify all who are directly contributing to the child's plan of care; may be multiple sites or providers

C.   **Identify the existing spiritual and/or religious influences and supports for the child, siblings and parents belief system**

1.   Evaluate spiritual needs and concerns for sick child, siblings and each parent

D.   **Treatment/intervention goals**

1.   Discuss with child's primary MD and parents (and child as developmentally appropriate/ physically capable)

a)   Goals for treatment therapies or interventions

b)   Goals that each person has, including the child to the extent possible

c)   Use each change in condition or new symptom as an opportunity to review child/ family goals and response to same

2.   This discussion is essential to articulate as much as possible, the intent, benefit, burden and *meaning* of the treatments/interventions for all involved

3.   Upon discussion it may become evident that the understanding and perceptions of the goals of treatments/interventions may be shared, divergent or conflicting among those involved

a)   Some interventions may be considered for continuation

b)   Others may be "titrated" down in intensity

c)   Other interventions may not be consistent with mutually agreed upon goals or are no longer contributing to quality of life for the child

4.   When creating a plan of care with the child/family, it is very important to place emphasis on the parent's *desired intensity of care* and symptom management for the child

a)   This requires a thoughtful, planned discussion with consideration of timing and the readiness of parents

b)   Key caregivers must participate

c)   Provide an appropriate time and setting for the discussion. Arrange so both parents can be present and their support system if appropriate

d)   Be sure that adequate information is available

E.   **Pain and symptom management: this section specifically highlights those distinctly different issues related to children and suggestions for helpful approaches**

1.   Thoroughly assess medical, psychosocial, spiritual needs and issues of the sick child, parents, siblings and even grandparents when involved directly

2.   **QUESTT**[4]

a)   **Q** = Question the child. Verbal statement/description of pain is most important factor in pain assessment

b)   **U** = Use pain rating scales. Provides subjective quantitative measure of pain intensity

c)   **E** = Evaluate behavior. Common indicators of pain in children and are especially valuable in assessing pain in non-verbal children, including infants

d)   **S** = Secure parent's involvement because they know their child best

e)   **T** = Take cause of pain into account because pathology or procedure may give clues to expected intensity and type of pain

f)   **T** = Take action to meet the established goal (child's acceptable pain level) because the only reason to assess pain is to be able to relieve it through use of analgesic/ adjuvant drugs and/or non-pharmacological methods

3.   GOLDEN RULE: Whatever is painful to an adult is painful to a child or an infant! Identify the appropriate scale to be used routinely and be consistent and document! A sleeping or playing child does not mean they are pain free

4.   Utilize topical anesthetic cream for blood draws or IV insertion to decrease distress or fears. Adhere to routine that comforts and reassures child

5.   Detailed guides for pain and symptom management in hospice and palliative care are found in Chapters IV and V

6.   Safe consistent and effective pain management is essential regardless of age and size of infant or child

7.   Parents may need help translating their child's behavior to indicate comfort or distress; need to increase pain medication etc.

8.   Ongoing monitoring of child's weight is critical for accurate dosing on pediatric patients. They continue to grow and may need dose adjustment with weight gain or general growth

F.   **After-hours coverage and continuity of care**

1.   Needs and expectations of child/family should be thoroughly assessed prior to admission to either hospice or palliative care program

a)   Consider if and how the individual hospice/palliative care program can meet anticipated needs and skill level based on current resources available

b)   Be sure family is clear on their expectations and realistic response times/approaches/ resources

c)   Consider back up plan for rural settings, contact EMS dept in local area

d)   If needs cannot safely and realistically be met with the present resources, identify additional or alternative resources in the community best equipped to handle and meet the pediatric patient/family needs or expectations. Avoid situations where patient/referral source expectation cannot be realistically met

e)   Attempt to create a collaborative framework to meet the needs of patient and family with all providers involved with child's care/family needs, including faith community

2.   For children and their families, a high priority must be placed on continuity of care

a)   Fragmented or poorly coordinated care for the child and family can exacerbate an already strained coping pattern

i.   The nurse can facilitate communication between the providers and the family in order to maintain the established plan of care for the child/family and to avoid frustration, confusion and duplication of efforts

ii.   Maximizing opportunities to communicate between providers and ensure continuity between settings (home, clinic, hospital, school etc.) is an important and primary role of the nurse

b) As a "case manager" the nurse can keep the team and other healthcare providers updated on the evolving plan of care for the child and keep the existing support system intact for the benefit of the family

c) Regular reports to referral sources can maintain optimal contact with the child's care team

V. **Developmental Considerations in Pediatric Assessment**

A. **Special considerations for examining and interpreting assessment information are necessary for clinicians dealing with infants and children[5]**

B. **Appraisal of the child's developmental level is the first step toward a positive interaction, which reinforces the child's sense of security, mastery and self-esteem**

1. *Infant (0–1 year)*

a) Stranger anxiety is prevalent at 7 months of age and older; do physical examination with parent holding baby or within close view; smile; approach should be unhurried and gentle, use high pitched, soft voice; avoid abrupt jerky movements

b) Pain related behaviors: increased irritability, changes in crying patterns, handling/feeding changes, usual comfort measures less effective, facial expression is vigilant or angry, withdraws affected body part

i. In the first few months there is no apparent "understanding" of pain but baby has response to painful stimuli

ii. Children eventually develop anticipatory fear related to perceived painful situations and as verbal skills develop uses descriptive words for pain such as "owie, boo-boo, ouchie"

iii. Ask parent/child how pain/hurt is referred to; utilize the familiar words for pain in the family; plan supportive interventions with parents; child may withdraw from social or play activity if pain persists[5]

2. *Toddler (1–3 years)*

a) Separation and stranger anxiety decreases by age two

b) Examine child in parent's lap, complete physical assessment through playful interactions (i.e., "Simon Says . . ." and puppet play) and minimize initial physical contact

c) Praise for cooperative behavior

d) Identify words used for pain and discomfort

e) Offer choices when appropriate

3. *Preschool Child (3–5 years)*

a) Likes being a "helper," having choices and trying out equipment for him/herself; fearful of bodily harm

b) Examine with parent close by

c) Needs positive reinforcement and praise

d) Less tentative than toddlers

   e) Identify words used by child to describe pain

   f) Offer choices when appropriate and incorporate measures that the child believes will work such as warm wash cloth on abdomen[5]

  4. *School-age Child (5 years+)*

   a) Able to understand simple explanations regarding illness and body functioning

   b) Developing understanding of "cause and effect," understands relationship between pain, other symptoms and disease process

   c) Provide age appropriate information and teaching regarding pain regimen and rationale

   d) Answer questions briefly and honestly

   e) Include child in decision-making process when possible

   f) Identify words to describe pain used by child

   g) Utilize dolls for "parallel" assessment and intervention

   h) Use appropriate picture books for aiding in explanation of bodily functions or changes

   i) Offer choices when appropriate and incorporate measures that the child believes will work

  5. *Adolescent*

   a) More privacy and independence needed, prefers being included in explanation/findings

   b) More introspective; increasing use of mental/cognitive coping strategies; has capacity for coherent understanding of physiologic processes

   c) Allow for adolescent's input, insight and choices

   d) Attention needs to be given to self esteem and personal image as it changes over time, related to peers and develop strategies to assuage distress in this area, reinforce the positives and choices available

   e) Participation in decision-making may be influenced by culture, age and religious norms of family

VI. General Care Issues for Child/Family

A. Symptom management approaches

  1. Nurse needs to be familiar with the child's developmental level to engage in any discussion on how they are physically feeling, for teaching related to care or disease progression, selection of pain assessment tools

  2. Give child and parents choices in planning medication, treatments or procedures and their daily living regimen to fit family lifestyle and goals for comfort

  3. An important element of care for children and their families is the maintenance of NORMALCY in as many areas of life as possible and the incorporation of attention to physical appearance/self-esteem into daily routines

4. CONTROL is a most important aspect of approaching care for both the child and parents

    a) The sick child may demonstrate an increased need for structure and routine as their scope of control diminishes

    b) This is normal and should be accommodated with an ongoing attempt to give choices and respect their need for routine that reinforces a sense of safety and security

5. Nursing visits typically involve some socialization activities with the child and siblings to create a therapeutic and relaxed environment prior to doing physical exam as a means of transitioning focus of time together

    a) Child will be more at ease when related to as a child first and as a sick child last

    b) Incorporate play into methods of communication

    c) Assume a relaxed posture, perhaps sitting beside the child on the floor, at his/her level, having "child friendly" clothes and demeanor

B. Planning care for the pediatric patient

1. This patient population requires familiarity with and a planned response to any potential symptoms for the child's disease process and diagnosis (See Appendix 3: Standards of Hospice Care for Children)

2. Identify those symptoms or perceived "emergencies" which the child and parents fear most and have a plan in place to respond quickly to treat them across possible settings (home, hospital, school, palliative care unit, inpatient hospice)

3. Nurses need to *anticipate* and *prepare* a plan for these to *prevent* and minimize experience of suffering fear or pain

4. Examples may include

    a) Seizure management: have necessary medications in appropriate routes on hand for children with any neurological component to their disease to respond to any possible seizure symptoms, which may cause physical or emotional distress (suggestions include: lorazepam, gabapentin, phenobarbital, phenytoin, diazepam or compounded suppository)

    b) Pain management is essential for **all** ages

        i. Select appropriate routes and dosages *based on weight (mg/kg)* for infants and children

        ii. Discuss with and provide education to parents and child on safe use, benefits of narcotics/opioids for pain relief and what to expect

            (a) Assist them to create a schedule that fits their lifestyle and maintains desired level of relief

            (b) Consider cultural and ethnic influences as well as the exposure to education in schools related to illegal drug use (DARE programs etc.), which may influence perception of the use of therapeutic medications

        iii. Always evaluate need for combined strategies and/or methods for complex pain and multiple types of pain

iv.   Assess for pain in the non-verbal child with behavioral indicators and facial expressions, appropriate pain assessment tools. Examples include[4]

(a)   Poker chip tool (how many pieces of pain do you have?)

(b)   Eland color tool (selection of colors to represent intensity of pain applied to outline image of child's body)

(c)   Faces scale (series of 5 faces to represent range of pain ratings); Numeric scales (usually 1–5 or 1–10)

v.   Pain in children can be approached with the principles of the WHO ladder as it applies to all patients

c)   Anxiety and agitation

i.   Minimizing stress and anxiety in the child relieves the suffering and anxiety of parents as well

ii.   Agitation may arise related to tests and procedures, strangers, previous experiences, untreated/under-treated pain and from fears related to his/her condition, one's future, concerns for self or family, what will happen as they are dying, etc.

iii.   Pharmacologic and non-pharmacologic interventions should be used such as relaxation/soothing strategies; lorazepam, diazepam, reassess pain regimen for efficacy

d)   Respiratory difficulties, dyspnea, congestion

i.   These can be very distressful to caregivers/parents and cause restlessness in the child

ii.   Using medication to decrease secretions may benefit the child (glycopyrrolate, scopolamine patch)

iii.   Assess fluid intake versus volume tolerated

(a)   May need to adjust feedings if congestion continues

(b)   Parents may need education on the symptoms of fluid overload, the inability to tolerate routine feedings in the child's current condition

(c)   Gradually decreasing fluids based on demand and tolerance is easier for parents than an all or none approach

(d)   Trial use of oxygen may be beneficial if it does not increase agitation (use pediatric cannula or mask or blow by)

e)   Elimination

i.   Maintain bowel function and prevent the acute stress and distress associated with constipation and the need for invasive remedies

ii.   Invasive efforts to relieve constipation are very traumatic and risky for the child especially the oncology patient with bleeding precautions

iii.   PREVENTION is very important via nutrition, hydration and a preventative bowel regimen to avoid painful stooling/constipation. Hydration as long as possible to maintain urination, avoid indwelling catheters and maintain general comfort and hygiene

    f)   Blood products/transfusions

        i.   Pediatric patients often benefit from continuing intermittent transfusions if they add to or maintain a desired quality of life; may help the child to accomplish specific personal goals, i.e., graduation, birthday, significant outing or other milestone etc.

        ii.   These interventions may prevent a traumatic dying experience if it is expected that the child may actually hemorrhage or will die at home with that possibility

        iii.   The balance of benefit/burden for these therapies and the decision whether or not to provide them is a discussion to plan ahead for and review over time as the child's condition changes to review the goals for care

    g)   Depression

        i.   May not be anticipated in the dying child or adolescent, but needs to be assessed when symptoms appear

        ii.   Children show the same symptoms as adults, i.e., becoming more withdrawn, increase desire for sleep; apathy for known interests, decreased tolerance to change and increased labile emotions, irritability, sleep disorders, etc.

        iii.   Consult with physician, psychologist or psychiatrist to determine the best pharmacologic approach and social worker for follow up communication on assessment of need and counseling needs as well

        iv.   Reassure parents and child that this type of "situational" depression is treatable and not uncommon

        v.   Utilize immediate onset medications for a more rapid therapeutic effect

C.   Preparation for the last days of life

    1.   Utilize hopeful language in context of condition

        a)   Negative and consistently "death oriented" discussions are not palatable for most children and their families on a regular basis

            i.   Parents of young children are often not prepared to make final arrangements until death is imminent or afterwards

            ii.   This may not be denial, but rather a personal decision reflecting the parents' needs and beliefs

        b)   "Titrate" family's ability to handle these discussions, as trust and readiness are apparent

            i.   Forcing them may lead to conflict and hostility or even rejection of care

            ii.   Hope is always present in some form and some expression for these families

    2.   As much as possible, plan where the death will take place

        a)   With the help and support of the interdisciplinary team, discuss with patient and parents where they would prefer last days of living to take place

        b)   Explore any fears or concerns—realistic or not—related to the decisions for place of death and dispel if appropriate

c) If transfer to another unit i.e., hospice unit or other setting, suggest a pre-transfer visit. For ICU patients, inpatient staff may need additional information and education about what is possible for discharge to home setting and advocate for what parent's wishes are

d) Communicate the plan to all staff involved, especially those that cover after hours, at change of shift or assignments etc.

3. Explore and discuss the spiritual dimension of the child's life as it relates to coping with their illness and life changes

a) Have similar discussions with each parent and the sibling(s) and grandparents, if present

b) Collaborate with chaplain/spiritual counselor to address the needs and concerns that arise during these discussions

i. Discuss what would bring comfort at this time and what continues to be a source of strength to each of them

ii. Facilitate obtaining the desired spiritual and/or religious support

iii. Provide for rituals requested

4. Prepare family members and child as he/she desires for what to expect as the dying process nears

a) Providing this in a written form is particularly helpful for them to refer to and to use with other relatives

b) Use language that is gentle, informative and based on child's level of understanding

VII. Counsel/Provide Emotional Support for Child's Grief

A. **Important to consider developmental stages as the context upon which to base explanations, education, needs assessment and relevant approaches**

1. If children have a sibling or a parent, significant grandparent etc. who is dying, the issues of their grief need to be assessed and addressed by the interdisciplinary team

2. Interdisciplinary team members, including the nurse have significant opportunities to make the child feel included, to validate concerns and anticipatory grief, their desire to help and participate fulfilled—PRIOR to the death of their loved one

3. Grieving begins upon the realization something is seriously wrong/has changed in the family and that "someone is not getting better"

B. **Eric Erikson's stages of human development; all stages are considered a "crisis" that must be overcome and mastered; non-resolution of a stage may handicap a person in later life; most marked effect on later life is the non-resolution of stage one: trust versus mistrust[6]**

1. Trust versus mistrust (infancy)

2. Autonomy versus shame and doubt (early childhood)

3. Initiative versus guilt (preschool)

4. Industry versus inferiority (childhood)

5.   Identity versus diffusion (adolescence); directed toward dating and social roles

6.   Intimacy versus isolation (young adulthood)

7.   Generativity versus self-absorption (adulthood); most potential to change society

8.   Integrity versus despair (maturity)

C.   **Piagetian stages**[7,8]

1.   Sensory-motor (birth to 3 years): Infant goes through several substages that lead from complete self involvement to learning through trial and error to use certain acts to affect an object or a person; by age 2, toddler learns that certain actions have a specific effect on the environment; thinking is egocentric (for instance, if mother leaves, child thinks it is because of his/her action)

2.   Pre-operational (3–7 years): Thought is intuitive and prelogical (magical); thinking remains egocentric with conclusions based on what child feels or would like to believe

3.   Concrete operational thought (7–12 years): Conceptual organization becomes more stable and rational; child develops a conceptual framework that is used to evaluate and understand objects in the world around him/her

4.   Formal operational thought (12–18 years): Adolescent is increasingly able to deal effectively with reality, abstract thinking and future thinking; deductive reasoning develops; important ideals and attitudes develop in late adolescence

D.   **Children and grief responses by age (note: children and adolescents do not grieve in a linear pattern but rather in a "clumping pattern" of sometimes intense periods separated by long intervals where they apparently are not affected by the loss)**[9]

1.   The infant: birth to 2 years (pre-verbal)

a)   Grief reactions: irritability, change in crying or eating patterns, bowel or bladder disturbances, emotional withdrawal and slowing of development; clinginess; do not tolerate changes in daily living routines

b)   How to help: provide secure and stable environment, lots of TLC; follow a schedule, hold and play with the child often; a consistent caregiver and maintaining routines is critical

2.   The preschool child: age 3 to 5 years

a)   Grief reactions: grasp of SOME concepts related to death, time and permanence are limited and often see death as temporary; may ask seemingly inappropriate questions ("Why can't we just go out and get another mom?"), indifference, physiological symptoms (sleeping, eating, stomachaches), regression, fears, imagined guilt/feelings of responsibility, wide-ranging emotions

b)   How to help: same as above; understand and accept the behavior as normal; use the correct terminology; BRIEF EXPLANATIONS; reassure the child he/she had nothing to do with CAUSING the ILLNESS or the death

3.   The grade school child: age 6 to 10

a)   Grief reactions: a child of this age gradually begins to understand death, but may still believe that it only happens to other people; may feel guilt (magical thinking) and blame self for death; may see on again, off again grieving, problems in school (including socially inappropriate behavior, anger towards teacher or classmates, poor grades, physical ailments), anger; at this age children are at the most risk for complicated grief—they intellectually understand death, but lack coping skills to deal with the emotions

  b)   How to help: same as above; provide simple, honest and accurate information, accept behavior as normal, contact and ask for help from school counselors and teachers, acknowledge normalcy of anger and teach ways to constructively express it

4.   The pre-adolescent and adolescent: age 10 to 18

  a)   Grief reactions: typically, by age 12 to 14, children have a complete view of mortality; they may, however, deny that death can happen to them or one of their peers; may view death as punishment; grief at this developmental stage may interfere with the child's development of identity; may see hidden or denied emotions, so called "common and normal adolescent behaviors" may be made worse by a loss at this stage (fighting, unruliness at school, rebellion, using drugs, sexual activity, suicidal tendencies)

  b)   How to help: same as above; acknowledge that adolescents are not adults and do not need to act or think like adults; evaluate supports available and informed at school; engage school and other trusted adults for support, be aware of destructive behaviors and set limits. Continue discipline parameters to maintain appropriate behavioral limits—this actually enhances security in the adolescent. Due to the inherent ambivalence and duality of feelings, intense emotions and desires for independence and tentativeness to release feelings; peer influences; may be interested in journaling, peer groups, tape recording, artistic expression, art therapy modes of expression

5.   Young adult: age 19 and over

  a)   Grief reactions: fully formed notion of death including how death affects him/her and changes in the family structure; may experience ambivalence and confusion about what is next for them, including the feeling of responsibility to take on some of the roles of the dead family member

  b)   How to help: urge the young adult to focus on their needs and be able to express them to adults around them as well as peers so that others can support them; may be interested in support groups (not easy in the midst of the pain of grief!)

E.   Ten Needs of Grieving Children[a,10]

  1.   **Adequate Information**

    a)   Children need information that is clear and comprehensible

    b)   When they don't have sufficient information, they'll make up a story to fill in the gaps

    c)   If possible children should be informed about an impending death; they already know something is taking place

    d)   They can become anxious, maybe feel responsible or may even wonder if they can "catch" whatever the cause of the person's death

---

[a] Adapted by San Diego Hospice

2. **Fears and Anxieties Addressed**

   a)   Children need to know they will be cared for; many children who lose one parent fear the other will die too; they fear for their own safety as well

   b)   Research has also shown that bereaved children who were given consistent discipline after parental death were less anxious than those for whom discipline became lax

3. **Reassurance That They Are Not to Blame**

   a)   Bereaved children may wonder, "Did I cause it to happen?" They need to know they didn't cause the death out of their anger or shortcomings

   b)   Younger children especially may experience "magical thinking" and may have difficulty in this area

4. **Careful Listening**

   a)   Children need to have a person who will hear out their fears, fantasies and questions and not minimize their concerns

   b)   Some of their questions may be uncomfortable for adults, yet they need answered as valid things kids wonder about

5. **Validation of Individual's Feelings**

   a)   It is sometimes a temptation to tell a child how he or she should feel, but children's feelings must be acknowledged and respected as valid

   b)   Children also need to express their thoughts and feelings in their own way

   c)   Adults must remember each child's personality is unique as well as their relationship with the deceased

6. **Help with Overwhelming Feelings**

   a)   Children need help in dealing with emotions that are too intense to be expressed

   b)   The most common feelings expressed by bereaved children are sadness, anger, anxiety and guilt

   c)   Sometimes these feelings are acted out and adults can help kids express them in safer ways through play activities and/or writing

7. **Involvement and Inclusion**

   a)   Children need to feel important and involved before the death as well as afterward

   b)   It is recommended that children over age 5 be allowed to make an informed decision as to whether or not they want to attend the funeral, for example

   c)   Children may want to have something special they have made buried with the person

   d)   Children also need to be included in rituals around anniversaries or other special times when it's appropriate to remember the deceased in a more formal way

8. **Continued Routine Activities**

   a)   Children need to maintain age appropriate interests and activities

   b)   Adults sometimes need to be reminded that children cope and communicate through play activity (kids are kids first and grievers second)

9. **Modeled Grief Behaviors**

   a)   Learning theory tells us that modeled behavior is one of the most effective sources of learning; children learn how to mourn by observing mourning behavior in adults

   b)   Encouraging children to think about, to remember and to talk about the deceased is a rather simple but effective way that adults can influence the course of bereavement in children

   c)   Acknowledging and sharing feelings with the child in this way is very important

10. **Opportunities to Remember**

   a)   Children need to be able to remember and to memorialize their lost loved one not only after the death but also continuously as they go through the remaining stages of life

   b)   Pictures and objects belonging to the deceased can be useful reminders of who the person was and the things that were important in the relationship; shared reminiscences can also be helpful

Cited References

1. Berry P, Zeri K, Egan K. *The Hospice Nurses Study Guide: A Preparation for the CRNH Candidate.* 2nd ed. Pittsburgh, PA: Hospice Nurses Association; 1997.

2. American Cancer Society. *Cancer facts and figures 2000.* American Cancer Society; 2000.

3. Children's Hospice International. *Children's Hospice International: 2001 Informational Overview.* Alexandria, VA: Children's Hospice International; 2001.

4. Wong DL. *Wong & Whaley's Clinical Manual of Pediatric Nursing.* 5th ed. St. Louis, MO: Mosby; 2000.

5. Clark E. *Palliative Pain and Symptom Management for Children and Adolescents.* Alexandria, VA: Children's Hospice International and Division of Maternal and Child Health—US Department of Health and Human Services; 1985.

6. Erikson E. *Childhood and Society.* New York, NY: W.W. Norton & Co; 1963.

7. Wadsworth B. *Piaget's Theory of Cognitive Development.* New York, NY: David McKay Co.; 1971.

8. Petrillo M, Sanger S. *Emotional Care of Hospitalized Children: An Environmental Approach.* 2nd ed. Philadelphia, PA: J.B. Lippincott; 1980.

9. Volker B, ed. *Hospice and Palliative Nurses Practice Review.* 3rd ed. Dubuque, IA: Kendall/Hunt Publishing; 1999.

10. Worden JW. *Children and Grief: When a Parent Dies.* New York, NY: The Guilford Press; 1996.

Additional References and Resources

Armstrong-Daily A, Zarbock S, ed. *Hospice Care for Children.* 2nd ed. New York, NY: Oxford University Press; 2004.

Carter B, Levetown M, ed. *Palliative Care for Infants, Children and Adolescents: A Practical Handbook.* Johns Hopkins Press: Baltimore, MD; 2004.

ChIPPS. *Compendium of Pediatric Palliative Care: Professional Development and Resource Series.* Alexandria, VA: NHPCO; 2000.

Davies B, Brenner P, Orloff S, Sumner L, Worden W. Addressing Spirituality in Pediatric Hospice and Palliative Care. *Journal of Palliative Care* 2002;18:1:59–67.

Davies B, Gudmundsdottir M, Worden W, Orloff S, Sumner L, Brenner P. Living in the dragon's shadow: fathers' experience of a child's life threatening illness. *Journal of Death Studies.* 2004; March 28(2):111–135.

Doka K, ed. *Children Mourning/Mourning Children.* Washington, DC: Hospice Foundation of America; 1995.

Doyle D, Hanks GWC, MacDonald N, ed. *Oxford Textbook of Palliative Medicine.* 3rd ed. New York, NY: Oxford University Press; 2004.

Ferrell BR, Coyle N, ed. *Textbook of Palliative Nursing.* New York, NY: Oxford University Press; 2001.

Field M, Behrman R, ed. *When Children Die: Improving Palliative and End of Life Care for Children and Their Families.* Washington, DC: Institute of Medicine of the National Academies, National Academy Press; 2003.

Foley G, Fochtman D, Mooney K, ed. *Nursing Care of the Child with Cancer.* 2nd ed. Philadelphia, PA: W.B. Saunders; 1993.

Hames CC. Helping infants and toddlers when a family member dies. *Journal of Hospice and Palliative Nursing.* 2002:5(2):103–110.

Hess CS. *The child in pain.* In: *Wong DL. Wong and Whaley's Clinical Manual of Pediatric Nursing.* 4th ed. St. Louis, MO: Mosby; 1996:314-331.

Glazer HR, Clark MD, Stein DS. The impact of hippotherapy on grieving children. *Journal of Hospice and Palliative Nursing.* 2002:6(3):171–175.

Levetown M, Gerri F. UNIPAC 8: The hospice/palliative medicine approach to caring for pediatric patients. In: Storey P, Knight C, eds. *UIPAC Book Series: Hospice/Palliative Care Training for Physicians, A Self Study Program.* New York, NY: Mary Ann Liebert, Inc. Publishers; 2003.

Sumner L. Lighting the way: improving the way children die in America. *Caring Magazine of the NAHC.* May 2003.

Sine D, Sumner L, Gracy D, Von Gunten C. Pediatric Extubation: "pulling the tube." *Journal of Palliative Medicine.* 2001;4(4):519–524.

Texas Cancer Council. *End of Life Care for Children.* Austin, TX: Author; 2000.

Tobin D, Hilden J. *Shelter from the Storm: Caring for a Child with a Life Threatening Condition.* Cambridge, MA: Perseus Publishing; 2003.

ORGANIZATION AND INTERNET RESOURCES

Children's Hospice International: Resources and publications, www.chionline.org.

Compassionate Passages: Video and discussion guide for training healthcare professional on the needs and experience of parents when a child is dying. Video: When a Child is Dying. www.compassionatepassages.org.

End-of-Life Nursing Education Consortium (ELNEC): Pediatric Palliative Care-Pediatric train the trainer course and curriculum. Information and registration, materials available at: www.aacn.nche.edu/elnec.

Initiative for Pediatric Palliative Care: www.ippcweb.org. Curriculum for interdisciplinary approach to implementing palliative care and changing one's institutional support and includes voice of parents. Regional retreats being offered.

National Hospice and Palliative Care Organization: Pediatric resources and publications, www.nhpco.org.

Society of Pediatric Nurses: 1-800-723-2902 Member list serve for pediatric nurses. www.pedsnurses.org.

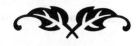

CHAPTER IX

INDICATORS OF IMMINENT DYING

Jeanne Martinez, RN, MPH, CHPN®

First Edition Authors
Kathy Kalina, RN, BSN, CHPN®
Joanne E. Sheldon, RN, MEd, CHPN®, CIC

I.   **Introduction/Overview**

   A.   **Care at the time of dying, includes the support and education needed to allow a comfortable, natural death in any healthcare setting or the patient's home**

   B.   **Nursing has the opportunity to optimize each person's quality of life and comfort in the last stages of life. Nurses are often responsible for the care given directly before and after death**

   1.   Facilitating the patient and family's transition to the actively dying phase of care requires open communication among patient, family and the healthcare team[1]

   2.   There is only one chance to do this well and "get it right" for each person

   C.   **Providing effective care at the time of dying includes emotional support and preparation of family members, as well as patients**

   1.   Listen and be present as they grieve their losses

   2.   Prepare and educate patients and families about the dying process, grieving, available information and support resources

   3.   Facilitate patient and family communication with each other and with members of the healthcare team

   D.   **Any care environment can be enhanced to improve care at the time of dying**

   1.   Ensure that the physical environment is as comfortable, private and personal as possible

   2.   Work with the healthcare team to maintain patient goals and avoid burdensome care

   3.   Care of dying persons and their families can be improved in every care setting

E. **Recognize that professional caregivers need self-care**

1. To provide optimal care to the dying and their grieving family members, professionals need to be attentive to their own emotional coping and grieving

2. Professionals need to be attentive and assistive to the emotional responses and coping of their colleagues, as well

F. **When done well, care at the time of dying can be amongst the most rewarding of nursing experiences**

II. **Guiding Principles to Facilitate Natural Dying**

A. **Anticipate and manage physical, emotional and spiritual needs of patients and families**

B. **Honor patient's wishes and current goals of care, including, when possible, the patient's preference for the place of death**

C. **Provide care that neither hastens death, prolongs life nor is burdensome to the patient**

D. **Adjust policies, care routines and the physical care environment to support the dying process**

III. **Indicators of Imminent Death**

A. **Physical signs that death is very near (hours or days) include**

1. Changes in mentation

    a) Psychological and physical withdrawal

    b) Increased periods of sleeping

    c) Decreased consciousness

2. Decreased and concentrated (dark) urinary output resulting from decreased blood circulation to the kidneys

3. Skin coolness, usually beginning with the extremities—hands, arms, feet and legs become increasingly cool

4. Changes in skin color; especially paleness and/or blue to purple areas of color, called mottling

5. Incontinence of urine and/or bowels

6. Dyspnea—difficulty breathing, feeling short of breath. This can be very distressing to families and may cause the patient discomfort

    a) Position the patient with the head of the bed up, with pillows behind the patient's head; and if possible, sit the patient up in a reclining chair

        i.   Short acting opioids usually provide most effective relief

        ii. Suggest that the patient move more slowly; keep still, lay quietly; and use pursed-lip or deep, slow breathing

       iii.   Direct a fan to the face or open a window (or both) to move air through the patient's room

       iv.   Use relaxation or distraction techniques with conscious patients

7.   Breathing pattern changes

   a)   The following breathing patterns are common in the final stages of dying and are not to be confused with dyspnea and although may be frightening to family members, generally do not cause discomfort in patients

   b)   Regular breathing pattern may change and become irregular, e.g., shallow breaths with periods of no breathing for 5 to 30 seconds, up to a full minute, known as Cheyne-Stokes breathing

   c)   Noisy, wet respirations (sometimes referred to as 'death rattle'). Interventions may include a change in position (i.e., high side-lying with the head of the bed elevated) and anticholinergic medications may help to decrease the secretions and thus, the noise

   d)   Apnea, defined as no breathing, ranging from short periods to longer periods as death approaches

B. Hydration and Nutrition in the Final Days or Hours

1.   Attempts at maintaining body weight, a level of caloric intake and/or reversing weight loss, are not reasonable or achievable goals in the final weeks and days of life. Dehydration is also a normal part of the process of a natural death, as the patient's oral intake decreases and body systems are slowly shutting down. It is helpful to discuss feeding and hydration with patients and families early in the disease process when reviewing preferences for care and advance directive documents, so that patient's desires can be known and respected. Thus, all involved can be prepared when these decisions need to be made. Goals for nutrition and hydration in the final stages of life should be directed at comfort

   a)   Allow patients to eat and drink for comfort and the social pleasure of sharing meals. If swallowing is not a problem, conscious patients should be offered frequent sips of liquids and soft food. The ability to swallow without aspiration needs to be continually assessed as the patient's condition declines. In the final weeks or days before death, artificial feeding, whether parenteral nor enteral, is rarely appropriate and is initiated only for reasons related to comfort. Providing fluids at end stage often creates more discomfort than benefit and increases the risk of many complications[2]

   b)   Prevent or correct metabolic problems, when possible. Artificial hydration may have limited benefit in a conscious, ambulatory patient with metabolic imbalance. A trial of hydration can determine the comfort vs. burden of such intervention[3]

   c)   Prevent fluid overload and other problems related to artificial feeding and hydration. At the very end of life, artificial hydration can cause fluid overload resulting in pulmonary congestion, cardiac overload, increasing ascites and creating or exacerbating edema

   d)   Attend to any symptoms created by dehydration or limited nutritional intake. Feed patients when hungry, rather than imposing scheduled meals. Provide frequent oral hygiene for symptoms related to thirst

   e)   Educate families about the physiologic rationale for not providing artificial feeding or hydration in the final stages of life. Recognize however, that feeding is a very emotional issue. These emotions need to be addressed with family members as well

C.   Pain during the Active Phase of Dying

1.   Patients who have not experienced pain during their illness are unlikely to experience pain from the disease during its final stages. If pain suddenly occurs or increases, a new problem (e.g., a pathologic fracture) should be suspected

2.   Pain assessment in the final stages often depends on caregiver observation, if the patient is no longer verbal or able to self-report

   a)   Patients may need to use an alternate pain reporting scale. Those who can no longer report verbally on a 0–10 scale, may be able to point on a visual scale or may only be able to nod 'yes' or 'no' in response to a verbal question of whether they have pain. If an alternate reporting scale is used, communicate this to the healthcare team and other caregivers and use consistently

   b)   For an unresponsive patient, behavior change is the most reliable sign of pain. Restlessness may indicate many other things such as agitation, early delirium, urinary retention or constipation. However, once those underlying causes are ruled out, assume the behavior change is related to pain

   c)   When pain has been managed with oral analgesics, anticipate the need for changing drug routes as the patient declines and may be unable to swallow

   d)   Managing pain at the very end of life requires careful assessment and observation. It is generally thought that continuing an opioid pain medication at the same dose is appropriate unless signs of toxicity related to impaired renal or hepatic function appear. These may include increasing somnolence and myoclonus. Rather than discontinuing the medication altogether, a reduction in dose and/or choice of another opioid may be appropriate. Regardless, as persons near death often can no longer reliably swallow, a change in the route of administration may also be necessary

D.   Anxiety, Agitation and Delirium

   a)   Few patients retain complete mental clarity during the dying experience. Changes in mentation range from mild anxiety to occasional agitation and confusion, to severe delirium. Causes and severity vary widely and require careful assessment. Changes in mentation can be caused by metabolic changes, medications such as opioids and in particular benzodiazepines, pain, other physical symptoms, full bladder and unresolved spiritual issues. The most effective treatment depends on identifying the cause. For many dying patients this may be difficult to determine. Therefore treatments often need to be by trial and may include hydration, medications and control of environmental stimuli [3]

IV.   Psychosocial and Spiritual Issues

A.   Allow patients as much control over their environment and caregiving as possible

B.   Maintain patient dignity

1.   Assume that the patient can hear all conversations; speak directly to the patient, even if she or he doesn't respond

2.   Be mindful of preserving patient dignity, especially as he/she is no longer able to control urine and stool, for example, using the term "padding" instead of diapers

   a)   Avoid having conversations with others as if the patient were not present

C.   Be aware of possible patient fears commonly experienced at the end of life including fear of

1.   The unknown

2.   Being abandoned

3.   Being a burden to one's family or support system

D.   Communication/support

1.   Listen carefully and address the patient's current concerns

2.   Orient the patient frequently, even if patient is non-communicative

3.   Periodically assess the non-verbal patient's ability to communicate by other means, such as squeezing hands or blinking

4.   When multiple family members are involved and the patient is no longer decisional and/or able to communicate, the healthcare team should consult with the person who the patient has designated as the healthcare proxy, if such a person has been so designated

5.   Respect patient desires about what information is shared with family and friends

6.   Spiritual issues

E.   Saying goodbye—patients and families should be encouraged to take the opportunity to say their good-byes and anything else each feels needs to be said to loved-ones

1.   Dying alone—some families have the goal of being with their loved one at the moment of death. However, there are deaths that seem to occur when all family have left the room. In this instance, families often need support to view the importance of all of their support over the entire illness and not feel that their absence at the time of death was a failure

2.   Permission to "go"—sometimes patients need explicit permission or encouragement to let go and die. Helping families express their sadness over the impending death but assuring the patient they will be fine and look after one another, for example, is often the role of the nurse

3.   Symbolic language—patients may talk about "preparing to go home," "going on a trip," "standing in line." Although the patient may seem confused, some refer to this phenomenon in dying as "near-death awareness." This may be accompanied by the patient either reporting or actually seeing and/or having conversations with previously deceased family and friends[4]

4.   Request for euthanasia or physician-assisted suicide (PAS). The patient or family may ask about euthanasia or assisted suicide. In the actively dying phase, this is most likely to come from a distressed family member, rather than the patient. In either case, the healthcare team should be prepared to respond in the following ways

     a)   Respond to the request in a non-judgmental and supportive manner

     b)   Assess for the underlying reason for the request—is it suffering? Need for information? Fatigue on the part of the patient and/or caregiver? Spiritual distress? Unmanaged symptoms? Unfinished business?

     c)   Know your agency policy or local guidelines for such a request. PAS is illegal in the United States, except in the state of Oregon

     d)   Collaborate with the healthcare team to develop a plan for a comprehensive, consistent approach to address the source of the patient or family's suffering

V.   **Family Caregiver Support and Teaching**

    A.   **Listen carefully and address family concerns**

    B.   **Allow the family as much control over the environment as possible**

        1.   Some families want to be present throughout the period when the patient is dying, whereas others are uncomfortable being near the person; respect these individual preferences, which may change over time. Discuss the possible scenarios with the family, emphasizing that there are wide variations. This is especially important when a family member absolutely wishes to be present at the time of death as this is not always possible

        2.   Common family fears at the time of the death of a loved one

            a)   The patient will suffer from a painful death

            b)   Being alone with the patient, especially at the time of death

            c)   One's own grief responses

            d)   Not knowing when the patient is dead

            e)   Causing the patient's death by giving medications (in home care setting)

    C.   **If the family desires, encourage them to participate in care giving**

    D.   **If a family member does not wish to provide care or is emotionally or physically tired of caregiving, give them permission to take a break and allow others to provide patient care**

    E.   **Reinforce to family members that breathing patterns such as Cheyne-Stokes, congestion and apnea are an expected part of the natural dying process and typically are not distressful to patients**

    F.   **Prepare family members about the anticipated processes of natural dying, emphasizing that each experience is individual and many physical processes may not be observed in every person**

    G.   **Anticipate if after the death, families will be approached to give permission for autopsy, organ or body donation. If so, the healthcare team should take the opportunity to discuss these requests in advance of the death, in order to give family members time to consider them. If approached sensitively by the healthcare team, some family members will view these requests as something positive they can contribute in the face of the tragedy of losing a loved one**

    H.   **A caring, attentive approach by the healthcare team at the end of life eases the grieving process for the family**

VI.   **Grief Coaching and Resources**

    A.   **Encourage families to communicate with the patient before death, even when the patient appears unresponsive**

B. **Suggest that family members may wish to say good-bye when leaving the person, as death is often unpredictable**

C. **Provide resources for available bereavement support**

D. **Assess spiritual and cultural needs regarding death early in order to provide appropriate and timely resources**

E. **Consult with chaplains and community clergy, for spiritual support as appropriate**

F. **Assess family members for high-risk or complicated grieving. This is primarily a question of the grieving person's ability to function, but the following are among some of the factors to assess**

   1. History of depression or other mental illness

   2. Extreme grief reaction

   3. Self-destructive behavior

   4. Increased use of alcohol and/or drugs

   5. Inadequate or perceived lack of social support[5]

VII. The Death Event

A. **Recognize that even with expected deaths, family and even professional caregivers will often express feeling unprepared when the death actually occurs**

B. **The following signs indicate that death has occurred**

   1. No respirations

   2. No audible heartbeat

   3. Bowel and/or bladder incontinence sometimes occurs

   4. Unresponsive

   5. Eyelids slightly open

   6. Pupils fixed and dilated

   7. No blinking

   8. Jaw relaxed and mouth slightly open

C. **Prepare family members about what they should do if they are alone with the patient at the time of death**

   1. The death of a hospice patient or a patient on an inpatient setting (with a Do Not Resuscitate or No Code order), is expected. Such a natural death does not require any emergency or heroic medical intervention. What is needed is calm and competent support and interpretation of what they will observe for the friends and family members who are at the bedside or coming to view the body

2.   The family or the nurse should notify the team (hospice, on-call or unit staff)

3.   The nurse is often the one to verify the absence of vital signs and notify the physician, the next-of-kin if not present and the funeral home. In most hospital settings, only a physician may pronounce a death. In home care settings, nurses may pronounce a death in some jurisdictions. Nurses should know the policies and laws that govern procedures around expected deaths in their specific care settings, in order to guide grieving family survivors through the necessary tasks

VIII.   Aftercare Rituals and Family Support

A.   Assist with facilitating any cultural or religious rituals that the family desires, if appropriate

B.   Position the body in a dignified way for family viewing

C.   Encourage family to spend time with the body, saying good-byes, prayers or other rituals meaningful to them

D.   Ask if other family, friends or clergy need to come to view or attend to the body before post-mortem care is performed

E.   Offer chaplain or other staff support, being mindful of maintaining the family's need for support and privacy

F.   Generally, the body should not be moved until the family is ready and feel they have been given enough time to say good-bye. However, nurses should know if local laws or customs are in conflict with this

G.   Reinforce teaching to family about what to expect

1.   Rigor mortis (stiffening of the body after death) occurs 2 to 4 hours after death

2.   Air may escape from the lungs, especially when turning the body; assure the family that this does not mean the patient is still alive

3.   Bowel and bladder incontinence commonly occur following death

H.   Post-mortem care of the body after death

1.   Handle the body with the same respect you would if the person were alive

2.   Bathe body and groom as appropriate; place either an adult diaper or a waterproof pad under the patient to catch urinary and bowel leakage and to minimize odor

3.   Ask if the family would like to participate in post-mortem care; some family members find it comforting to perform this last act of care for a loved one; in some cultures and for some relationships (such as the death of a child), family participation in preparation of the body may be very important for the grieving process[6]

4.   Prepare family members for the removal of the body from the room or home, as this is often a difficult process to observe. Give families the option of leaving the area prior to the body being removed

5. For a home death, arrange for the removal of durable medical equipment and medical supplies as soon as possible

6. Giving post-mortem care provides a good opportunity for nurses and other caregivers to say their "good-byes" to the patient

IX. Professional Coping with Care of the Dying

A. Recognize the importance of professional coping and self-care when working with the dying

1. Reframe your view of dying, so that death is an expected part of your practice and not considered a professional 'failure'

2. Develop and promote healthy coping mechanisms

   a) Acknowledge and explore your personal feelings about patients who die as the first step in discovering what works best for your emotions

   b) Create your own rituals to acknowledge the deaths of patients or provide a form of closure. This may include such things as private reflection, attending a patient's funeral service or writing a final note to the family

3. Recognize your emotional limits and seek assistance when you need it

X. Be Aware of the Emotional Needs of Colleagues Caring for Dying Patients

A. Reach out to colleagues who are having difficulty coping

1. Encourage colleagues to acknowledge their feelings on a regular basis

2. Promote the availability of resources for professionals to help them in processing their feelings

3. Develop organizational strategies to improve the coping of the healthcare team such as educational seminars, availability of consultant psychiatric or counselor professionals and formal debriefings of patient deaths

4. Assist colleagues in acknowledging the excellent care strategies and outcomes that they have provided

CITED REFERENCES

1. National Consensus Project for Quality Palliative Care. *Clinical Practice Guidelines for Quality Palliative Care*. Pittsburgh, PA: National Consensus Project for Quality Palliative Care; 2004:18. Available at www.nationalconsensusproject.org. Accessed July 29, 2004.

2. Kedziera P. Hydration, thirst and nutrition. In: Ferrell BR, Coyle N, eds. *Textbook of Palliative Nursing*. New York, NY: Oxford University Press; 2001:161.

3. Kubler KK, English N, Heidrich DE. Delirium, confusion, agitation and restlessness. In: Ferrell BR, Coyle N, eds. *Textbook of Palliative Nursing*. New York, NY: Oxford University Press; 2001:299.

4. Callahan M, Kelley P. *Final Gifts: Understanding the Special Awareness, Needs and Communications of the Dying*. New York, NY: Bantam Books; 1993.

5. Corless IB. Bereavement. In: Ferrell BR, Coyle N, eds. *Textbook of Palliative Nursing*. New York, NY: Oxford University Press; 2001:359.

6. Berry P, Griffie J. Planning for the actual death. In: Ferrell BR, Coyle N, eds. *Textbook of Palliative Nursing*. New York, NY: Oxford University Press; 2001:390.

ADDITIONAL REFERENCES AND RESOURCES

Forbes MA, Rosdahl DR. The final journey of life. *Journal of Hospice and Palliative Nursing*. 2002:5(4):213–220.

Gauthier D. The meaning of healing near the end of life. *Journal of Hospice and Palliative Nursing*. 2002:4(4):220–227.

Kruse BG. The meaning of letting go: the lived experience for caregivers of persons at the end of life. *Journal of Hospice and Palliative Nursing*. 2002:6(4):215–222.

Ternestedt BM, Andershed B, Eriksson M, Johansson I. A good death: development of a nursing model of care. *Journal of Hospice and Palliative Nursing*. 2002:4(3):153–160.

Woods AB. The terror of the night: posttraumatic stress disorder at the end of life. *Journal of Hospice and Palliative Nursing*. 2002:5(4):196–204.

CHAPTER X

ECONOMIC AND POLICY ISSUES IN HOSPICE AND PALLIATIVE CARE

Barbara Volker, RN, MSN, CHPN®
Patricia Berry, PhD, APRN, BC-PCM

First Edition Authors
Barbara Volker, RN, MSN, CHPN®
Ashby Watson, RN, MS, CS, OCN

I. **Economic Outcomes for End-of-Life Care**

   A. **Why measure economic outcomes?**

      1. To promote quality of care

      2. To control costs

      3. To benchmark for creative management

   B. **Economic issues affecting the provision of healthcare**

      1. Treatment costs and spending continue to rise

      2. High technology care is costly (1/2 of all Medicare spending occurs in the last six months of life)

      3. Increased consumer demand for sophisticated and expensive care

      4. Explosive growth of elderly population, who will survive longer with more chronic diseases

      5. Current insurance system rewards high technology interventions but does not reimburse for effective low technology interventions

   C. **Worldwide allocation of resources currently greatly favors curative care with less resources allocated to palliative care**

      1. World Health Organization (WHO) proposes[1]

         a) Greater allocation of palliative care resources to developing countries (survival not as great and palliative care needs are greater)

         b) More equal distribution of curative and comfort care resources in developed countries

D. Justification of Economic Outcomes[2]

1. Benefits should be weighed against toxicity and costs

2. Treatment justified if

   a) Improvement in overall survival

   b) Improvement in disease-free survival

   c) Improvement in quality of life

   d) Improvement in cost effectiveness

   e) Less toxicity occurs

3. Treatment should not be based on:

   a) Cost alone

   b) False hope that disease will improve or be cured

E. Economic evaluation of therapies for palliation

1. Hospice or Palliative Care may be a good economic choice[1]

   a) Symptom relief

   b) Prolongation of survival

   c) If quality time is still available to the patient

2. Example: chemotherapy for non-small cell lung cancer

   a) Small benefit of 2–4 months survival[3]

   b) May prevent hospitalizations late in disease course[2,4]

   c) Benefit can be shown at reasonable cost[5,6]

F. The following factors also may influence cost outcomes

1. Less expensive the setting, the less costly the intervention

   a) Home opioid infusions are less expensive than hospital infusions[7]

   b) Outpatient chemotherapy is cheaper than inpatient chemotherapy[8]

   c) Costs of home chemotherapy administration is less expensive than outpatient chemotherapy, making home chemotherapy a safe and economically realistic alternative to traditional hospital treatment[9]

   d) Exception to this "rule" occurs in home health where IV medications may sometimes be given instead of oral because Medicare will pay for IV home infusion, but won't pay for oral medications

2. Care coordination[10,11]

   a) Doesn't improve survival or symptom management outcomes, but can reduce costs by shortening hospital stays

   b) Patient and family satisfaction increased[10,11]

3. Pain management coordination programs

    a) Reduction in admissions and re-admissions

    b) Can lead to marked cost savings[12]

4. Advance Directives (refer to Chapter 12 for a complete discussion of advance care planning and goals of care)

    a) Research conflicting on cost-savings

        i. No positive or negative impact on costs[13]

        ii. Patients who sign advance directive may have lower costs at last hospitalization[14]

        iii. If every person who died in 1988 executed an advance directive that was honored, selected hospice, refused aggressive in-hospital care, the total savings would have been $18.1 billion dollars (3.3% of all healthcare spending)[15]

5. Ethics and Teaching Consultations[16]

    a) Surgical Intensive Care Unit (SICU) staff taught about dying and ethics of futile care

        i. Reduced length of stay

        ii. SICU days significantly reduced

    b) Ethics consultations[17]

        i. On all mechanically ventilated patients

        ii. Reduction in futile care

        iii. Increased transfers from ICU to lesser-intensity beds

        iv. Decreased costs because of less use of ICU

        v. Ethics teaching and consultations

        vi. Palliative care consultations

II. Access to Healthcare Systems at the End of Life

A. Factors may vary from state to state

1. Scope of healthcare benefits limited

2. Incentives for practitioners to provide less care

3. Pre-authorization requirements

4. Restricted eligibility

5. Poor access of under-served populations

6. Uninsured population, i.e., working poor, is growing

7. Delayed referral to hospice and palliative care

8. Cultural issues

B.   Factors originating within the healthcare system

1.   Patients discharged earlier and sicker

2.   Functionally disabled and cognitively impaired are increasingly admitted to long-term care facilities

3.   Stress on ambulatory services and home care services to meet needs of growing populations

C.   Financial impact

1.   Medicare, Medicaid, Social Security are being pressured to cut costs

2.   Families taking on more of the burden

   a)   Lost work hours

   b)   Out of pocket expenses

   c)   Care hours by family members not reimbursed

   d)   Caregiver stress and resultant poor health outcomes lead to increased use of healthcare system[18]

3.   Reported healthcare savings and costs may not reflect the actual cost of care for the full length of the illness

III.   Reimbursement Sources for End-of-Life Care

A.   Common payor sources for end-of-life care in the United States[18]

1.   Medicare

2.   Medicaid

3.   Veterans and defense health programs

4.   Employer sponsored programs

5.   Private insurance plans

6.   Uninsured

B.   Medicare is the most common source of payment for end-of-life care

1.   80.9% had Medicare as primary payment source[19]

2.   13% of Medicare beneficiaries also receive Medicaid

3.   28% of all Medicare payments is for care in the last year of life with nearly 50% of those costs incurred in the last 2 months of life[19]

4.   For all beneficiaries, Medicare covered less than half of all healthcare expenses[20]

   a)   Medicaid paid 14%

   b)   Private insurance paid 10%

   c)   Family out of pocket expenses paid 10–20%[19]

   d)   Other resources paid 3%

5.   Coverage limited for long term care, outpatient medications, supportive services

6. 3/4 of beneficiaries have supplemental policies for medications, but those policies cover only 25% of prescription services (60% is paid out of pocket)

7. Those who qualify for Medicare hospice benefit may receive some medications and non-medical services

8. Hospice accounts for 2.7% of Medicare spending, 1/10 of 1% of Medicaid spending[21]

   a) Time to death—more money spent in year prior to death

   b) Cause of death—payments influenced by disease and its treatment

   c) Age at death—payments per decedents dropped the older the person was at death, but those who survived may have had more chronic illnesses, thus increasing costs

   d) Cost offsets—for those persons who had both Medicare and Medicaid, lower Medicare costs may be offset by higher Medicaid costs

   e) Family costs—families may be assuming a larger part of the financial responsibility for care

C. Medicare hospice reimbursement via the Medicare Hospice Benefit[22]

   1. Under Medicare Part A (is seen as an alternative to hospitalization)

   2. Patient must be Medicare eligible

   3. Electing the hospice Medicare benefit requires that the patient give informed consent. If the patient lacks decision-making capacity, a surrogate decision-maker must give the informed consent

      a) Essential elements of an informed consent for hospice admission; patient/surrogate must be informed of

         i. Palliative nature of services and definition of the services

         ii. Service settings, home care, acute inpatient care, respite, residential settings

         iii. Bereavement services

         iv. Services covered and not covered

         v. Financial responsibility

         vi. Withdrawal or discharge criteria

      b) If the patient has capacity to make healthcare decisions, he/she must sign the consent form

      c) In any situation where the patient does not sign the consent and/or benefit election form, the reason must be clearly documented

   4. Terminally ill with less than 6 month prognosis (if the disease runs its usual course)

   5. Prognosis certified by primary physician and hospice medical director for first benefit period; by hospice medical director for subsequent benefit periods

   6. The scope of service is defined as palliative treatment related to the terminal illness

   7. Benefit periods

      a) There are two 90 day benefit periods and unlimited 60 day periods, as long as the patient remains appropriate for hospice care[23]

b) Patients may sign off of or **revoke** the Medicare hospice benefit and resume traditional Medicare coverage for the terminal illness. Any remaining days in that benefit period are forfeited

8. **Important note:** the Medicare hospice regulations *apply to the care of all patients* in a Medicare certified hospice

   a) Except for the 80/20 rule (see below) and requirement that the hospice continue to provide services regardless of ability to pay or bill a third party payer

   b) **Therefore, Medicare defines the delivery of hospice care in the U.S.**

9. "Core services" is a term used by Medicare to designate those team members that must be provided by the agency and not arranged for by contract (nurses, medical social services and counseling); this in no way negates the requirement for a more comprehensive team; other team members may be employees of the agency or their services may be arranged by contract

10. Must also provide therapy services (PT, OT, speech-language pathology), physician, volunteer, home health aide and homemaker services, medical supplies and equipment; acute and respite inpatient care, medications related to terminal illness, bereavement services; can be provided under contract

11. Levels of care in Medicare hospice program

   a) Routine home care day: a day in which a hospice patient receives care at home and is not receiving continuous care

   b) Continuous home care day: a day in which a hospice patient receives care at home for brief periods of crisis necessary to maintain the patient at home

      i. Continuous care is furnished during brief periods of crisis and only as necessary to maintain the terminally ill patient at home

      ii. Care is provided for at least 8 hours a day in order to qualify for the continuous home care reimbursement rate (Medicare defines the "day" as one that starts and ends at midnight)

      iii. Care must consist of predominantly (more than 50%) skilled nursing care (RN or LP/VN)

   c) Inpatient respite care: a day in which a hospice patient receives care in an approved facility on a short-term basis for respite of family or other caregivers

      i. The hospice will not be reimbursed for respite care more than 5 days consecutively

      ii. Payment to the hospice program for the sixth and any subsequent day of respite care is made at the routine home care rate

   d) General inpatient care: a day in which a hospice patient receives care in an approved facility for pain control or symptom management when care is not feasible in other settings (home or continuous care)

      i. Inpatient caps

         (a) Medicare has established a limit to the number of total patient care days that will be reimbursed at either the general inpatient or inpatient respite care rates

(b) The total inpatient days for Medicare patients may not exceed 20% of the total days for all those patients who elect the Medicare hospice benefit in any Medicare fiscal year (this is sometimes described as the 80/20 rule)

e) Change in level of care within the Medicare Hospice benefit

    i. Transfer to another level of care is based on the medical needs of the patient (e.g., uncontrolled pain)

    ii. Change in level of care requires a discussion with the patient and family and the IDT, changes in the plan of care, the primary physician's order, documentation in the patient's record

12. Volunteer Services

a) Volunteer service hours must account for 5% of all direct patient care hours for all paid hospice employees and contract staff in a Medicare certified hospice program

b) The volunteer hours may be accumulated as direct patient care hours or indirect, administrative support hours

13. Issues associated with the *discontinuation* of hospice care (other than by death of the patient and the completion of the bereavement period for the family)

a) Patient/family initiated actions

    i. Transfer: hospice care is transferred when a patient moves out of the service area of one hospice and into another hospice's service area or chooses a different provider in the area: patient remains in the current benefit period and loses no days in that period

        (a) Role of the hospice in facilitating patient transfer to a different care setting is to

            (i) Coordinate with the other hospice/palliative care service in order to provide continuity of care

            (ii) Notify the physician of the change in service area and/or service provider

        (b) Hospice Medicare/Medicaid benefit patients may transfer only once per benefit period

    ii. Withdrawal: any patient/family can choose to discontinue all services of the hospice for any reason

        (a) Role of the hospice in facilitating patient/family withdrawal from service

            (i) Notify primary physician of change and initiate any paperwork necessary for the change

            (ii) Coordinate any referrals for provision of on-going medical care

        (b) The choice to withdraw from hospice care requires the patient/legal representative to **revoke** the hospice benefit

    iii. Revocation of the Medicare Hospice Benefit is an option that may be chosen by the patient/family in order to receive treatment not covered under the hospice plan of care, to receive care from a different service provider, e.g., skilled nursing facility, non-contracted hospital or because of dissatisfaction with the service being provided

(a) Revocation: may occur any time during a benefit period; a patient may choose to revoke his/her Medicare hospice (note: the hospice program may not instruct the patient and family to revoke)

(b) Notify the physician of the change from hospice

(c) Have patient sign the Revocation statement/form on the date he/she revoked

(d) Be sure to indicate the date and time the form was signed

b) Hospice program initiated actions

    i. Discharge: a patient who no longer meets the Medicare criteria may be discharged; otherwise, this action is only used in extraordinary circumstances

       (a) Example: a patient may be discharged if continuing to provide care poses a serious threat to the safety of staff

       (b) A patient MAY NOT be discharged because of inability to pay for services, if the management of the illness and palliative treatment is too expensive for the hospice, if the primary physician orders expensive, "high tech" palliative care or if they are "difficult" to care for

    ii. Non-recertification: also referred to as "decertification." At the end of a benefit period, the Hospice Interdisciplinary Team, with the patient's primary physician, determines the patient no longer has a prognosis of 6 months or less (if the disease runs its normal course); a change in the status of the patient's terminal condition is the ONLY consideration justifying non-recertification

c) Role of the hospice program in discontinuation of care; the hospice program is responsible to

    i. Notify the patient and family of the reasons for discontinuation of services

    ii. Inform the patient and family that the hospice benefit is still available to them if the need arises later

    iii. Provide for continuity of care when transferring patient and family care to another agency

14. Actual and potential problems inherent in the Medicare Hospice Benefit

a) Medicare Hospice Benefit criteria may cause delayed hospice referrals, limiting access to care

b) However, trend, since 2001, is increased length of stay; average length of stay is 55 days, up from 48 days in 2001; mean length of stay is now 22 days, up from 20.5 days in 2001[19]

c) With short length of stays, however

    i. Crisis care mode with emphasis on just getting pain and symptoms under control

    ii. Rarely time for hospice team to form therapeutic relationships with families

    iii. Effective palliative care efforts so close to death may increase costs and negatively impact on quality of care

d) Expenses for patients who desire costly life-prolonging treatment may negatively impact hospice's bottom line

e) Current hospice *per diem* reimbursement has the potential to result in negative outcomes

   i. Could discourage the use of effective, but more costly pain medications even when less expensive drugs fail[24,25]

   ii. Might discourage nursing visits (especially after hours) to help families in crisis

   iii. Might discourage the appropriate application of high-tech equipment

   iv. Might discourage extensive counseling that may be useful for particularly distressed patients

f) Increased family costs—data has begun to indicate that families are shouldering not only the physical burden of care, but an increasingly larger portion of the financial burden[1]

g) Requirement for primary caregiver may deny access to hospice or cause financial hardship

   i. 75% of single-parent households headed by women who work[26]

   ii. To access benefit[27] a caregiver may have to

      (a) Take leave of absence

      (b) Use family medical leave (12 weeks without pay)

      (c) Quit job

h) Residents and families of residents in skilled nursing facilities who are appropriate both for the Medicare hospice benefit and for Medicare skilled care days may be negatively impacted

   i. Because it is to the economic advantage of the skilled nursing facility to have the resident on Medicare skilled care days, facility staff may not fully inform resident and family of their right to receive hospice care

   ii. A resident and family who chose hospice care instead of Medicare skilled days must bear the economic burden of paying room and board for the resident because Medicare does not provide that as part of the hospice benefit; this often creates a forced choice by families between Medicare skilled care in the nursing home (which does pay for room and board) and Medicare Hospice, (which does not pay for room and board)

D. Medicaid reimbursement under the Medicaid Hospice Benefit

1. In most states with a Medicaid hospice benefit the hospice benefit and reimbursement for care is modeled after the Medicare Hospice Benefit

2. The hospice nurse is responsible for knowing any differences between the Medicare hospice benefit and the Medicaid benefit as it is established in the geographical area served by the hospice

3. This is especially important to keep in mind if the hospice serves more than one state

    4.   Actual and potential problems inherent in the Medicaid Hospice Benefit

        a)   Hospice is an optional benefit under the Medicaid program

        b)   Not all states choose to provide it

E.   Reimbursement for palliative care under Medicare

    1.   No formal reimbursement system for palliative care therapies exist[28]

    2.   Palliative Care DRG[29]

        a)   DRG codes are used by Health Care Financing Administration to define how Medicare funds are reimbursed

        b)   *Reimbursement for palliative care is limited*

        c)   *In 1996 an ICD-9-CM "v66.7" code for palliative care was developed; does not actually bring reimbursement, but allows data to be collected about the provision of palliative care services to determine if new code is needed to pay hospitals to determine if it is feasible to reimburse for palliative care*

    3.   Demonstration projects and innovative programs developed to integrate palliative care approaches and to improve quality of end-of-life care

        a)   Robert Wood Johnson Initiative on Improving Care at the End of Life

        b)   Project Safe Conduct

        c)   City of Hope Pain Resource Center

        d)   The Institute for Healthcare Improvement Collaborative

        e)   United Hospital Fund's Hospital Palliative Care Initiative

F.   Reimbursement for hospice and palliative care under private insurance benefit plans

    1.   Hospice reimbursement under private insurance benefit plans

        a)   About 80% of private insurance plans have a hospice benefit; most others will negotiate a rate for hospice; some use a home health benefit

            i.   Many hospices refuse to "unbundle" hospice services even when insurance companies only pay for some aspects of the program

            ii.   If a program is Medicare certified, all patients must receive all the services available to a Medicare beneficiary whether or not the insurance company pays

        b)   Types of plans

            i.   Per Diem—reimbursement to the hospice is similar to Medicare/Medicaid in that it is on a daily basis and includes all services

            ii.   Per visit—insurance company authorizes the number of visits and the disciplines visiting

                (a)   Services not involving visits such as bereavement and participation in interdisciplinary team meetings are not reimbursed

                (b)   The insurance company may not authorize other services such as spiritual counseling

                (c)   Many hospices will not accept per visit reimbursement

   iii. Dollar caps—the patient has a benefit with a limited amount of money; for example, $5,000 lifetime maximum per patient for hospice

     (a) The hospice may be at financial risk if the cost of care exceeds the cap

     (b) Many hospices continue the care when the cap is exceeded and provide services without compensation

   iv. Negotiated rates—rate of reimbursement is individualized according to the plan of care and agreement reached between the hospice and the insurance provider

2. Palliative care reimbursement under private insurance benefit plans

  a) Palliative care services (non-hospice benefits) generally are reimbursable under various parts of the patient's medical insurance, e.g., hospital medical services, physician medical services, etc. (part of the specialty consult process)

   i. Determined by the IDT to be necessary

   ii. Follow agency/provider guidelines and reimbursement requirements for obtaining medications, medical equipment and supplies

3. Actual and potential problems inherent in the provision of care under private insurance

  a) Availability and type of insurance affect the use and provision of healthcare[30–33]

  b) Managed healthcare plans have limited scopes and levels of benefits

   i. Use can ease the financial burden of illness and encourage people to obtain beneficial care[34]

   ii. Utilization increases costs, so insurance companies use a variety of means to discourage use of their resources

  c) Uninsured patients

   i. Cannot be turned away if they have acute or life-threatening problems[18]

   ii. Care paid for by special public or charitable funds, application for public insurance

  d) Penalizes those with advanced disease[34]

  e) Bias risk selection—purpose is to attract healthy participants, not sick ones

   i. Exclude pre-existing conditions

   ii. The sicker one is, the more one has to pay out of pocket for care

   iii. Additional caps

     (a) Outpatient prescription medications excluded

     (b) Deductibles, coinsurance payments

     (c) Caps on visits or days of care, dollar amounts of payments, defined time periods

     (d) No upper limits on beneficiary liability for cost-sharing

  f) Financial incentives for clinicians to provide less care[34]

   i. Fixed payments per day, per case, per capita

   ii. Plans may vary in capitation of services

iii.   Pre-authorization requirements

    (a)   Require approval prior to obtaining service

    (b)   "Gatekeepers" to approve specialist visits

iv.   Protocols developed by the insurance companies require

    (a)   Specific services to be given for certain diseases

    (b)   Specific medications from designated formularies

v.   Productivity standards for physician appointments

    (a)   Visits may be limited by plan expectations

    (b)   Impact may be less time spent with patients

vi.   Health plan "panel" limitations

    (a)   Patient may use only designated physicians

    (b)   Out-of-plan costs are greater

    (c)   Limitations on specialized services such as pain management specialists

    (d)   Both access and length of time to appointment can be affected

    (e)   Frequent denials from insurance companies due to lack of knowledge about palliative care and/or equating it with hospice care

IV.   Relevant Economic Issues in End-of-Life Care

A.   In the hospital setting

1.   DRG prospective payment system[34]

    a)   Assumes that hospitals get a mix of patients so costs can be averaged out over all patients

    b)   Hospital stays are paid on a prospectively determined, diagnosis-related basis

    c)   If hospitals can discharge patients ahead of time, they get to keep any money they've made

    d)   Outlier patients are high cost patients; hospital costs for these patients must reach certain designated levels before the hospital is reimbursed

2.   Actual or potential effect of the prospective payment system on end-of-life care in the hospital setting

    a)   Shorter hospital stays have not been offset by increased admissions

    b)   Shorter stays have put increased burden on the family

        i.   Drug costs

        ii.   Huge burden on those with dying family members

    c)   Early studies showed early discharge, but no negative impact on mortality[35-39]

    d)   Premature discharge from hospital may leave families without adequate support systems to manage care

        i.   Home care system not in place or inadequate

      ii.   Symptom management expertise may vary

      iii.   Hospice coverage for inpatient care is limited

   e)   Issues for palliative care in the hospital setting

      i.   How to identify homogeneous care resources (not tied to diagnosis) that can be reimbursed and monitored

      ii.   Not intended to discourage referral to hospice

      iii. No data yet released on the palliative care ICD-9 code

B.   Issues for physicians who care for the dying

1.   Importance of coding visits for "evaluation and management" vs. procedures and tests

2.   Different codes exist for brief, limited, extended and other classes

3.   Codes do not differentiate between classes of patients[40-41]

   a)   May discourage care of those with special needs

      i.   Hearing/sight/cognitively impaired

      ii.   Those requiring special symptom management

      iii. Those with needs for emotional support

   b)   Restrictive interpretation of codes may limit physician time spent with these patients[18]

4.   Nursing home visits not reimbursed at same level as hospital visits

C.   Issues in the skilled nursing facility where most funding comes from Medicaid

1.   7 of 10 residents receive some funding from Medicaid[42]

2.   12% of beneficiaries accounted for 33% of total expenditures, much accounted for by nursing home use[43]

3.   Not all states adjust payments based on nursing home case mix[44]

   a)   Discourages nursing homes from accepting sicker patients

   b)   Discourages nursing homes from providing adequate level of care

4.   Nursing home populations are more severely ill and impaired and more demanding of resources due to

   a)   Reduced hospital lengths of stay

   b)   More sophisticated technological care; nursing home staff are not usually able to provide such care; systems not in place

   c)   Increasing resident age and disability

5.   Recent data on Medicare hospice care in skilled nursing facilities in five states from 1992 to 1996[45] demonstrated

   a)   Hospice care is associated with less hospitalization for Medicare hospice patients

   b)   Diffusion of palliative care philosophy and practices to care of non-hospice residents resulted in lower rates of end-of-life hospitalizations as well

D. Provision of hospice services

1. Hospice benefit was originally adopted after years of increased Medicare spending;[18] it was designed to control costs

    a) Limit number of qualifying beneficiaries (6 month life expectancy)

    b) Encourage efficient and economical home care

    c) Four levels of per diem payment rates

    d) Overall cap on payments

    e) Discourage inpatient care with per diem payment for inpatient care and 20% cap on aggregate hospital payments

    f) Required use of volunteers limits Medicare liability for some care

2. Capitation of hospice is characterized by many as "high-risk"[18]

    a) Lack of data on incidence and variability of terminal illness

    b) Variability across populations

    c) Lack of effective tools to detect and deflect inappropriate early referrals to hospice

    d) Lack of other information needed to set rates and manage financial risk

3. Medicare HMO beneficiaries' election of hospice benefit

    a) Not limited only to HMO-selected hospice

    b) HMO's not required to provide hospice benefits themselves

    c) HMO's cannot deny access to HCFA-certified hospice

4. Hospice coverage for those not eligible for Medicare or Medicaid varies greatly—80% of large and medium-size companies offer hospice coverage[46]

E. Issues for Home Healthcare in providing palliative care services

1. Eligibility requirements

    a) Patient must be homebound

    b) Patient must need part-time or intermittent skilled nursing care or physical or speech therapy

2. Growth in home care expenditures[47]

    a) Changes in Medicare home care policies

    b) Growing supply of providers

    c) Earlier discharge from hospitals

    d) Increased feasibility of providing advanced technology in the home

3. Demonstration projects currently examining quality of care, efficiency and cost control due to past evidence of fraud and abuse[48]

4. Cost shifting in home care has been documented[49]

    a) Savings from averted hospital care may be offset by increased financial burden on family

b) Clauser reported that Medicare home care users were more likely to be disabled, living alone, poor and receiving Medicaid when compared to nonusers[18]

5. Medication coverage issues in palliative home care pose significant problems for patients and families[25,50]

a) Medicare home care benefit does not cover medications in most cases

b) Some supplemental policies cover outpatient prescriptions (programs vary)

c) Some cover prescriptions but limit refills, number of prescriptions covered in a month or quantity of medication

F. Economic value of the Advanced Practice Nurse (APN) in hospice and palliative care settings

1. APN definitions

a) Application of an expanded range of practical, theoretical and research-based therapeutics to phenomena experienced by patients within a specialized clinical area of the larger discipline of nursing

b) Advanced practice registered nurses manifest a high level of expertise in the assessment, diagnosis and treatment of the complex responses of individuals, families or communities to actual or potential health problems, prevention of illness and injury, maintenance of wellness and provision of comfort[51]

c) The advanced practice registered nurse has a master's or doctoral education concentrating in a specific area of advanced nursing practice, had supervised practice during graduate education and has ongoing clinical experiences[51]

d) Advanced practice registered nurses continue to perform many of the same interventions used in basic nursing practice; the difference in this practice relates to a greater depth and breadth of knowledge, a greater degree of synthesis of data and complexity of skills and interventions[51]

2. Practice Models

a) Should provide clarity and direction to the field

b) Purposes served are determined by the concepts delineated in the framework, i.e., practice competencies

c) Competency is core concept in several APN practice models

i. Model of Expert Practice[52,53]

ii. Expert Practice Domains of the CNS and NP[54,55]

iii. Model of Advanced Nursing Practice[56]

iv. Model of Nurse Practitioner Practice[57]

3. Factors indicating a need for advanced practice nurses who specialize in end-of-life care

a) Our evolving healthcare system places more emphasis on integration of care across different settings and over a continuum of life

b) Studies increasingly are demonstrating the APN role can improve quality of life in a cost-effective way[58–69]

4. As a member of the interdisciplinary palliative care team, the Advanced Practice Nurse assumes many roles as he/she interfaces with families, staff, colleagues and communities[61]

    a) Advanced clinician

    b) Educator

    c) Researcher

    d) Consultant

    e) Role Model

    f) Mentor

5. Advanced practice nurses who specialize in end-of-life care should be

    a) Resourceful and flexible in interactions with dying patients and families

    b) Accepting of a broadened definition of palliative care that includes earlier service to a population with life-threatening illness

    c) Comfortable with technologies that employ both drug and non-drug technologies for pain and symptom control

    d) Advocates for patient and family self-determination

    e) Able to accommodate and advocate for family needs while negotiating with multiple healthcare professionals in a variety of settings

CITED REFERENCES

1. Coyne P, Lyckholm L, Smith TJ. Clinical interventions, economic outcomes and palliative care. In: Ferrell BR, Coyle N, eds. *Textbook of Palliative Nursing*. New York, NY: Oxford University Press; 2001:317–327.

2. American Society of Clinical Oncology Outcomes Working Group (ASCO), c.m., Outcomes of cancer treatment for technology assessment and cancer treatment guidelines. *Journal of Clinical Oncology*. 1995;14:671–679.

3. Souquet PJ, Chauvin F, Boissel JP, Cellerino R, Cormier Y, Ganz PA, Kaasa S, Pater JL, Quoix E, Rapp E, et al. Polychemotherapy in advanced non-small cell lung cancer: a meta-analysis. *Lancet*. 1993;342:19–21.

4. Jaakkimainen L, Goodwin PJ, Pater J, Warde P, Murray N, Rapp E. Counting the costs of chemotherapy in a National Cancer Institute of Canada randomized trial in non-small cell lung cancer. *Journal of Clinical Oncology*. 1990;8(8):1301–1309.

5. Le Chevalier T, Brisgand D, Douillard JY, Pujol JL, Alberola V, Monnier A, Riviere A, Lianes P, Chomy P, Cigolari S, et al. Randomized study of vinorelbine and cisplatin versus vindesine and cisplatin versus vinorelbine alone in advanced non-small cell lung cancer: results of a European multicenter trial including 612 patients. *Journal of Clinical Oncology*. 1994;12(2):360–367.

6. Smith TJ, Hillner BE, Neighbors DM, McSorley PA, Le Chevalier T. An economic evaluation of a randomized clinical trial comparing vinorelbine, vinorelbine plus cisplatin and vindesine plus cisplatin for non-small cell lung cancer. *Journal of Clinical Oncology*. 1995;13(9):2166–2173.

7. Ferris FD, Wodinsky HB, Kerr IG, Sone M, Hume S, Coons C. A cost-minimization study of cancer patients requiring a narcotic infusion in hospice and at home. *Journal of Clinical Epidemiology*. 1991;44(3):313–327.

8. Wodinsky HB, DeAngelis C, Rusthoven JJ, Kerr IG, Sutherland D, Iscoe N, Buckman R, Kornijenko M. Re-evaluating the cost of outpatient cancer chemotherapy. *Canadian Medical Association Journal*. 1987;137(10):903–906.

9. Lowenthal RM, Piaszczyk A, Arthur GE, O'Malley S. Home chemotherapy for cancer patients: cost analysis and safety. *Medical Journal of Australia*. 1996;165(4):184–187.

10. Addington-Hall J.M, MacDonald LD, Anderson HR. Randomized controlled trial of effects of coordinating care for terminally ill patients. *British Medical Journal*. 1992;305:1317–1322.

11. Raftery JP, Addington-Hall JM, MacDonald LD, Anderson HR, Bland JM, Chamberlain J, Freeling P. A randomized controlled trial of the cost-effectiveness of a district co-coordinating service for terminally ill cancer patients. *Palliative Medicine*. 1996;10:151–161.

12. Grant M, Ferrell BR, Rivera LM, Lee J. Unscheduled readmissions for uncontrolled symptoms: a health care challenge for nurses. *Nursing Clinics of North America*. 1995;30:673–682.

13. SUPPORT, S.P.I., A controlled trial to improve care for seriously ill hospitalized patients: A study to understand prognoses and preferences for outcomes and risks of treatments (SUPPORT). *Journal of the American Medical Association*, 1995. 274: p. 1591–1598.

14. Weeks WB, Kofoed LL, Wallace AE, Welch HG. Advance directives and the cost of terminal hospitalization. *Archives of Internal Medicine*. 1994;154(18):2077–2083.

15. Emanuel EJ, Emanuel L. The economics of dying: the illusion of cost savings at the end of life. *New England Journal of Medicine*. 1994;330(8):540–544.

16. Holloran SD, Starkey GW, Burke PA, Steele G Jr, Forse RA. An educational intervention in the surgical intensive care unit to improve ethical decisions. *Surgery.* 1995;118(2):294–298.

17. Dowdy MD, Robertson C, Bander JA. A study of proactive ethics consultation for critically and terminally ill patients with extended lengths of stay. *Critical Care Medicine.* 1998;26(2):252–259.

18. Field MJ, Cassel CK. *Approaching Death: Improving Care at the End of Life.* Washington, DC: Institute of Medicine Task Force; 1997.

19. National Hospice and Palliative Care Organization, NHPCO *Facts and figures (Updated February 2004),* National Hospice and Palliative Care Organization; 2004.

20. Gornick M, McMillan A, Lubitz JA. A longitudinal perspective on patterns of Medicare payments. *Health Affairs.* 1996;12(2):140–150.

21. U.S. Department of Health and Human Services. *2003 CMS Statistics.* Available at: http://www.cms.hhs.gov/researchers/pubs/03cmsstats.pdf. Accessed on April 27, 2005.

22. Health Care Financing Administration (HCFA). *Transmittal #256: Medicare state operations manual.* Baltimore, MD: HCFA; 1994:Sections 2080–2087.

23. *Balanced Budget Act.* In: *Congressional Record.* 1997.

24. Brown G. *Statement before the IOM committee on care at the end of life on behalf of hospice of the Blue Grass.* In: *IOM Committee on Care at the End of Life.* Washington, DC; 1996.

25. Joranson DE. Are health-care reimbursement policies a barrier to acute and cancer pain management? *Journal of Pain and Symptom Management.* 1994;9(4):244–253.

26. Emanuel EJ, Fairclough DL, Slutsman J, Alpert H, Baldwin D, Emanuel LL. Assistance from family members, friends, paid care givers and volunteers in the care of terminally ill patients. *New England Journal of Medicine.* 1999;341(13):956–63.

27. Covinsky KE, Goldman L, Cook EF, Oye R, Desbiens N, Reding D, Fulkerson W, Connors AF Jr, Lynn J, Phillips RS. The impact of serious illness on patients' families. SUPPORT Investigators. Study to understand prognoses and preferences for outcomes and risks of treatment. *Journal of the American Medical Association.* 1994;272:1839–1844.

28. Whedon MB. Hospital care. In: Ferrell BR, Coyle N, eds. *Textbook of Palliative Nursing.* New York, NY: Oxford University Press; 2001:584–608.

29. Cassel C. *Letter to Colleagues about New Medicare Palliative Care Code.* New York, NY: Milbank Memorial Fund: 1996.

30. Hadley J, Steinberg EP, Feder J. Comparison of uninsured and privately insured hospital patients: Condition on admission, resource use and outcome. *Journal of the American Medical Association.* 1991;265(3):274–279.

31. Manning WG, Newhouse JP, Duan N, Keeler EB, Leibowitz A, Marquis MS. Health insurance and the demand for medical care: Evidence from a randomized experiment. *American Economic Review.* 1987;77(3):251–277.

32. Braveman P, Oliva G, Miller MG, Reiter R, Egerter S. Adverse outcomes and lack of health insurance among newborns in an eight-county area of California. *New England Journal of Medicine.* 1998;321:508–513.

33. Newhouse JP, Group IE. *Free for all? Lessons from the Rand Health Insurance Experiment.* Cambridge, MA: Harvard University Press; 1993.

34. Millman M. *Access to Health Care in America*. Washington, DC: Institute of Medicine—National Academy Press; 1993.

35. ProPAC, P.P.A.C., *Medicare and the American Health Care System: Report to the Congress*. Washington, DC: ProPac; 1985.

36. ProPAC, P.P.A.C. *Medicare and the American Health Care System: Report to the Congress*. Washington, DC: ProPac; 1989.

37. Kahn KL, Keeler EB, Sherwood MJ, Rogers WH, Draper D, Bentow SS, Reinisch EJ, Rubenstein LV, Kosecoff J, Brook RH. Comparing outcomes of care before and after implementation of the DRG-based prospective payment system. *Journal of the American Medical Association*. 1990; 264(15):1984–1988.

38. Kosecoff J, Kahn KL, Rogers WH, Reinisch EJ, Sherwood MJ, Rubenstein LV, Draper D, Roth CP, Chew C, Brook RH. Prospective payment system and impairment at discharge. The 'quicker-and-sicker' story revisited. *Journal of the American Medical Association*. 1990;264(15):1980–1983.

39. Rubenstein LV, Kahn KL, Reinisch EJ, Sherwood MJ, Rogers WH, Kamberg C, Draper D, Brook RH. Changes in quality of care for five diseases measured by implicit review, 1981–1986. *Journal of the American Medical Association*. 1990;264(15):1974–1979.

40. PPRC, P.P.R.C., *Annual Report to Congress*. Washington, DC: PPRC; 1991.

41. PPRC, P.P.R.C., *Annual Report to Congress*. Washington, DC: PPRC; 1992.

42. American Health Care Association. *Facts and Trends: The Nursing Facility sourcebook*. Washington, DC; American Health Care Association, (AHCA); 1995.

43. PPRC, P.P.R.C., *Annual Report to Congress*. Washington, DC: PPRC; 1993.

44. Swan JH, Dewit S, Harrington C. *State Medicaid Reimbursement Methods and Rates for Nursing Homes, 1993*. Wichita, KS: Wichita State University; 1994.

45. Miller SC, Gozalo P, Mor V. Hospice enrollment and hospitalization of dying nursing home patients. *American Journal of Medicine*. 2001;111(1):38–44.

46. Snow C. New hospice horizons: HMO expansion could boost provider's popularity. *Modern Healthcare*. 1997;27(9):90, 92.

47. Health Care Financing Administration (HCFA). Trends in Medicare home health agency utilization and payment: Cys 1974–94. *Health Care Financing Review*. 1996;Statistical Suppl:76–77.

48. Clauser SB. Recent innovations in home health care policy research. *Health Care Financing Review*. 1994;16(1):1–6.

49. Weissert WG. A new policy agenda for home care. *Health Affairs*. 1991;10(2):67–77.

50. Soumerai SB, Ross-Degnan D, Avorn J, McLaughlin T, Choodnovskiy I. Effects of Medicaid drug-payment limits on admission to hospitals and nursing homes. *New England Journal of Medicine*. 1991;325(15):1072–1077.

51. American Nurses Association. *Scope and Standards of Advanced Practice Registered Nursing*. Washington, DC: American Nurses Association; 1996.

52. Benner P. *From Novice to Expert*. Menlo Park, CA: Addison-Wesley; 1984.

53. Benner P. The oncology clinical nurse specialist as expert coach. *Oncology Nursing Forum*. 1985;12(2):40–44.

54. Fenton MV. Identifying competencies of clinical nurse specialists. *Journal of Nursing Administration.* 1985;15(12):31–37.

55. Fenton MV, Brykczynski KA. Qualitative distinctions and similarities in the practice of clinical nurse specialists and nurse practitioners. *Journal of Professional Nursing.* 1993;9:313–326.

56. Calkin JD. A model for advanced nursing practice. *Journal of Nursing Administration.* 1984;14(1):24–30.

57. Shuler PA, Davis JE. The Shuler nurse practitioner practice model: a theoretical framework for nurse practitioner clinicians, educators and researchers. Part I. *Journal of the American Academy of Nurse Practitioners.* 1993;5:11–18.

58. Rich MW, Beckham V, Wittenberg C, Leven CL, Freedland KE, Carney RM. A multidisciplinary intervention to prevent the readmission of elderly patients with congestive heart failure. *The New England Journal of Medicine.* 1995;333(18):1190–1195.

59. Stuck AE, Aronow HU, Steiner A, Alessi CA, Bula CJ, Gold MN, Yuhas KE, Nisenbaum R, Rubenstein LZ, Beck JC. A trial of annual in-home comprehensive geriatric assessments for elderly people living in the community. *The New England Journal of Medicine.* 1995;333(18):1184–1189.

60. Naylor MD, Brooten D, Campbell R, Jacobsen BS, Mezey MD, Pauly MV, Schwartz JS. Comprehensive discharge planning and home follow-up of hospitalized elders. A randomized clinical trial. *Journal of the American Medical Association.* 1999;281:613–620.

61. Krammer LM, Ring AA, Martinez J, Jacobs MJ, Williams MB. The nurses' role in interdisciplinary and palliative care. In: Matzo ML, Sherman DW, eds. *Palliative Care Nursing: Quality Care to the End of Life.* New York, NY; Springer Publishing Co; 2001.

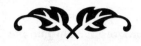

CHAPTER XI

TRENDS FOR THE FUTURE

Betty Rolling Ferrell, PhD, RN, FAAN

First Edition Authors
Patricia Murphy, RN, MA
Betty Rolling Ferrell, PhD, RN, FAAN

I. **Issues Affecting Healthcare Delivery in the Next 20 Years**

A. **Labor shortages, especially shortages of nursing personnel**

1. By the year 2005 there will be a shortage of 400,000 Registered Nurses in the United States

B. **Increase in chronic disease population**

1. It is anticipated that by 2020 there will be 14 million individuals with Alzheimer's disease as opposed to 4 million in 2001

2. Other chronic diseases, including heart and lung disease have a similar demographic profile

C. **Increase in population of those over the age of 65**

1. The death rate of all humans is 100% although the overall life expectancy is increasing

2. The median age nationally is 35.3 years, up from 28 years in 1990

3. Average life expectancy is 74 years for males and 79 years for females

4. 40 million baby boomers will begin to reach the age of 65 in 2009

D. **Healthcare cost containment**

1. In 2000, healthcare costs were 18% of the gross national product having risen nearly 1% per year over the past decade

2. One out of eight Medicare dollars is spent on patients in the last three weeks of life

E. **New family structures/elder caregiver issues will continue to evolve as the population ages**

1. The number of traditional nuclear families has decreased by 3.7% from 1990 to the year 2000

2. 70% of children live in a household where a single parent or both parents are employed outside of the home

3. The number of individuals living alone is 20.6%, one-third of whom are over the age of 65

4. Nearly 26 million Americans spend an average of 18 hours a week caring for frail relatives or friends suffering from progressive chronic medical conditions

5. 73% of family caregivers are women

F. Consumer awareness of health and wellness

1. Consumer advocacy groups have formed in response to managed care cost containment strategies, pain management and other health issues

2. The media continues to produce more public information related to health and healthcare

3. 60% of web users access healthcare information on the Internet

G. Medicare Trust at risk

1. Government predictions are that bankruptcy of the Medicare Trust may occur by 2020

H. Multi-Culturalism

1. The nation is becoming more culturally diverse

2. There was an 11% rise in the Latino population and 6% rise in Asian population in the years from 1990 to 2000

I. Increasingly sophisticated technology

1. The utilization of the laser, computerized axial tomography, nuclear magnetic resonance devices, micro-surgery and gene therapy are revolutionizing medicine

2. Telemedicine applications such as interactive video are in use currently with more products being created

J. Bio-technology/the Genome project

1. The human genome project is slated to complete its work in 2005 leading to major change in the modification of disease

K. Broadened use of advance directives and advance care planning

1. Advance care planning can facilitate greater access to palliative care and hospice

II. Goals for Reform of End-of-Life Care in 10 Years

A. The development of a cost effective care management model from diagnosis of chronic illness onward that would combine disease modifying therapies, palliative care and hospice

B. Consumer education and public engagement about choices in treatment services and advanced healthcare directives

C. Education of physicians and other professionals about clinical, psychological, social, spiritual, cultural, economic and ethical aspects of palliative care and hospice

D. Funding for demonstration projects of new models for end-of-life care

E. Medicare funding for palliative care and long-term care and continued and enhanced funding of hospice care

F. Applying telemedicine technology to the care process

G. Bereavement services for survivors

III. Actualizing a New Model for Reform of End-of-Life Care

A. Change will occur as a result of an effective interface of public policy, legislation, the development of standards of care, research and adequate reimbursement

B. Hospice and palliative care leaders will lead the development of new end-of-life care models and will advocate for demonstration projects, standards and funding

C. The Federal government will create demonstration projects that will study hospice and palliative care, case management models, long-term care models and reimbursement methodologies

IV. Legislation as a Component of Reform

A. Major Statements Will Guide Reform of End-of-Life Care

1. The SUPPORT Study[1]

a) Funded by the Robert Wood Johnson Foundation the study focused on decision making and medical practice at the end of life

b) A major study involving over 9,000 patients in acute care settings with the goal of evaluating end-of-life care

c) Findings revealed serious deficiencies in care, use of advance directives and relief of pain

2. Institute of Medicine Report—(1997)

a) In 1993, the Institute of Medicare embarked on a survey of end-of-life care nationwide which culminated in a report that identified steps that can be taken to improve care at the end of life

b) A consensus document addressing the needs for the nation to improve end-of-life care

3. National Comprehensive Cancer Network (NCCN at http://www.nccn.org/patients/patient_gls/_english/_palliative/index.htm) Guidelines for Palliative Care, 2003: leading cancer centers addressing end-of-life care

4. Institute of Medicine (IOM)/National Cancer Policy Board (NCPB) Report for End-of-life Care/Cancer Centers (2001): a consensus document on improving care in cancer centers

5. Institute of Medicine (IOM) Pediatric Report, (2001): builds on the earlier IOM report to address pediatric needs

6. National Hospice Work Group (NHWG): Access and Values Project[2]

   a) The NHWG is a group of hospice leaders who convened a series of meetings with influential decision makers to discuss expansion of the hospice model of care into the delivery of palliative care.

   b) A consensus project to evaluate the current access and services of hospice and need for reform.

B. Barriers to Hospice Care Will Be Lessened

1. The six-month prognostic requirement will be changed increasing access to hospice for chronically ill individuals nearing life's end

2. The Hospice clinical and leadership model will be fully integrated across the continuum of care into hospitals, nursing homes, daycare and home healthcare

3. Additional reimbursement will enable hospice to develop palliative care programs for the chronically ill

V. Reimbursement as a Component of Reform

A. The security of the Medicare Trust will be a central goal

B. Reimbursement methodology for palliative care and hospice care will reflect innovative care delivery such as case management and telehealth

C. Managed care entities will be held to distinct standards for end-of-life care case management and payment

D. Medical groups and third party payer organizations will utilize the most cost effective and ethical end-of-life care models

VI. Standards of Care as a Component of Reform

A. The healthcare industry will apply uniform standards for end-of-life care across the continuum of care

B. A tiered system of centers of excellence in end-of-life care offering hospice and palliative care will be developed

C. Standards and certification for all disciplines involved in end-of-life care will be developed and promulgated

D.   Quality end-of-life care will be measured against clinical performance indicators developed by hospice and palliative care professionals

E.   Bench marking of individual programs and models that offer end-of-life care will occur

F.   Education of healthcare professionals about quality end-of-life care, including pain management, symptom control, client-family focus, psychosocial spiritual issues, self-diversity and communication will occur as part of a program and discipline specific certification initiative nation-wide

VII. Research as a Component of Reform

A.   Research will be identified as a critical component in the development of new models

B.   Critical areas of research are

1.   Pain management

2.   Symptom management

3.   Communication

4.   Roles and needs of the primary family caregiver

5.   Professional education approaches

6.   Health policy studies

7.   Cost analysis

8.   Bereavement

9.   Effectiveness of varied models of care

10. Psychosocial and spiritual end-of-life care

11. Quality of life closure

VIII. Key Partnerships as Component of Reform

A.   Provider organizations

B.   Public interest groups

C.   The federal and state governments

D.   The business community

E.   Private foundations

F.   Related human service organizations

G.   Healthcare professionals

H.   Elder care associations and advocacy groups

I.   The disabled

J.   Multi-cultural advocacy groups

K.   Consumer advocacy

IX.   Future Professional Roles in Hospice/Palliative Care

A.   Role of Hospice/Palliative Care Certified Nurse

1.   Skilled assessment, intervention, care coordination, case management and program leadership

2.   Management with the goal of providing care and services to patients with advanced illness along the continuum of care in a variety of settings

3.   Supportive care to survivors

4.   Education of consumer and professional community

5.   Support of research and public policy

B.   Roles for Advanced Practice Nurses (Clinical Nurse Specialist and Nurse Practitioner)

1.   Primary care model

2.   Utilization of advanced practice skills focused on care and referral to meet comprehensive needs of patients with advanced medical illness

3.   Advanced Practice Nurse competencies—there are six core competencies essential to advanced practice nursing

a)   Expert guidance and coaching of patients, families and other care providers

b)   Consultation

c)   Skills including research utilization, conduct and evaluation

d)   Clinical and professional leadership; competence as a change agent

e)   Collaboration

f)   Ethical decision-making skills

C.   Roles for Nurse Researchers Prepared at the Doctoral Level

1.   Identification of areas for research in advanced disease

2.   Design and implementation of human subject research based on sound clinical practice and ethical principles

3.   Design and implementation of organizational and public policy research to improve systems

D. Role of Unlicensed Personnel

1. NBCHPN® certification for nursing assistants

2. Provides physical care that assists activities of daily living and promotes quality of life

3. Provides emotional support and respite for primary caregivers

4. Assists with nutrition

5. Reports status changes to the RN, NP or CNS

X. Model Programs

A. Models that extend/integrate hospice and palliative care into active treatment

1. Project Safe Conduct, a demonstration project, features collaboration between a community-based hospice (Hospice of the Western Reserve) and an NCI cancer center (Ireland Cancer Center of Case Western Reserve University/University Hospitals of Cleveland), which led to pioneering a groundbreaking model of palliative care, funded by the Robert Wood Johnson Foundation

   a) Project's premise entails vertically integrating the principles of palliative/end-of-life care into the acute care setting rather than creating a separate team

   b) Patients are not required to abandon life-prolonging care including experimental therapy protocols in order to receive palliative care

   c) If treatment fails, a seamless transition occurs from the acute care program to the hospice program. Primary oncologists remain involved through the entire course of the disease

2. Simultaneous Care (UC Davis, Fred Meyers PI)—a model of care to integrate palliative care with clinical trials for advanced cancer. Initial study completed at UC Davis with multisided study now in progress

3. Hospice of the Bluegrass—provides palliative care consultation in an inpatient and outpatient setting

B. Models integrating palliative care into home care and other settings

1. HOPE is a National Cancer Institute funded project (Betty Ferrell, PhD, PI) to incorporate palliative care into non-hospice home care settings

2. Hospice Palliative Care Center of the North Shore—is a hospital based palliative care unit operated by a certified hospice program

XI. Clinical Practice Guidelines for Quality Palliative Care

A. Developed by the National Consensus Project for Quality Palliative Care

B. HPNA is one of five palliative care organizations who developed these guidelines

C. **Domains of the guidelines include**

1. Domain 1: Structure and Processes of Care

2. Domain 2: Physical Aspects of Care

3. Domain 3: Psychological and Psychiatric Aspects of Care

4. Domain 4: Social Aspects of Care

5. Domain 5: Spiritual, Religious and Existential Aspects of Care

6. Domain 6: Cultural Aspects of Care

7. Domain 7: Care of the Imminently Dying Patient

8. Domain 8: Ethical and Legal Aspect of Care

D. **These guidelines can be used as a framework for clinical programs, education and research**

CITED REFERENCES

1. SUPPORT, A controlled trial to improve care for seriously ill hospitalized patients: a study to understand prognoses and preferences for outcomes and risks of treatments (SUPPORT). *Journal of the American Medical Association.* 1995;274:1591–1598.

2. Field MJ, Cassell CK, eds. *Approaching Death: Improving Care at the End of Life. Report of the Institute of Medicine Task Force.* Washington, DC: National Academy Press; 1997.

3. Foley KM, Gelband H, eds. *Improving Palliative Care for Cancer Summary and Recommendations.* Washington, DC: National Academy Press; 2001.

4. Field MJ, Behrman RE. *When Children Die: Improving Palliative and End-of-Life Care for Children and their Families.* Washington, DC: National Academy Press; 2003.

5. Ryndes T, et al. *Just Access and Human Values in Hospice and Palliative Care: Building an End-of-Life Care System for the 21st Century.* The Hastings Center and the National Hospice Work Group; 2001.

6. Hamric AB. A definition of advanced nursing practice. In: Hamric AB, Spross JA, Hanson CM, eds. *Advanced Nursing Practice.* 2nd ed. Philadelphia, PA: W. B. Saunders Company; 2000:53–73.

7. National Consensus Project for Quality Palliative Care. *Clinical Practice Guidelines for Quality Palliative Care.* Pittsburgh, PA: National Consensus Project for Quality Palliative Care; 2004. Available at www.nationalconsensusproject.org.

ADDITIONAL REFERENCES AND RESOURCES

Administration on Aging. *Older population by age: 1900 to 2050.* 2000 Can be accessed at http://www.aoa.dhhs.gov./aoa/stats/AgePop2050Chart-numbers.html.

American Association of Colleges of Nursing. *Peaceful death: Recommended Competencies and Curricular Guidelines for End-of-life Nursing Care.* Washington, DC: Report from the Robert Wood Johnson End-of-Life Care Roundtable; 1997.

Coyle N. Introduction to palliative nursing care. In: Ferrell BR, Coyle N, eds. *Textbook of Palliative Nursing.* New York, NY: Oxford University Press; 2001:3–6.

Egan KA, Labyak MJ. Hospice care: A model for quality end-of-life care. In: Ferrell BR, Coyle N, eds. *Textbook of Palliative Nursing.* New York, NY: Oxford University Press; 2001:7–26.

Ferrell B, Virani R, Grant M, Coyne P, Uman G. Beyond the Supreme Court decision: nursing perspectives on end-of-life care. *Oncology Nursing Forum.* 2000;27(3):445–455.

Ferrell B, Virani R, Grant M. Analysis of end-of-life content in nursing textbooks. Oncology *Nursing Forum.* 1999;26(5):869–876.

Heller BR, Oros MT, Durney-Crowley J. The future of nursing education: ten (10) trends to watch. *Nursing & Health Care Perspectives.* 2000;21(1):9–13.

Last Acts. *Means to a Better End: A Report on Dying in America.* 2002.

Last Acts Palliative Care Task Force. *Precepts of Palliative Care.* Princeton, NJ: Robert Wood Johnson Foundation; 1997. Available at http://www.lastacts.org.

National Hospice and Palliative Care Organization. *Medicare Benefit Reform Task Force Report.* Alexandria, VA: Author; 1999.

National Hospice and Palliative Care Organization (NHPCO). *Delivering Quality Care and Cost-Effectiveness at the End of Life: Building on the 20-year Success of the Medicare Hospice Benefit.* Alexandria, VA: Author; 2002. Available at: http://www.nhpco.org.

CHAPTER XII

ADVANCE CARE PLANNING: THE ROLE OF THE NURSE

Linda Briggs, MA, MSN, RN

I. **Introduction**

    A. **Respecting an individual's choices for future healthcare is required by federal and state legislation and is considered essential to respecting the integrity of the individual within ethical and professional arenas. These choices are only possible, however, if individuals are adequately informed of the wide range of healthcare options available and provided guidance on the decision-making process. To assist individuals in making decisions about their future healthcare, individuals can benefit extensively from skilled professionals who provide timely and appropriate information and facilitation. As one member of a team of professionals who may provide this guidance, nurses have unique opportunities to engage in effective Advance Care Planning (ACP) activities with patients and families. As patient advocate in the ACP process, nurses must embrace the roles and responsibilities inherent in assisting individuals to articulate preferences for care and make plans to attain the care desired**

II. **Goals of Advance Care Planning**

    A. **Ensure clinical care is consistent with patient preferences when capacity is lost, i.e., the patient receives all the care and only the care desired**

    B. **Improve the decision-making process by facilitating shared decision-making among those the patient wishes to involve in this process and the attending physician; preparing surrogate decision-makers to speak on behalf of patient and providing education that meets the needs of the patient**

    C. **Improve patient well being by reducing frequency of over or under treatment. Reduce patient concern regarding possible burden placed on family and others**

        1. These goals are unlikely to be accomplished by simply assisting an individual to complete an advance directive document and will often require facilitating an ACP discussion. The clear and important distinctions between "advance directive" and "advance care planning" must be understood to appreciate the roles and responsibilities of the nurse in achieving quality ACP outcomes

III. Clarifying Terminology: Advance Directives and Advance Care Planning

A. Advance Directive

1. A plan for healthcare for a time in the future when the patient may lack capacity to make healthcare decisions

2. This plan may be communicated orally (verbal expressions to loved ones, friends or healthcare providers; in formal written documents that meet statutory requirements (living will, power of attorney for healthcare) or informal documents (letter to physician, values history) that may not meet statutory requirements, but provide evidence of preferences

3. Written plans that meet statutory requirements are typically recommended (although openness to patient's preferred mode of communication must be supported). The two most common statutory written plans are

   a) Living Will: a document that provides a set of narrow guidelines for life-sustaining treatment under specific conditions, i.e., terminal illness or persistent vegetative state with no reasonable expectation for recovery

   b) Power of Attorney for Healthcare (POAHC): a document that allows a person to express preferences for future healthcare under a wide range of conditions as well as assign a surrogate decision-maker (healthcare agent, proxy) to assume all heathcare decisions in the event the patient looses decision-making capacity. A POAHC is the recommended written plan for most individuals who have a trusted individual to rely upon to make decisions if needed and to allow flexibility in decision-making

B. Advance Care Planning

1. A process of assisting individuals to

   a) *Understand* why ACP is important, how it relates to the individuals' current state of health or illness, the range of choices available and the associated risks and benefits of these choices

   b) *Reflect* upon personal beliefs, values, cultural or religious norms and goals

   c) *Discuss* these choices, beliefs, values and goals with others who might be helpful in the decision-making process and

   d) *Develop* a plan for communicating preferences, i.e., an advance directive

2. ACP is a dynamic process that is important to initiate for a young, healthy adult as a component of routine medical care. It is also important to keep this conversation alive and assist individuals to revisit and reexamine healthcare choices as illness occurs and becomes progressive over time

3. ACP requires the professional to translate important clinical knowledge required to assist an individual in making decisions for future medical care and to integrate critical communication skills of listening, exploring, clarifying and improving understanding

IV. The History of the Advance Directive Movement in the United States

A. The Karen Quinlan case in 1976 raised awareness of end-of-life decision-making and introduced the concept of ethics committee review of such cases

B.   California passed the first Natural Death Act in 1976 that allowed patients and surrogates to develop written directives to forgo life-sustaining treatment

C.   In 1977 in the Massachusetts Saikewicz case, rights to self determination were extended to individuals who never had the capacity for decision-making

D.   The President's Commission for the Study of Ethical Problems in Medicine and Biomedical and Behavioral Research in 1983 published a document that, among other critical issues, offered the notion of a durable power of attorney to act as substitute decision-maker for patients who lose decision-making capacity

E.   A variety of legal rulings in the 1980's applied the rights of individuals to forgo unwanted treatment to such routine interventions as CPR, medications and artificial nutrition and hydration

F.   In 1990 the United States Supreme Court ruled in the Nancy Cruzan case that the most a state can require in honoring patient preferences is clear and convincing evidence of what the patient would want, whether written or verbal. This decision led to the Patient Self-Determination Act of 1991 that required all health institutions receiving federal aid to inquire on admission if patients had a written advance directive, provide information about patient's right to self determination and provide education to staff and community

G.   Currently all 50 states have statutory documents recognized as legal tools for documenting patients' preferences. However these documents are not always honored across state lines. Few Americans have completed any type of written advance directive and there is little evidence that advance care planning discussions are occurring

V.   Advance Care Planning: The Nurses Role

A.   ACP is not a "one size fits all" intervention. The knowledge needed to participate in effective planning will vary with an individual's state of health, stage of chronic illness, coping mechanisms, among other variables. The nurses' role in ACP is multifaceted and includes the following competencies

   1.   Recognize the unique nursing opportunities to initiate conversations about advance care planning

      a)   The admission assessment process provides opportunities to not only inquire into the existence of an advance directive, but to explore patient's knowledge and provide information about the importance of discussion

      b)   Through repeated contact with patients, e.g., clinic visits, frequent admissions, care management teams

      c)   When patients' chronic illness progresses, symptoms or frequency of hospitalizations/emergency visits increase and/or function declines

      d)   When patients express concern about the care received and their quality of life ("I'm not sure I can take this anymore")

2. Initiate ACP discussions

    a) Decide when to initiate routine discussions

        i. It's never too early to "plant a seed"

        ii. Encourage discussions in non-stress times, e.g., outpatient setting, community or church groups

        iii. Weave discussions in over time, especially when repeated contact with patient is expected, e.g., care management teams, clinics

    b) Decide when to initiate urgent discussions

        i. Person you suspect could likely die within the next 6–12 months

        ii. Person recently hospitalized for progression of illness/complications

        iii. Person with poor prognosis, increased suffering; aggressive treatment is no longer effective

        iv. Person expressing interest in discussing advance care planning

3. Determine if patient has decision-making capacity

    a) The legal right to make informed choices and execute a written advance directive is granted to all adults age 18 years and older who possess decision-making capacity

    b) An advance directive document is only valid if completed by a person with decision-making capacity

    c) An advance directive document only becomes activated in the event a person is assessed to have lost decision-making capacity

    d) Professionals must assess decision-making capacity or make referrals to others who can provide this assessment

4. Develop a trusting, therapeutic relationship

    a) Emphasize that discussions are becoming part of routine medical care for all adults who need to plan for an unexpected accident or complication that might leave them unable to make their own medical decisions

    b) Begin by encouraging discussion and understanding rather than making specific decisions

    c) Assist patient in appreciating the benefit of these conversations with loved ones who may need to assume the burden of surrogate decision-making

5. Assess understanding of medical condition

    a) Explore understanding of illness, if appropriate

    b) Assist in developing questions for healthcare provider when understanding of illness/increased symptoms is unclear

    c) Provide information on disease progression as appropriate

6. Explore attitudes and experiences

    a) Assess attitude, knowledge and beliefs about advance care planning

        i. Explore reasons for lack of planning, e.g., feeling too ill, fear of talking about end of life, desire to not burden family with discussion or responsibility for making decisions, belief that stated preferences will be ignored, cultural or religious beliefs, among others

 b) Allow person to discuss and explore personal experiences in making healthcare decisions for self, family and/or friends

 c) Assess what was learned through these experiences

 d) Explore and clarify statements or ambiguous terms

7. Assist person in the selection and preparation of an appropriate surrogate decision-maker

 a) Review characteristics of an appropriate surrogate decision-maker, i.e., willing and trustworthy; understands patient's goals/values; able to make decisions under sometimes stressful conditions and willing to understand role and responsibilities

 b) Assist surrogate in understanding the roles and responsibilities of making decisions for a loved one

  i. Include surrogate in discussions and planning

  ii. Provide written information on role of surrogate

8. Maintain awareness of and sensitivity towards individuals from diverse cultures, ethnic, religious or socioeconomic groups

 a) Avoid assumptions regarding individual beliefs

 b) Identify potential barriers with individual in discussing ACP, i.e., distrust of authority/professionals, fear of loss of control, superstitions, reading/language barriers, cultural mores.

 c) Determine patient's preferred mode of communication

 d) Enlist non-medical assistance/support

 e) Facilitate discussion in a non-hurried manner

 f) Focus on value of discussion rather than premature decisions

 g) Engage in values clarification for self and appreciate how personal values may interfere with facilitation of ACP discussions

9. Assist the healthy adult to understand the importance of advance care planning

 a) Remind healthy adult that everyone needs to plan for a sudden, unexpected event e.g., car accident that might leave him/her unable to make own healthcare decisions, thus requiring a surrogate decision-maker

 b) Assist healthy adult to think about goals for medical treatment if a sudden event were to occur that left him/her incapacitated with no reasonable expectation of recovery. In this situation, would the individual prefer to continue life-sustaining treatment or forego such treatment and allow death to occur?

 c) Assist in the selection of an appropriate surrogate decision-maker

 d) Explore religious, spiritual, cultural or personal beliefs that might influence healthcare decisions

10. Assist the person with a life-limiting illness to make choices about future medical care

 a) Understand the unique and often complex advance care planning needs of patients who have end-stage or terminal illness or those who "we would not be surprised if they died in the next 1–2 years"

b)   Explore the concept of "hoping for the best" as well as "planning for the worst" with the goal of providing the patient with the opportunity to participate in disease-specific decision-making

c)   Explore concept of "living well" or the individuals life goals or how their life has meaning

   i.   Explore with individual what gives life meaning

   ii. Explore what activities are important for a person to maintain the individual's meaning of life, achieve life goals or to "live well"

   iii. Inquire if there are spiritual, cultural, religious or personal beliefs that may influence decision-making

d)   Assist person to understand the need to begin to make disease-specific healthcare decisions; that they have an illness that is difficult to predict when a complication may occur that might leave them unable to make own healthcare decisions. In this situation, the burden of decision-making falls to a loved one, who is often unprepared for this stressful role

e)   Explore persons' understanding of the potential complications that may occur given his/her current progressive illness e.g., person with end stage heart failure is at risk for cardiac arrest and sudden death; person with end stage lung failure is at risk for progressive breathing difficulty leading to respiratory arrest, etc.

f)   Assist person to understand the medical choices that need to be made in relation to his/her progressive illness, e.g., CPR, intubation, artificial nutrition, hydration, antibiotics, etc.

g)   Assist person to understand the benefits as well as burdens of each life-sustaining intervention under consideration

h)   Provide information on outcome statistics if known and available or make a referral to attending physician

i)   Assist person to explore the multiple non-medical choices that may be critically important for individual to achieve a quality end-of-life experience. Make referrals as necessary, e.g.,

   i.   Meaning of and options for comfort care

   ii. Psychosocial, religious, spiritual choices

   iii. Environmental options, e.g., home care, hospice, long-term care facility

j)   Develop a list of specific patient questions and concerns that have emerged during the conversation and assist the patient in getting these questions answered, e.g., make referrals to attending physician, schedule appointment with clergy or financial advisor

11. Provide emotional support and ongoing discussions as needed over time

12. Advocate for a plan of care consistent with patient's preferences, e.g.,

a)   Communicate person's concerns/goals/values to other healthcare providers

b)   Facilitate family and healthcare provider care conferences to improve shared understanding and decision-making

c)   Make referrals when person needs further assistance

13. Document discussion and interventions

   a) Record conversations regarding ACP discussions in appropriate location in medical/electronic record

   b) Include interventions in routine care planning conferences, discussions and reports, noting any changes or amends the individual has made to their ACP

14. Comply with organizations' policies/practices related to future medical decision-making

   a) Do-not-resuscitate

   b) Withdrawing/withholding life-sustaining treatment

   c) Assessment of decision-making capacity

   d) Advance directives/advance care planning

   e) Ethics consultation

15. Assist individual in creating a plan to communicate preferences for future medical care (or make appropriate referral)

   a) Assess person's understanding of options for creating a plan and assist in choosing an acceptable option

   b) Recommend the preferred written plan (for most individuals), i.e., an advance directive noting a Power of Attorney for Healthcare that meets the state statutory requirements

   c) Confirm that the person understands the statutory requirements for completing an advance directive to include:

      i. Knowledge of living will document and related qualifications i.e., under what conditions does the living will become activated?

      ii. Knowledge of the Power of Attorney for Healthcare document and its related power and authority given to the appointee to make healthcare decisions

      iii. Identifies surrogate decision-maker

      iv. Identifies method of including option for documenting specific preferences for life-sustaining treatment within document

      v. Explains the criteria for making the document legal, e.g., witness/notarization, signatures, dates, contact information, etc.

      vi. Understands the systems for making changes to plan, entering plan into medical record and transferring plan throughout the continuum of care

      vii. Identifies the name of the pre-hospital do-not-resuscitate order, if one exists and system for utilization/application

The content in this chapter is based on material presented in the Respecting Choices® Facilitator Manual (see Hammes and Briggs 2002).

ADDITIONAL REFERENCES AND RESOURCES

Back AL, Arnold RM, Quill TE. Hope for the best, and prepare for the worst. *Annals of Internal Medicine,* 2003;138:439–443.

Briggs L. Shifting the focus of advance care planning: using an in-depth interview to build and strengthen relationships. *Innovations in End-of-Life Care.* 2003;5. On-line peer reviewed journal available at http://www.edc.org/lastacts/.

Briggs L, Colvin E. The nurse's role in end-of-life decision making for patients and families. *Geriatric Nursing.* 2002;23:302–310.

Briggs L, Kirchoff K, Hammes B, Song M, Colvin E. Patient-centered advance care planning in special patient populations: a pilot study. *Journal of Professional Nursing.* 2004;20:47–58.

Communication, Truth-telling and advance care planning. An interview with Bud Hammes. *Innovations in End-of-Life Care.* 1999;1. On-line peer reviewed journal available at http://www.edc.org/lastacts/.

Ersek M, Kagawa-Singer M, Barnes D, Blackhall L, Koenig BA. Multicultural considerations in the use of advance directives. *Oncology Nursing Forum.* 1998;25:1683–1690.

Fins JJ. Commentary: from contract to covenant in advance care planning. *Journal of Law, Medicine, and Ethics.* 1999;27:46–51.

Fried TR, Bradley EH, Towle VR, Phil M, Allore H. Understanding the treatment preferences of seriously ill patients. *New England Journal of Medicine.* 2002;346:1061–1066.

Hammes BJ, Rooney BL. Death and end-of-life planning in one Midwestern community. *Achieves of Internal Medicine.* 1998;158:383–390.

Hammes BJ. What does it take to help adults successfully plan for future medical decisions? *Journal of Palliative Medicine.* 2001;4:453–456.

Hammes BJ, Briggs LA. *Respecting Choices Facilitator's Manual.* La Crosse, WI: Gundersen Lutheran Medical Foundation; 2002.

Lynn J, Nolan K, Kabcenell A, Weissman D, Milne C, Berwick D. Reforming care for person near the end of life: the promise of quality improvement. *Annals of Internal Medicine.* 2002;137:117–122.

Molloy DW, Guyatt GH, Russo R, et al. Systematic implementation of an advance directive program in nursing homes: a randomized controlled trial. *Journal of the American Medical Association.* 2000;283:1437–1444.

Schwartz CE, Wheeler HB, Hammes B, et al, and the UMass End-of-Life Working Group. Early intervention in planning end-of-life care with ambulatory geriatric patients. *Archives of Internal Medicine.* 2002;162:1611–1618.

Stewart AL, Teno J, Patrick DL, Lynn J. The concept of quality of life of dying persons in the context of health care. *Journal of Pain and Symptom Management,* 1999;17:93–108.

Teno JM, Lynn J. Putting advance-care planning into action. *Journal of Clinical Ethics.* 1996;7:205–213.

Tilden VP, Tolle SW, Nelson CA, Fields J. Family decision-making to withdraw life-sustaining treatments from hospitalized patients. *Nursing Research.* 2001;50:105–115.

Tolle SW, Tilden VP. Changing end-of-life planning: the Oregon experience. *Journal of Palliative Medicine.* 2002;5:311–317.

CHAPTER XIII

ETHICAL ISSUES IN END-OF-LIFE CARE

Mary Ersek, PhD, RN

I. Introduction

A. What Is Ethics?[1]

1. General term for methods used to understand and examine the moral life; also a branch of philosophy that focuses on the moral life

2. Morality: social customs, norms and rules that define "right" and "wrong" behavior; does not encompass systematic reflection or study of what's right and wrong

3. Healthcare ethics (also called bioethics, medical ethics): the study of moral obligations of healthcare providers and society in preventing and treating disease and injury and in caring for the people with illness and injuries

4. Nursing ethics: the reflection on and study of the moral norms for the practice, tradition and institutions of nursing

5. Ethics and legality

    a) Ethics can guide the development and enforcement of laws

    b) Some legal actions are considered immoral by some people (e.g., capital punishment, apartheid)

    c) Some illegal actions can be viewed as moral by some people (e.g., active, voluntary euthanasia)

6. Ethics is not static; it is influenced by societal norms and change over time; although the principles and methods generally are fairly constant, sociocultural trends and scientific advances alter the way ethical principles are applied to a given situation

B. Ethical Principles[1]

1. Principles: concepts used to evaluate and decide the morality of an action, commonly used to frame and deliberate about bioethical issues

2. Four major bioethical principles

    a) Autonomy

        i. From the Greek—*autos* (self) and *nomos* (rule, law, governance); person's right to choose freely

        ii.   In American society, which is based on individual rights, autonomy influences greatly how healthcare decisions are made

        iii.   Autonomy depends on

            (a)   Liberty: ability to make a choice that is not overly influenced or coerced by others

            (b)   Agency: capacity (agency) to understand relevant information, consider the options, evaluate risks and benefits, make and communicate a decision

            (c)   Having information necessary to make the decision (e.g., information about diagnosis, prognosis, treatment options)

        iv.   Informed consent depends on autonomy

        v.   Autonomy includes the right to choose or refuse therapies

    b)   Beneficence

        i.   Obligation to "do good," to act for another's benefit

        ii.   In clinical practice, it is usually necessary to consider benefits, burdens and costs of a particular action (treatment) to ensure beneficence

    c)   Nonmaleficence

        i.   Obligation not to inflict harm; is the basis for the phrase, "first, do no harm"

        ii.   Doing what helps patients and prevents harm

        iii.   In palliative care, nonmaleficence is most commonly invoked when deliberating about life-prolonging therapies that can harm patients by causing increased suffering without increasing patient's quality of life; nonmaleficence offers justification for withholding/withdrawing futile treatments

        iv.   Futility

             (a)   Clinician's determination that a therapy offers a patient no benefit and therefore should not be prescribed[2]

            (b)   Used to justify withholding/withdrawing of therapies

            (c)   Determining futility involves making a judgment based on both values and scientific evidence[1,3]

            (d)   Because the value judgment is based on clinician's or societal perspectives, determining the patient's goals for treatment and values should *precede* any judgment about the futility of a particular therapy whenever possible[3]

    d)   Justice

        i.   "Fair, equitable and appropriate treatment in light of what is due or owed to persons"[1, p. 226]

        ii.   Distributive justice

             (a)   Distribution of societal rights and responsibilities

            (b)   Allocation of scarce healthcare resources

(c)   Concept offers support for policies that restrict access to intensive care and other costly, aggressive therapies that are seen as futile; that is, if the therapy will likely not benefit the patient, then the cost to society is not justified

(d)   Decisions about just allocation of scarce resources are best made at an institutional or societal level rather than one provider making the decision for a particular patient[4]

e)   Bioethical principles guide reflection and discussion about ethical issues but do not provide answers; sound ethical reasoning and action depends on clinicians who understand and evaluate their beliefs and values in light of societal norms, laws, professional obligations and values and goals of patients and families

II.   Ethical Dilemmas and Conflicts

A.   Dilemmas arise when evidence suggests that a particular act is both morally right and morally wrong (e.g., abortion) or when a person is uncertain whether or not a particular act is morally right (e.g., giving large opioid doses to imminently dying people)[1]

B.   Ethical conflicts[5]

1.   Arise when there is disagreement

a)   About goals of care (e.g., aggressive, curative treatment vs. comfort care)

b)   Whether or not specific medical treatments are futile

c)   About what the incapacitated patient would want

2.   Involve disagreements between or among

a)   Healthcare team members

b)   Family members

c)   Patient (or surrogate)

C.   Process to resolve ethical dilemmas and conflicts is similar to other problem-solving methods[6]

1.   *Identify the issue:* what is it about the clinical situation that is causing distress or conflict?

2.   *Gather data:* seek information on the following

a)   Information about the clinical situation—patient's clinical status (e.g., diagnosis, prognosis), burdens and benefits of all the treatment options

b)   Patient and family's understanding of the situation and their values, goals of care and wishes; if the patient is unable to voice preferences and values seek information from patient's advance directives, if available or from others who know the patient well

c)   Who are the decision-makers in the situation and what are their opinions, beliefs and values? Who else will be affected by the decision and what are their opinions, beliefs and values?

d)   What are the ethical principles and/or values that are in conflict?

3. What are all the possible courses of action? What are the possible outcomes of these actions?

4. Evaluate the possible courses of action with input from

    a) Statutory law

    b) Case law

    c) Ethics and healthcare literature

    d) Position and consensus statements from professional organizations (e.g., Hospice and Palliative Nurses Association, American Nurses Association, American Medical Association)

    e) Institutional or agency policies

    f) Formal ethics consultation

5. Make a decision and implement the plan

6. Evaluate the plan—were acceptable outcomes achieved? Does the plan need to be changed?

7. Open and respectful communication that reflects cultural sensitivity, negotiation and consensus building must occur throughout the process of resolving conflicts[7]

III. Common Ethical Issues at the End of Life

A. Truth-telling

1. Current ethical and legal obligations require that healthcare providers ensure that patients are fully informed about their conditions, including diagnosis, prognosis and potential risks and benefits of all treatment options (e.g., no active, curative treatment)

2. Providing complete, accurate information is necessary to ensure that patients and families are able to make informed decisions and provide informed consent or refusal

3. There sometimes is tension between what healthcare providers need to tell patients and families and what they want to hear

    a) Some patients do not wish to be burdened with all the information or wish to have others (family or healthcare providers) make decisions

    b) Some families do not want the patient to know the details of the illness for fear of having the patient become upset or hopeless

    c) Some families, especially those from nonEuropean-American cultures, consider it the responsibility of the adult children to receive information and make decisions for their elderly parents

    d) In some cultures, giving ill people negative information about their condition is considered rude and/or emotionally destructive

    e) In cases where tension exists about disclosure of health-related information

        i. Clinicians must "offer" truth rather than "inflict" truth; patient should be offered information but if s/he freely chooses not to receive the information, that wish should be honored

        ii. Clinicians should continue to offer information, always giving the patient the option to refuse it and/or request that the information be given to others whom the patient trusts[8]

B.   Withholding and withdrawing life-sustaining therapies

1.   Also referred to as letting or allowing a patient to die, as death would naturally occur without the therapy; terms distinguish these actions from actions that are generally seen as ethically *unjustified* (see section on Assisted Death)[9]

2.   Generally, therapies may be withheld/withdrawn if the patient (or designated surrogate) refuses it and/or if the treatment is medically futile; ideally, the concept of futility is not invoked without consent of the patient/family.[10] This may vary based on individual state law as state law may be more narrow; understanding the law of the state in which you practice is critical

3.   Courts, professional healthcare organizations and many religions recognize patients' ethical and legal right to refuse life-sustaining therapies[10–14]

4.   Two highly publicized court cases, those involving Karen Ann Quinlan[15] and Nancy Cruzan[16] were instrumental in establishing the legal right to withhold/withdraw life-prolonging therapies

5.   The Patient Self-Determination Act of 1991 reaffirmed the right of patients to choose or refuse therapies, requiring healthcare agencies to inform patients of this right

   a)   Advance directives: state law governs the use of advance directives, a mechanism through which persons can communicate their wishes in the event they are unable to communicate them directly. It is also referred to as a plan for future medical care created for some yet uncertain future. This plan can be communicated orally (verbal expressions to loved ones, friends or healthcare providers); in formal written documents that meet statutory requirements (living will, power of attorney for healthcare) or informal documents (letter to physician, values history) that may not meet statutory requirements, but provide evidence of preferences

   b)   Advance care planning (ACP): a process of assisting individuals to understand why ACP is important, reflect on personal beliefs, cultural or religious norms and goals, discuss these choices, values, beliefs, with others and develop a plan for communicating preferences, i.e., an advance directive

   c)   Refer to Chapter 12, *Advance Care Planning: The Role of the Nurse*, for an indepth discussion of this topic

6.   Life-prolonging treatments include

   a)   CPR

   b)   Mechanical ventilation

   c)   Dialysis

   d)   Enteral and parenteral nutrition

   e)   Antibiotics (note: antibiotics can be used, when appropriate, for the provision of comfort)

7.   Withholding vs. withdrawing therapies

   a)   No moral or legal differences between withholding and withdrawing treatments

   b)   Some clinicians and family caregivers report greater emotional distress when *withdrawing* therapy

c) To alleviate distress around initiating and withdrawing life-prolonging therapies, experts recommend initiating a time-limited trial, which involves starting a treatment only with specific criteria and a timeline for achieving clinical goals; at established times, treatment efficacy, burdens and benefits are evaluated vis-à-vis criteria; if goals are not met therapy is discontinued[17]

d) There is variation according to state law regarding withholding and withdrawing therapies

C. Administering opioids at the end of life: risk of hastening death[18]

1. Healthcare workers are legally and ethically required to treat patients' pain adequately, including aggressive pain therapy at the EOL; this obligation has been voiced by professional nursing organizations[8,18–21]

2. Despite the fear that administering opioids to seriously ill patients can hasten death, there is *no* empirical evidence to justify this concern[18,22–27]

3. If concerns remain despite the lack of evidence, administering aggressive opioid therapy is ethically and legally justified through the Rule of Double Effect (RDE)[1,18,28]

4. RDE: derived from the principle of nonmaleficence, RDE provides ethical justification for actions that have positive intended effects and negative unintended but foreseen effects[1]

5. RDE justification for administering opioids when there is a risk of hastening death involves four conditions

a) The action in question must be good or at least morally neutral—relieving pain by administering opioids is a morally and clinically accepted act

b) The clinician must intend only the good effect—the nurse must administer the opioid with the intention of relieving pain (and not to end the patient's life)

c) The bad effect must not be the means to the good effect—that is, it is not necessary to end the patient's life in order to relieve pain

d) The good effect must outweigh the bad effect—that is, the good involved in relieving pain outweighs the minor (unproven) risk of hastening death[1]

6. The clinical and ethical justifications for providing palliative sedation are similar to those for administering opioids

7. The moral obligation to relieve pain and suffering should be the primary issue in administering palliative therapies at the EOL[18]

D. Assisted Death[9]

1. Term includes

a) Euthanasia: acting to end the life of a patient to relieve the patient's suffering; also called "mercy killing"; usually involves administration of a lethal injection[29]

b) Assisted suicide: providing a person with the means (usually a prescription for a lethal amount of a medication) knowing that the person intends to kill himself or herself by taking an overdose of the medication[30]

2. Unlike withholding/withdrawing life-prolonging therapies, assisted death is generally not seen as ethically acceptable or justified

3. Currently, euthanasia is illegal throughout the U.S. and Canada and assisted suicide is legal only in the state of Oregon

4. Arguments for and against assisted death (see Table 1)

5. Many professional organizations have published position statements against the legalization of assisted suicide and euthanasia[29–34]

6. Oregon Nurses Association position statement addresses nursing roles where assisted suicide is legal[35] (see Table 2)

IV. **Cultural Issues in EOL Ethical Decision-Making**

   A. **Bioethics and healthcare system generally reflect European-American values**

   B. **In a diverse society, important to recognize variations in values and perspectives that can cause distress and conflict**

   C. **Major differences between European-American values and those of the cultures that may influence decision-making**

Table 1. Summary of Arguments For and Against Assisted Death[40–42]

Bioethical Concept/Principle	Argument in Support of Assisted Death	Argument Against Assisted Death
Autonomy: "Respect for the individual's right to choose"	Patients have a right to make their own decisions to preserve free choice and human dignity	Honoring the sanctity of life overrides the right of individuals to choose how and when they will die. Autonomy does not include the right to engage others (e.g., clinicians) in immoral acts[30]
Beneficence: "Doing good"	Assisting a suffering patient to maintain control and end his/her suffering is an ethical, merciful (beneficent) act	Aid in dying constitutes abandonment
Professional Integrity Nonmaleficence: "Do no harm"	Inability (or refusal) to relieve suffering destroys trust between the healthcare professional & the patient	Assisting a patient to die destroys trust & violates the ethical traditions of healthcare professionals
Societal consequences "slippery slope"	We can provide safeguards to ensure safe, ethical practice of assisted death; assisted death already occurs, without any safeguards	The "slippery slope" argument: there is a risk to vulnerable groups, e.g., elderly, underinsured, that they might feel compelled to request assisted death to avoid being a "burden" to family and/or society

Reprinted from Ersek, M. The continuing challenge of assisted death. *J Hospice and Palliative Nursing.* 2004;6(1):46–59. Used with permission.

Table 2. Oregon Nurses Association Provides Guidance on Nurses' Dilemma—Position Statement on the Nurses' Role in the Death with Dignity Act

Nurses Who Choose to Be Involved:
If as a nurse, your own moral and ethical value system allows you to be involved in providing care to a patient who has made the choice to end his/her life, within the provisions of the Death with Dignity Act, the following guidelines will assist you:

You may:
- Provide care and comfort to the patient and family through all stages of the dying process. Teach the patient and family about the process of dying and what they may expect.
- Maintain patient and family confidentiality about the end-of-life decisions they are making.
- Explain the law as it currently exists.
- Discuss and explore with the patient options with regard to end-of-life decisions and provide resource information or link the patient and family to access the services or resources they are requesting.
- Explore reasons for the patient's request to end their life and make a determination as to whether the patient is depressed and whether the depression is influencing his/her decision; or whether the patient has made a rational decision based on the patient's own fundamental values and beliefs.
- Be present during the patient's self-administration of the medication and during the patient's death to console and counsel the family.
- Be involved in policy development within the healthcare facility and/or the community.

You may not:
- Inject or administer the medication that will lead to the end of the patient's life; this is an act precluded by law.
- Breach confidentiality of patients exploring or choosing assisted suicide.
- Subject your patients or their families to unwarranted, judgmental comments or actions because of the patient's choice to explore or select the option of assisted suicide.
- Subject your peers or other healthcare team members to unwarranted, judgmental comments or actions because of their decision to continue to provide care to a patient who has chosen assisted suicide.
- Abandon or refuse to provide comfort and safety measures to the patient.

Nurses Who Choose Not to Be Involved:
If as a nurse, your own moral and ethical value system does not allow you to be involved in providing care to a patient who has made the choice to end his/her life, within the provisions of the Death with Dignity Act, the following guidelines will assist you.

You may:
- Provide ongoing and ethically justified end-of-life care.
- Conscientiously object to being involved in delivering care. You are obliged to provide for the patient's safety, to avoid abandonment, and withdraw only when assured that alternative sources of care are available to the patient.
- Transfer the responsibility for the patient's care to another provider.
- Maintain confidentiality of the patient, family and healthcare providers continuing to provide care to the patient who has chosen assisted suicide.
- Be involved in policy development within the healthcare setting and/or the community.

You may not:
- Breach confidentiality of patients exploring or choosing assisted suicide.
- Inject or administer the medication that will lead to the end of the patient's life; this is an act precluded by law.
- Subject your patients or their families to unwarranted, judgmental comments or actions because of the patient's choice to explore or select the option of assisted suicide.
- Subject your peers or other healthcare team members to unwarranted, judgmental comments or actions because of their decision to continue to provide care to a patient who has chosen assisted suicide.
- Abandon or refuse to provide comfort and safety measures to the patient.

From: Oregon Nurses Association. *ONA Provides Guidance on Nurses Dilemma's.* 1995. Available at: http://www.oregonrn.org/associations/3019/files/AssistedSuicide.pdf. Accessed May 27, 2005.

1. Autonomy is highly valued in American society but less so in other cultures; for example, needs and wishes of the family or community may be more important than individual's rights and wishes; family/community may expect to play a greater role in decision-making than is typical in American culture

2. Truth-telling is a moral and ethical imperative in American healthcare system; however, some cultures view full disclosure disrespectful and/or harmful

3. Personal control is desired by many patients, but some cultures and religions value trust in a deity, the healthcare team or family over the need for personal control

4. Patients/families from racial and cultural groups who have a history of discrimination and oppression, including African-Americans,[36–38] may distrust the healthcare team and value aggressive therapy even in hopeless situations

D. **Clinicians must never make assumptions about patient/family values and preference based on patient's/family's culture, religion, age or gender; individual assessment always is necessary[8]**

V. **Nursing Roles**

A. **Practice self reflection: awareness of one's values and beliefs and understanding how they influence one's behavior, particularly responses to patients, families and other healthcare team members**

B. **Maintain clinical competence**

C. **Demonstrate moral integrity: the consistent application of ethical norms; in other words, one's *basic* approach to ethical decision making does not change depending on the situation or the specific patient or family[1]**

D. **Practice conscientious objection responsibly**

1. Conscientious objection: the right of persons to refuse to participate in acts that they deem unethical; examples of clinical situations in which nurses may practice conscientious objection include abortion, capital punishment and assisted suicide

2. Clinicians may morally refuse to participate in care, but only on the grounds of a moral objection to a specific type of intervention; they may not refuse care on grounds of discomfort, lack of knowledge or discrimination

3. Clinicians who refuse to provide specific care based on moral beliefs must assure that decisions of patient/family are respected and they are not abandoned if their goals differ from that of the healthcare team.[35,39] (see Table 2)

E. **Keep current with ethical and legal issues related to EOL care**

F. **Provide information to assist in decision making and resolving ethical conflicts**

G. **Advocate for patients and families**

H. Participate in patient/family conferences that address ethical issues

I. Ensure informed consent for clinical care and research participation

J. Participate in institutional/agency committees and boards, e.g.,

1. Institutional Review Boards (IRB) for Human Subjects Protections

2. Ethics committees

K. Seek resources and assistance as needed when dealing with ethical concerns, questions and dilemmas

CITED REFERENCES

1. Beauchamp TL, Childress JF. *Principles of Biomedical Ethics*. 5th ed. New York, NY: Oxford University Press; 2001.

2. Cantor MD, Braddock CH, 3rd, Derse AR, et al. Do-not-resuscitate orders and medical futility. *Archives of Internal Medicine*. 2003;163(22):2689–2694.

3. Bailey S. The concept of futility in healthcare decision making. *Nurs Ethics*. 2003;11(1):77–83.

4. Shafazand S, Crawley LM, Raffin T, Koenig B. Withholding and withdrawing treatment: the doctor-patient relationship and the changing goals of care. In: Beger A, Portenoy R, Weissman D, eds. *Principle and practice of palliative care and supportive oncology*. 2nd ed. Philadelphia, PA: Lippincott Williams & Wilkins; 2002:880–890.

5. Schneiderman LJ, Gilmer T, Teetzel HD, et al. Effect of ethics consultations on nonbeneficial life-sustaining treatments in the intensive care setting: a randomized controlled trial. *JAMA*. 2003;290(9):1166–1172.

6. Scanlon C. Ethics in palliative care. In: Panke J, Coyne P, eds. *Conversations in Palliative Care*. Pensacola, FL: Pohl Publishing; 2004:163–187.

7. Way J, Back AL, Curtis JR. Withdrawing life support and resolution of conflict with families. *BMJ*. 2002;325(7376):1342–1345.

8. Wilson S, Ersek M, Kraybill B. Culture. In: Panke J, Coyne P, eds. *Conversations in Palliative Care*. Pittsburgh, PA: HPNA; 2004:41–57.

9. Ersek M. The continuing challenge of assisted death. *J Hospice and Palliative Nursing*. 2004;6(1):46–59.

10. Luce JM, Alpers A. Legal aspects of withholding and withdrawing life support from critically ill patients in the United States and providing palliative care to them. *American Journal of Respiratory & Critical Care Medicine*. 2000;162(6):2029–2032.

11. deBlois J, O'Rourke KD. Issues at the end of life: the revised ethical and religious directives discuss suicide, euthanasia, and end-of-life procedures. *Health Progress*. 1995;76(8):24–27.

12. Clarfield AM, Gordon M, Markwell H, Alibhai SM. Ethical issues in end-of-life geriatric care: the approach of three monotheistic religions—Judaism, Catholicism, and Islam. *Journal of the American Geriatrics Society*. 2003;51(8):1149–1154.

13. Barilan YM. Revisiting the problem of Jewish bioethics: the case of terminal care. *Kennedy Institute of Ethics Journal*. 2003;13(2):141–168.

14. Pauls M, Hutchinson RC. Bioethics for clinicians: 28. Protestant bioethics. *Canad Med Assoc J*. 2002;166(3):339–343.

15. In re Quinlan. *755 A2A 647*: (New Jersey); 1976.

16. Cruzan v. Director of Missouri Department of Health. *397*: DS 261; 1990.

17. Scanlon C. Ethical concerns in end-of-life care. *American Journal of Nursing*. 2003;103(1):48-55; quiz 56.

18. Hospice and Palliative Nurses Association. *Position Statement: Providing Opioids at the End of Life*. Available at: http://www.hpna.org/positions.asp. Accessed July 16, 2004.

19. American Nurses Association. Position Statement: Promotion of Comfort and Relief of Pain in Dying Patients. American Nurses Association, Task Force on the Nurse's Role in End-of-Life Decisions. December 5, 2003. Available at: http://www.ana.org/readroom/position/ethics/etpain.htm. Accessed July 16, 2004.

20. American Nurses Association. Code of ethics for nurses with interpretive statements. Washington, DC: American Nurses Association; 2001.

21. American Society of Pain Management Nurses. Position Statement on End of Life Care. *ASPMN.* Available at: http://www.aspmn.org/html/PSeolcare.htm. Accessed July 16, 2004.

22. Campbell ML, Bizek KS, Thill M. Patient responses during rapid terminal weaning from mechanical ventilation: a prospective study. *Critical Care Medicine.* 1999;27(1):73–77.

23. Morita T, Tsunoda J, Inoue S, Chihara S. Effects of high dose opioids and sedatives on survival in terminally ill cancer patients. *Journal of Pain & Symptom Management.* 2001;21(4):282–289.

24. Sykes N, Thorns A. The use of opioids and sedatives at the end of life. *Lancet Oncology.* 2003;4(5):312–318.

25. Walsh TD. Opiates and respiratory function in advanced cancer. *Recent Results in Cancer Research.* 1984;89:115–117.

26. Walsh T, Rivera N, Kaiko R. Oral morphine and respiratory function amongst hospice inpatients with advanced cancer. *Support Care Cancer.* 2003;11(12):780–784.

27. Wilson WC, Smedira NG, Fink C, McDowell JA, Luce JM. Ordering and administration of sedatives and analgesics during the withholding and withdrawal of life support from critically ill patients. *JAMA.* 1992;267(7):949–953.

28. Natural Death Act. *Washington State.* Vol RCW 70.122.010; 1992.

29. American Nurses Association. Position Statement: Active Euthanasia. *American Nurses Association, Task Force on the Nurses' Role in End-of-Life Decisions, Center for Ethics and Human Rights* December 8, 1994. Available at: http://www.ana.org/readroom/position/ethics/eteuth.htm. Accessed July 16, 2004.

30. American Nurses Association. Position Statement: Assisted Suicide. *American Nurses Association, Task Force on the Nurse's Role in End-of-Life Decisions, Center for Ethics and Human Rights* December 8, 1994. Available at: http://www.ana.org/readroom/position/ethics/etsuic.htm. Accessed July 16, 2004.

31. Hospice and Palliative Nurses Association. HPNA Position Statement: Legalization of assisted suicide. *Journal of Hospice and Palliative Nursing.* 2002;4(2):64–65.

32. American Society of Pain Management Nurses. *Position statement: Assisted suicide. ASPMN.* Available at: http://www.aspmn.org/html/PSassistsuicide.htm. Accessed July 16, 2004.

33. American Academy of Hospice and Palliative Medicine. *Position Statement: Comprehensive end-of-life care and physician-assisted suicide.* AAHPM. Available at: http://www.aahpm.org/positions/suicide.html. Accessed November 5, 2003.

34. National Hospice and Palliative Care Organization. *Statement of the national hospice organization opposing the legalization of euthanasia and assisted suicide:* NHPCO; 1999.

35. Oregon Nurses Association. ONA provides guidance on nurses' dilemma. *Oregon Nurses Assoc.* Available at: http://www.oregonrn.org/associations/3019/files/AssistedSuicide.pdf. Accessed July 19, 2004.

36. West SK, Levi L. Culturally appropriate end-of-life care for the Black American. *Home Healthcare Nurse*. 2004;22(3):164–168.

37. Crawley LM, Marshall PA, Lo B, Koenig BA. End-of-Life Care Consensus P. Strategies for culturally effective end-of-life care. *Annals of Internal Medicine*. 2002;136(9):673–679.

38. Born W, Greiner KA, Sylvia E, Butler J, Ahluwalia JS. Knowledge, attitudes, and beliefs about end-of-life care among inner-city African Americans and Latinos. [see comment]. *Journal of Palliative Medicine*. 2004;7(2):247–256.

39. Stanley K, Zoloth-Dorfman L. Ethical considerations. In: Ferrell B, Coyle N, eds. *Textbook of Palliative Nursing*. 2nd ed. New York: Oxford University Press; in press.

40. Thomasma DC. An analysis of arguments for and against euthanasia and assisted suicide: Part One. *Cambridge Quarterly of Healthcare Ethics*. 1996;5(1):62–76.

41. Thomasma DC. Assessing the arguments for and against euthanasia and assisted suicide: Part Two. *Cambridge Quarterly of Healthcare Ethics*. 1998;7(4):388–401.

42. Scanlon C. Assisted suicide: clinical realities and ethical challenges. *American Journal of Critical Care*. 1996;5(6):397–403; quiz 404–405.

ADDITIONAL REFERENCES AND RESOURCES

American Association of Colleges of Nursing and the City of Hope National Medical Center. Module 5: Legal/Ethical Issues. *End-of-life Nursing Education Consortium (ELNEC) Project*, 2003. Funded by the Robert Wood Johnson Foundation. For more information, see: http://www.aacn.nche.edu/elnec.

Ersek M. Ethical issues at the end of life. *Palliative Care Resource Education Team (PERT) Curriculum*. Seattle (WA): Swedish Medical Center; 2002. Accessed July 17, 2004. Available from: URL: http://www.swedishmedical.org/PERT/PERT_content.htm.

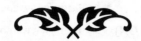

WEBSITE/INTERNET RESOURCES[1]

Agency for Healthcare Research and Quality	http://www.ahcpr.gov/
Aging with Dignity	http://www.agingwithdignity.org
American Academy of Hospice and Palliative Medicine	http://www.aahpm.org
American Academy of Pain Medicine	http://www.painmed.org
American Alliance of Cancer Pain Initiatives	http://www.aacpi.org/resource.html
American Association for Therapeutic Humor	http://www.aath.org
American Board of Internal Medicine— Care for the Dying, Physician Narratives	http://www.abim.org/pubs/narr001.htm
American Cancer Society	http://www.cancer.org
American Chronic Pain Association	http://www.theacpa.org/
American Council for Headache Education	http://www.achenet.org
The American Geriatrics Society	http://www.americangeriatrics.org
American Holistic Nurses Association	http://www.ahna.org
American Massage Therapy Association	http://www.amtamassage.org
American Medical Association	http://www.ama-assn.org.
American Medical Association Education of Physicians on End of Life Care (EPEC)	http://www.ama-assn.org/ama/pub/category/2719.html
American Music Therapy Association	http://www.namt.com
American Pain Foundation	http://www.painfoundation.org
American Pain Society	http://www.ampainsoc.org
American Society of Anesthesiologists	http://www.asahq.org
American Society for Bioethics and Humanities	http://www.asbh.org
American Society of Clinical Oncology (ASCO)	http://www.asco.org
American Society of Law, Medicine and Ethics	http://www.aslme.org
American Society of Pain Management Nurses	http://www.aspmn.org
Approaching Death: Improving Care at the End of Life	http://www.nap.edu/readingroom/books/approaching/
Arthritis Foundation	http://www.arthritis.org
Association of Cancer Online Resources, Inc.	http://www.acor.org

Association for Death Education and Counseling (ADEC)	http://www.adec.org
Association of Nurses in AIDS Care	http://www.anacnet.org
Association of Oncology Social Work (AOSW)	http://www.aosw.org
Association of Pediatric Oncology Nurses (APON)	http://www.apon.org
Before I Die: Medical Care and Personal Choices	http://www.wnet.org/archive/bid
Cancer Care®	http://www.cancercare.org
CancerLink	http://www.personal.u-net.com/~njh/cancer.html
National Cancer Institute Cancer Topics	http://www.cancer.gov/cancerinformation
Candlelighters Childhood Cancer Foundation	http://www.candlelighters.org
Caregiver Network Inc.	http://www.caregiver.on.ca/index.html
Catholic Health Association of the United States	http://www.chausa.org
Center to Improve Care of the Dying	http://www.gwu.edu/~cicd
Children's Hospice International	http://www.chionline.org
Choices	http://www.choices.org
City of Hope Pain/Palliative Care Resource Center	http://prc.coh.org
The Compassionate Friends Inc.	http://www.compassionatefriends.org/
U. S. Department of Health and Human Services, Healthfinder®	http://www.healthfinder.gov
Dying Well	http://www.dyingwell.org
Education for Physicians on End of Life Care Project (EPEC)	http://www.epec.net
The End of Life: Exploring Death in America	http://www.npr.org/programs/death/
End of Life / Palliative Education Resource Center (EPERC)	http://www.eperc.mcw.edu
FACCT—Foundation for Accountability	http://www.facct.org
Family Caregiver Alliance®	http://www.caregiver.org
Fibromyalgia Network	http://www.fmnetnews.com
Geronurse Online	http://www.geronurseonline.org
Growth House, Inc.	http://www.growthhouse.org
Hospice Association of America	http://www.hospice-america.org
Hospice and Palliative Nurses Association	http://www.hpna.org
Hospice Foundation of America (HFA)	http://www.hospicefoundation.org
Hospice Cares Pharmacy	http://www.hospice-cares.com
Institute for Healthcare Improvement	http://www.ihi.org
International Association for the Study of Pain®	http://www.iasp-pain.org/
Leukemia & Lymphoma Society®	http://www.leukemia.org
Make a Wish Foundation®	http://www.wish.org
Medical College of Wisconsin: Center for the Study of Bioethics	http://www.mcw.edu/bioethics/

Medical College of Wisconsin: Palliative Care Center	http://www.mcw.edu/pallmed/
Memorial Sloan-Kettering Cancer Center	http://www.mskcc.org
The Nathan Cummings Foundation	http://www.ncf.org/index.html
National Association for Home Care and Hospice (NAHC)	http://www.nahc.org/
The National Center for Health Statistics	http://www.cdc.gov/nchs/about.htm
National Conference of State Legislatures	http://www.ncsl.org/programs/pubs/endoflife.htm
National Family Caregivers Association	http://www.nfcacares.org/
National Hospice and Palliative Care Organization	http://www.nhpco.org
The National Institute on Aging	http://www.nih.gov/nia/
National Prison Hospice Association	http://www.npha.org
The Neuropathy Association	http://www.neuropathy.org
New York State Partnership for Long-Term Care	http://www.nyspltc.org/about/index.html#3
Not Dead Yet	http://www.notdeadyet.org/
On Our Own Terms	http://www.thirteen.org/onourownterms
OncoLink	http://www.oncolink.com
Open Society Institute	http://www.soros.org
Oregon Health Sciences University Center for Ethics in Health Care	http://www.ohsu.edu/ethics/
Oncology Nursing Society	http://www.ons.org
PainLink	http://www.edc.org/PainLink
Pain Net, Inc.	http://www.painnet.com
Partners Against Pain®	http://www.partnersagainstpain.com
Patient Education Institute	http://www.patient-education.com
Pediatric Pain	http://is.dal.ca/~pedpain/prohp.html
Pediatric Pain Education for Patients & Families	http://pedspain.nursing.uiowa.edu
Reflex Sympathetic Dystrophy Association of California	http://www.rsdsa-ca.org/
Regional Palliative Care Program in Edmunton Alberta	http://www.palliative.org
The Robert Wood Johnson Foundation	http://www.rwjf.org
Sickle Cell Disease Association of American, Inc.	http://www.sicklecelldisease.org
Southern California Cancer Pain Initiative (SCCPI)	http://sccpi.coh.org
Supportive Care of the Dying	http://www.careofdying.org
TMJ Association, Ltd.	http://www.tmj.org
TALARIA: The Hypermedia Assistant for Cancer Pain Management	http://www.stat.washington.edu/TALARIA/talariahome.html
Telemedicine Information Exchange	http://tie.telemed.org
Today's Caregiver Magazine	http://www.caregiver.com/
United Hospital Fund of New York	http://www.uhfnyc.org
University of Wisconsin Pain & Policy Studies Group	http://www.medsch.wisc.edu/painpolicy/

VistaCare	http://www.vista-care.com
Task Force on Life & the Law: When Death is Sought	http://www.health.state.ny.us/nysdoh/provider/death.htm
Wisconsin Pain Initiative	http://www.aacpi.wisc.edu/wcpi
World Health Organization	http://www.who.int/en

[1] From TEXTBOOK OF PALLIATIVE NURSING, edited by Betty Ferrell and Nessa Coyle, copyright © 2000 by Oxford University Press, Inc. Used by permission of Oxford University Press, Inc.

Editor's Note: Any URLs found to be non-functional or inaccurate at the time of publication have been either corrected or deleted.

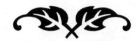

APPENDIX 2

COMMONLY USED MEDICATIONS
Trade and Generic Names

ALZHEIMER'S DRUGS

Aricept® . . . . donepezil
Cognex® . . . . tacrine
Exelon® . . . . rivastigmine
Namenda® . . . . memantine
Reminyl® . . . . galantamine

ANALGESICS

Actiq® . . . . fentanyl citrate
Avinza®/Kadian®/
MS Contin/
Oramorph®SR/
Roxanol® . . . . morphine sulfate
Dilaudid®/
Palladone™ . . . . hydromorphone
Dolophine® . . . . methadone
Duragesic® . . . . fentanyl transdermal system
Empirin w/Codeine®/
Tylenol w/Codeine® . . . . . . aspirin/codeine
Fiorinal® . . . . aspirin/caffeine/butalbital
Lidoderm HCL Topical® . . . lidocaine
Levo-Dromoran® . . . . levorphanol
Oxycontin®/
OxyFAST® . . . . oxycodone
Percocet®/Roxicet® . . . . oxycodone/acetaminophen
Percodan® . . . . oxycodone/aspirin
Tylenol® . . . . acetaminophen
Ultram® . . . . tramadol
Vicodin®/Lorcet® . . . . hydrocodone/acetaminophen

ANTACIDS/ANTIFLATULANTS/DIGESTANTS

Basaljel® . . . . aluminum carbonate gel
Carafate® . . . . sucralfate
Gelusil® . . . . aluminum hydroxide/magnesium hydroxide/simethicone

Maalox® . . . . magnesium hydroxide/aluminum hydroxide
Mylanta® . . . . magnesium hydroxide/aluminum hydroxide/simethicone
Mylicon® . . . . simethicone
Pancrease®/Viokase® . . . . . . pancrelipase

ANTIANGINAL
Calan®/Isoptin® . . . . verapamil
Isordil® . . . . isosorbide dinitrate
Cardizem® . . . . diltiazem
Persantine® . . . . dipyridamole
Procardia® . . . . NIFEdipine*

ANTIBIOTICS
Ancef® . . . . cefazolin
Augmentin® . . . . amoxicillin
Bactrim® . . . . trimethoprim/sulfamethoxazole
Biaxin® . . . . clarithromycin
Ceclor® . . . . cefaclor
Cefobid® . . . . cefoperazone
Ceftin® . . . . cefuroxime
Claforan® . . . . cefotaxime
Cleocin® . . . . clindamycin
Fortaz® . . . . ceftazidime
Garamycin® . . . . gentamicin
Rocephin® . . . . ceftriaxone
Timentin® . . . . ticarcillin/clavulanate
Unasyn® . . . . ampicillin/sulbactam
Zithromax® . . . . azithromycin
Zosyn® . . . . piperacillin/tazobactam

ANTICOAGULANTS
Coumadin® . . . . warfarin
Lovenox® . . . . enoxaparin

ANTICONVULSANTS
Depacon® . . . . valproate
Depakote® . . . . valproic acid
Dilantin® . . . . phenytoin
Keppra® . . . . levetiracetam
Klonopin® . . . . clonazepam
Lamictal® . . . . lamotrigine
Mysoline® . . . . primidone
Neurontin® . . . . gabapentin
Tegretol® . . . . carbamazepine
Topamax® . . . . topiramate
Zonegran® . . . . zonisamide

ANTIDEPRESSANTS
Adepin®/Sinequan® . . . . doxepin
Celexa® . . . . citalopram
Cymbalta® . . . . duloxetine

Desyrel®	trazodone
Effexor®	venlafaxine
Elavil®/Endep®	amitriptyline
Lexapro®	escitalopram
Luvox®	fluvoxamine
Norpramin®	desipramine
Pamelor®	nortriptyline
Paxil®	paroxetine
Prozac®	fluoxetine
Remeron®	mirtazapine
Serzone®	nefazodone
Surmontil®	trimipramine
Tofranil®	imipramine
Tofranil® PM	imipramine pamoate
Vivactil®	protriptylin
Wellbutrin®	buPROPion*
Zoloft®	sertraline

ANTIDIABETICS

Amaryl®	glimepiride
Diabinese®	chlorproPAMIDE*
Glucotrol®/	
Glucotrol XL®	glipiZIDE*
Glynase®/Micronase®	glyBURIDE*
Orinase®	TOLBUTamide*
Prandin®	repaglinide
Starlix®	nateglinide
Tolinase®	TOLAZamide*

ANTIDIARRHEAL

Donnagel®/Kaopectate®	kaolin/pectin
Imodium®	loperamide
Lomotil®	diphenoxylate/atropine
Pepto-Bismol®	bismuth subsalicylate
Paregoric®	camphorated opium tincture
Sandostatin®	octreotide

ANTIFUNGAL

Diflucan®	fluconazole
Flagyl®	metronidazole
Monistat	miconazole nitrate
Mycelex®/Lotrimin®	clotrimazole
Nizoral®	ketoconazole
Mycostatin®	nystatin
Sporanox®	itraconazole

ANTIGOUT

Benemid®	probenecid
Zyloprim®/Lopurin®	allopurinol

ANTIHYPERTENSIVES

Capoten®	captopril
Corgard®	nadolol
Inderal®	propranolol
Lopressor®	metoprolol
Prinivil®/Zestril®	lisinopril
Tenormin®	atenolol
Trandate®	labetalol
Vasotec®	enalapril

ANTIHYSTAMINES

Allegra®	fexofenadine
Atarax®	hydrOXYzine*
Benadryl®	diphenhydrAMINE*
Chlor-Trimeton®	chlorpheniramine
Clarinex®	desloratadine
Claritin®/Alavert®	loratadine
Tavist®	clemastine
Zyrtec®	cetirizine

ANTINAUSEA/ANTIEMETIC/PROMOTILITY

Aloxi®	palonosetron
Antivert®	meclizine
Anzemet®	dolasetron
Compazine®	prochlorperazine
Dramamine®	dimenhyDRINATE*
Emend®	aprepitant
Haldol®	haloperidol
Kytril®	granisetron
Phenergan®	promethazine
Reglan®	metoclopramide
Thorazine®	chlorproMAZINE*
Tigan®	trimethobenzamide
Torecan®	thiethylperazine
Trilafon®	perphenazine
Zofran®	ondansetron

ANTIPARKINSON AGENTS

Apokyn®	apomorphine
Artane®	trihexyphenidyl
Cogentin®	benztropine
Mirapex®	pramipexole
Parlodel®	bromocriptine
Permax®	pergolide
Sinemet®	carbidopa/levodopa
Stalevo®	carbidopa/levodopa/entacapone
Symmetrel®	amantadine

ANTIPRURITICS
Caladryl® . . . . calamine/diphenhydrAMINE*

ANTIPSYCHOTICS
Clozaril® . . . . clozapine
Haldol® . . . . haloperidol
Loxitane® . . . . loxapine
Mellaril® . . . . thioridazine
Moban® . . . . molindone
Navane® . . . . thiothixene
Prolixin® . . . . fluphenazine
Risperdal® . . . . risperidone
Seroquel® . . . . quetiapine
Stelazine® . . . . trifluoperazine
Thorazine® . . . . chlorproMAZINE*
Trilafon® . . . . perphenazine
Zyprexa® . . . . olanzapine

ANTISECRETORY/ANTICHOLINERGIC
Levsin® . . . . hyoscyamine
Transderm-Scop® . . . . scopolamine

ANTIVIRAL
Famvir® . . . . famciclovir
Valtrex® . . . . valacyclovir
Zovirax® . . . . acyclovir

ANXIOLYTIC/ANTIDEPRESSANT
Etrafon®/Triavil® . . . . perphenazine/amitriptyline

ANXIOLYTIC/SEDATIVE
Ambien® . . . . zolpidem
Ativan® . . . . lorazepam
Zydis®/Zyprexa® . . . . olanzapine
BuSpar® . . . . busPIRone
Dalmane® . . . . flurazepam
Halcion® . . . . triazolam
Klonopin® . . . . clonazepam
Librium® . . . . chlordiazepoxide
Nembutal® . . . . pentobarbital
Placidyl® . . . . ethchlorvynol
Restoril® . . . . temazepam
Seconal® . . . . secobarbital
Serax® . . . . oxazepam
Sonata® . . . . zaleplon
Tranxene® . . . . clorazepate
Valium® . . . . diazepam
Versed® . . . . midazolam

APPETITE STIMULANT
Megace® . . . . megestrol

BISPHOSPHONATES
Aredia® . . . . pamidronate
Zometa® . . . . zoledronic acid

CARDIAC GLYCOSIDES
Lanoxin® . . . . digoxin

H₂ BLOCKERS/PROTON PUMP INHIBITORS
Nexium® . . . . esomeprazole
Pepcid® . . . . famotidine
Prevacid® . . . . lansoprazole
Prilosec® . . . . omeprazole
Protonix® . . . . pantoprazole
Tagamet® . . . . cimetidine
Zantac® . . . . ranitidine

LAXATIVES
Benefiber® . . . . soluble fiber
CitroMag® . . . . magnesium citrate
Citrucel® . . . . methylcellulose
Chronulac® . . . . lactulose
Colace®/Surfak®/
Regutol® . . . . docusate sodium
Dulcolax® . . . . bisacodyl
Fiberall®/FiberCon® . . . . calcium polycarbophil
Fleet Enema® . . . . sodium biphosphate/phosphate
Metamucil® . . . . psyllium
MiraLax™ . . . . polyethylene glycol
Phillips' Milk of
Magnesia® . . . . magnesium hydroxide
Senokot® . . . . senna

MUSCLE RELAXANTS
Flexeril® . . . . cyclobenzaprine
Lioresal® . . . . baclofen
Norflex® . . . . orphenadrine
Robaxin® . . . . methocarbamol
Soma® . . . . carisprodol
Quinamm® . . . . quinine sulfate
Valium, Valrelease® . . . . diazepam

NSAIDs
Aleve®/Anaprox®/
Naprosyn® . . . . naproxen sodium
Celebrex® . . . . celecoxib
Indocin® . . . . indomethacin
Motrin® . . . . ibuprofen
Trilisate® . . . . choline magnesium trisalicylate

PSYCHOSTIMULANTS

Dexedrine®	dextroamphetamine
Provigil®	modafinil
Ritalin®	methylphenidate

STEROIDS

Decadron®	dexamethasone
Deltasone®	predniSONE*
Orapred®/Prelone®	prednisoLONE*
Medrol®/SoluMedrol®	methylPREDNISolone*
Solu-Cortef®	hydrocortisone

* "Tall Man" lettering as suggested by the FDA to differentiate look-alike medication names

REFERENCE

Skidmore-Roth L. *2005 Mosby's Nursing Drug Reference*. St. Louis, MO: Mosby, Inc.; 2005.

APPENDIX 3

CHILDREN'S HOSPICE INTERNATIONAL PROGRAM FOR ALL-INCLUSIVE CARE FOR CHILDREN AND THEIR FAMILIES™ (CHI PACC)

CHI PACC® STANDARDS OF CARE AND PRACTICE GUIDELINES

Principles of Care with Practice Guidelines

Access to Care

- **Principle:**

  Children and adolescents diagnosed with life-threatening conditions and the members of their families have ease of access to a comprehensive, coordinated, competent continuum of care in their communities.

- **Practice:**

  A.C.1.   Outreach plans are implemented across all geographic areas in which CHI PACC® programs are available, in order to ensure eligible families, providers, and community organizations have adequate information to facilitate referral to the program. Programs must be comprised of adequate professional medical, social, and supportive staff to serve the needs of those eligible families in the program's service area.

  A.C.2.   CHI PACC® services are culturally relevant, sensitive, and available to children/adolescents and families of the diverse cultures within the program's service area, and in language that is understandable.

  A.C.3.   CHI PACC® program provides communication supports to assist children/adolescents and family members that are sensory or cognitively impaired.

  A.C.4.   The CHI PACC® program provides organized outreach, ongoing education, accurate information about services, and timely resources to all potential referrers to the CHI PACC® palliative care program to enhance their ability to identify potentially appropriate children/adolescents and families for referral.

A.C.5: Children/Adolescents in CHI PACC® Programs have access to treatments and therapies aimed at cure, condition modification or life extension concurrent with and integrated with treatments and services aimed at palliative care goals throughout the entire course of their care.

Child/Adolescent/Family as Unit of Care

- **Principle:**

The CHI PACC® care continuum provides care that is consistently child/adolescent oriented and family-centered in its philosophy, values, practices and operation. All care seeks to support and enhance the life-experience and its quality for each child/adolescent/family unit as defined by their culture, values, beliefs, priorities, circumstances, choices and structure.

- **Practice:**

U.C.1. Care is provided to children/adolescents within the context of each one's age, developmental stage, level of understanding, communication ability, as well as severity of life-threatening condition and its symptomology. Each child/adolescent's own interest, hopes, fears, values, beliefs, and needs are solicited to ensure to the fullest degree possible the integration of the child/adolescent's own point of view and perspective in planning, implementing and evaluating services.

U.C.2. Care is available to all members of the family according to assessed needs and individual choice, including siblings, parents, grandparents and/or other individuals significant to the family unit.

U.C.3. Care affirms the uniqueness and distinctiveness of each family's own system of inter-relationships, roles, decision-making processes, and organizational structure.

U.C.4. Care is implemented to encourage and assist each child/adolescent/family unit to live as normal as is possible under existing circumstances, continue in their customary roles and activities as much as possible and participate in the communities of which they are a part.

U.C.5. Each family unit is assessed in order to establish a plan for meeting the ongoing family member's involvement in caregiving at home. Each family is provided education, training and support for its care giving activities and responsibilities. Careful attention is given to helping families be open to receiving additional support through volunteers, respite care, ancillary staff support, as well as assistance from others in the community.

Ethics

- **Principle:**

The CHI PACC® program operates its services for children/adolescents and family members according to generally accepted ethical standards.

- **Practice:**

E.1. CHI PACC® service staff respect and honor the individuality, uniqueness, and humanness of each child/adolescent and family member, ensuring their inclusion in decision-making to the full extent possible, and consistent with the beliefs and values of their culture, spirituality and family structure.

E.2.   CHI PACC® program staff ensures the appropriate, necessary, and responsible use of all information about each child/adolescent and family member, and protects the confidentiality of all communications, documents, records and materials from unauthorized exposure or use.

E.3.   CHI PACC® service staff ensures that each child/adolescent and family member receives information concerning the life-threatening conditions, diagnosis, condition trajectory, treatment options and their side effects, symptoms and their treatment options and side effects, and their quality of life implications in language understandable to them, and within a supportive respectful communication environment.

E.4.   CHI PACC® program staff ensures that its services are available and accessible to any child/adolescent diagnosed with any life-threatening condition and family members without discrimination for reason of age, gender, racial or ethnic origin, national origin, geographic location in service area, language, religion or spirituality, sexual orientation, diagnosis, disability, family structure or status, ability to pay or potential cost of care to the program.

E.5.   The CHI PACC® service staff implements treatments and services whose intentions are designed to achieve the maximum beneficial child/adolescent and family outcomes possible with the least amount of negative impact possible on quality of life goals.

E.6.   The CHI PACC® program staff insures that its resources provide adequate support for the services provided and the continuing development of the program and an appropriate system of accountability is in place.

E.7.   The CHI PACC® program staff provides an ethics consultation and educational service to assist program personnel, family members and the child/adolescent living with a life-threatening condition when there are conflicts about choices for services and treatments.

Management and Operations

- **Principle:**

The CHI PACC® program is a comprehensive integrated continuum of services operating according to nationally recognized standards of care, evidence based treatments, and best practices. It is accountable to all appropriate licensure, regulatory and accreditation bodies and to the communities in which the families and children/adolescents live.

- **Practice:**

M.O.1.   The CHI PACC® program establishes and maintains current, accurate, adequate and comprehensive management of all aspects of the program, provides all needed services, manages all personnel, coordinates all collaborative relationships, assures fiscal, clinical, and managerial accountability and ongoing evaluation and program improvement and development.

M.O.2.   The CHI PACC® program operates within the requirements all local, state and federal laws and regulations that govern the establishment and delivery of CHI PACC® services by various providers, as well as qualifications of professionals and volunteers delivering services.

M.O.3.   The CHI PACC® program provides a clear, accessible and responsive grievance procedure for children/adolescents and family members which outlines how to voice concerns or complaints about services and care without jeopardizing their relationship to the CHI PACC® program or access to needed services.

M.O.4.   The CHI PACC® program ensures that all personnel, including administrative, managerial, clinical, supportive and voluntary are qualified and oriented for their positions and responsibilities, operate with a current accurate job description, have a designated supervisor/administrator, have access to appropriate support and ongoing training and skills building, and are evaluated on a routine basis by criteria based on their job description and responsibilities.

Interdisciplinary Team

- **Principle:**

Children/adolescents living with life-threatening conditions and the members of their families have a wide range and intensity of ongoing and changing stresses, needs, problems and hopes requiring care. This complex need for care requires the expertise and competence of many disciplines, perspectives and skills working together as an integrated, comprehensive, coordinated team to provide effective care.

- **Practice:**

I.T.1.   The CHI PACC® core team is staffed by an appropriate and representative range of medical, nursing, psychosocial and spiritual professionals, ancillary and support personnel, and volunteers adequate to meet the need for care. The team incorporates and integrates members of many disciplines, and may include pediatricians, pediatric medical and nursing specialists, advance practice nurses, high tech nurses, physician specialists, physician assistants, nurse assistants, social workers, chaplains, home health aides, home makers, in-home respite workers, physical therapists, occupational therapists, speech and language therapists, nutritionists, art therapists, music therapists, play therapists, recreation therapists, pediatric psychiatrists and/or psychologists, massage therapists, and others according to their availability in the program service area.

I.T.2.   The CHI PACC® core team is responsible to provide ease of admission, comprehensive assessments, identification and clarification of goals of care, development and implementation of a current plan of care, facilitate continuity of care in all settings, provide effective symptom management, counseling and supportive services for those it serves, including end-of-life care as appropriate.

I.T.3.   The child/adolescent and family are included as members of the team assigned to their care, and encouraged to manage the care according to their desire and abilities.

I.T.4.   The CHI PACC® core team has a qualified medical director, nurse manager and psychosocial/spiritual care coordinator/supervisor, and a designated team coordinator.

I.T.5.   The CHI PACC® core team establishes and maintains an effective system to ensure timely sharing of information between all team members and the coordination of services.

I.T.6. The CHI PACC® core team collaborates and coordinates care with the professionals in other settings.

I.T.7. CHI PACC® core team members are qualified in their particular discipline, role and responsibilities by training and/or experience, and certification and/or licensure when appropriate or required.

I.T.8. CHI PACC® core team members receive educational, emotional and spiritual support appropriate to their roles and responsibilities, setting of care, and need.

I.T.9. Essential medical, nursing, psychosocial and spiritual services are available to children/adolescents and family members 24 hours a day, each day, in all settings of care.

I.T.10. In communities in which particular pediatric, medical or palliative care expertise is not available, the team has a documented plan and method to access that expertise.

Admission Process

- **Principle:**

The CHI PACC® program maintains a barrier-free process which facilitates ease of entry into the program for children/adolescents and their families, timely response to initial and presenting needs and problems, and access to on-call care at the time of admission.

- **Practice:**

A.P.1. The CHI PACC® program provides ease of entry into its services for children/ adolescents and their families and monitors the process of admission, recognizing that at the time of referral, many children/adolescents and families may be in crisis and need immediate care.

A.P.2. An initial plan of care is established promptly after admission to guide care and services, (recognizing that it may take time to develop a trusting relationship between the child/adolescent and family and CHI PACC® staff) to assess the comprehensive needs of the child/adolescent and each family member, respond to presenting needs or problems, negotiate goals of care, receive, disseminate and evaluate all relevant and necessary information from the child's/adolescent's primary medical team and/or hospital.

A.P.3. The CHI PACC® program acquires all necessary and needed demographic information, relevant medical history, and documentation about disease management and/or medical therapies at the time of referral and admission.

A.P.4. Admission to the CHI PACC® program is made on the basis of the need for care and criteria for CHI PACC® eligibility without regard to age, gender, racial or ethnic origin, national origin, geographic location in service area, language, religion or spirituality, sexual orientation, diagnosis, disability, family structure or status, ability to pay or potential cost of care to the program.

A.P.5. CHI PACC® program eligibility criteria are available in language and terminology understandable to nonprofessionals, and family members and available in the primary languages spoken in the service area.

A.P.6. Admission to CHI PACC® program is admission to the entire continuum of care and its comprehensive system of services.

Comprehensive Assessment Process

- **Principle:**

  Comprehensive interdisciplinary assessment instruments are utilized by the CHI PACC® care team to insure that the goals of care and plan of care are based on needs identified as important to the child/adolescent and family. This assessment process is ongoing as needs, circumstances and hopes change during the course of care in response to the progression of the child/adolescent's life-threatening condition and its symptomology.

- **Practice:**

  C.A.P.1.   CHI PACC® interdisciplinary staff members assess the comprehensive ongoing physical, psychosocial, emotional, spiritual, practical and financial situations, circumstances, needs, hopes, concerns and goals of each child/adolescent and family member, from the time of admission and continuing throughout the entire course of care, including end-of-life care and bereavement.

  C.A.P.2.   CHI PACC® team assessments take into consideration the child's/ adolescent's developmental stage, spirituality, diagnosis, trajectory of life-threatening condition, treatment choices and protocols, and progressive symptomology, whether caused by the progression of the condition or its treatments.

  C.A.P.3.   CHI PACC® team assessments are made within the understanding, language, culture, values, beliefs, hopes, family structure and social context of each child/adolescent and family.

  C.A.P.4.   CHI PACC® team assessments are utilized to gather all the information needed for implementing services, and to provide a means for CHI PACC® staff members to build relationships with each child/adolescent and family, offer education and information about choices and options, and provide support.

Goals of Care

- **Principle:**

  Consistent goals of care guide the establishment and implementation of all services in all care settings and by all providers of services. These goals reflect the culture, hopes, values, beliefs and quality of life needs of children/adolescents and their families in response to the assessed situation of the life-threatening condition. The goals are utilized to establish the integrated treatment of the disease or life-threatening condition along with the palliative care plan of care and array of services to be provided. All medical treatment goals and palliative goals are in response to the goals of the child/adolescent/family.

- **Practice:**

  G.O.C.1.   In order for children/adolescents/families to formulate reasonable, realistic goals of care within hope for cure, the most accurate truthful information is provided about the condition diagnosed, its symptomology, treatment options and their side effects and expectations, life expectancy, possible family burden, and opportunities for quality of life.

  G.O.C.2.   The CHI PACC® Interdisciplinary Team collaborates with the primary care/disease management personnel and palliative care personnel to assess each child/adolescent's and family's life goals to offer best practices and supportive services to the child/adolescent and family within the context of these goals.

G.O.C.3. The CHI PACC® Interdisciplinary Team establishes methods to evaluate, re-assess and adjust both the global and specific goals of care throughout the progress of the life-threatening condition and its care.

G.O.C.4. The CHI PACC® Interdisciplinary Team utilizes the child/adolescent's and family's goals to frame discussions, education, and decision-making regarding the progression of the life-threatening condition, its symptomology, treatment options and achievable results.

G.O.C.5. The CHI PACC® Interdisciplinary Team members who are directly responsible for the care of each child/adolescent and family unit, orient staff members in all settings of care to the child/adolescent and family's life goals, disease-treatment goals, and the palliative care goals as settings of care change.

G.O.C.6. The CHI PACC® Interdisciplinary Team members responsible for the care of each child/adolescent/family unit ensure that discussions concerning the goals of care and their implications for services are conducted with language and vocabulary understandable to them, are done in a way that empowers the decision making choices of child/adolescent and family, and provides emotional and spiritual support.

G.O.C.7. The CHI PACC® Interdisciplinary Team members responsible for the care of each child/adolescent/family unit recognize that there will be times and occasions in which the child/adolescent and family members will experience ambiguity, conflict and/or unrealistic expectations regarding the goals of care, treatment therapies, and choices available to them, as well as potential differences about those choices, and their potential results. This ambiguity and/or conflict also may be present in the CHI PACC® team members and/or disease treatment professionals as well. Every effort is made to resolve the occasions through processes of mediation, consensus building, and provision of support, counseling and education.

G.O.C.8. The CHI PACC® program provides support to and advocacy for the child/adolescent/ family when there is a disconnect between the culture, values, and goals of the child/ adolescent/family and those delivering services in any setting. A process of mediation and consensus building should be utilized to resolve occasions of conflict over the goals of care and their implications for services, procedures and treatments.

Plan of Care

- **Principle:**

  An up-to-date comprehensive written plan of care is individualized to meet the specific needs, hopes and goals of each child/adolescent and family, addresses the medical, nursing, psychosocial, spiritual, and practical concerns and problems they have identified with achievable outcomes and results, and integrates the activity of the team implementing *medical* treatment services and the team implementing *palliative* services.

- **Practice:**

  P.O.C.1. The CHI PACC® Interdisciplinary Team establishes a comprehensive plan of care appropriate for each child/adolescent and family based on comprehensive ongoing assessment of needs, hopes and goals identified by the child/adolescent and family unit.

  P.O.C.2. CHI PACC® Interdisciplinary Team members monitor the plan of care integrating treatment goals and procedures of the life-threatening condition and palliative care goals and services.

P.O.C.3. The CHI PACC® Interdisciplinary Team ensures that each child/adolescent and family has direct input into the creation and establishment of the plan of care.

P.O.C.4. The CHI PACC® plan of care identifies a family member and a CHI PACC® team member, as the point of contact for the coordination of services and care, and the resolution of problems.

P.O.C.5. The CHI PACC® Interdisciplinary Team monitors, reviews and revises each plan of care on a regular and ongoing basis as goals, needs and hope change and the disease and symptoms progress.

P.O.C.6. The CHI PACC® Interdisciplinary Team establishes mechanisms to ensure the portability of the plan of care in all settings of care and communication with staff members of the plan of care when a change in the setting of care occurs.

P.O.C.7. The CHI PACC® program ensures that appropriately signed consents are negotiated and documented for the initiation or withdrawal or withholding of treatment.

Continuity of Care

- **Principle:**

CHI PACC® service delivery is based on a therapeutic relationship between child/adolescent, family members, and CHI PACC® team members. It maintains an integrated coordinated continuum of community based home care, outpatient services, respite care, supportive services, primary medical and inpatient care, end-of-life care, and community services. The CHI PACC® team ensures continuity and consistency of care, in any setting, is provided from the time of admission to the conclusion of bereavement services or discharges from the program and provides a system of care management to assist each child/adolescent/family unit. This continuity also extends to relationships important to the child/adolescent and family, such as school, religious affiliation, and community activities.

- **Practice:**

C.C.1. CHI PACC® medical, nursing, psychosocial and spiritual care is available on a consistent basis, 24 hours a day in all settings of care, to child/adolescent and family members.

C.C.2. Appropriate members of the CHI PACC® program are available to children/adolescents and families at all times when the office is closed.

C.C.3. The CHI PACC® program has a communication system that ensures the confidentiality and privacy of child/adolescent and family information, can be used to update team members about each child/adolescent's and family's status, and facilitates a timely response to changing needs and or problems.

C.C.4. The CHI PACC® program has a functioning continuum of care that ensures the portability of goals of care and the plan of care, and access to needed services as settings of care change.

C.C.5. The CHI PACC® program maintains all required and appropriate documents and clinical records, maintains their confidentiality, ensures their safety, and appropriate clinical use.

C.C.6.   The CHI PACC® program has written policies and procedures for transitioning a child/adolescent who reaches adulthood and the family to the new legal status of the child/adolescent, which includes continuity with changes in providers, payer sources, status of legal documents, and treatment options and choices.

Symptom Management

- **Principle:**

The range and intensity of symptoms which cause distress to the child/adolescent and family are managed to achieve the most attainable quality of life for child/adolescent and family within the context of their culture, beliefs, values and goals. Children/adolescents and their families must have access to care which is both competent and compassionate.

- **Practice:**

S.M.1.   The CHI PACC® Interdisciplinary Team assesses all symptoms which cause distress or discomfort, whether as the result of progression of the life-threatening condition or its treatment.

S.M.2.   The CHI PACC® Interdisciplinary Team identifies each distressing symptom, such as pain, dyspnea, fatigue, loss of appetite, loss of body image, constipation, diarrhea, vomiting, and loss of sleep and assesses each for its etiology, best practice evidence-based treatments, and range of choices for treatment.

S.M.3.   The CHI PACC® Interdisciplinary Team members discuss, evaluate and implement complementary, alternative and culturally relevant therapies and treatments important to children/adolescents and their families as appropriate to enhance the therapeutic environment.

S.M.4.   Members of the CHI PACC® Interdisciplinary Team provide clear, accurate information about evidence-based treatments and alternatives as objectively as possible to each child/adolescent and family to assist them in making the most appropriate choices for treatment options according to their own values, beliefs and goals.

S.M.5.   The CHI PACC® Interdisciplinary Team encourages consistency of symptom management services and treatments in all settings of care by all providers of care.

S.M.6.   The CHI PACC® program has clinical expertise through a competent medical and nursing staff to provide effective state-of-the-art symptom management, and access to specialists as may be required or needed.

Counseling and Supportive Care

- **Principle:**

The diagnosis of a child/adolescent at any age or stage of development with a life-threatening condition initiates a life-changing crisis within the family that turns their world, customary roles, activities, assumptions and expectations of each member "upside down." These children/adolescents and family members must have access to a comprehensive, coordinated, competent continuum of counseling and supportive services to assist them with the physical, emotional and spiritual issues, interpersonal dynamics and psychosocial dimensions of their experience.

- **Practice:**

    C.S.C.1.   The CHI PACC® Interdisciplinary Team identifies the initial ongoing and changing physical, psychosocial, emotional and spiritual issues, concerns, conflicts, priorities and needs of each child/adolescent and family member, assesses and evaluates each for the most appropriate response, integrates this into the written goals and plan of care, and assigns appropriate team members to implement services.

    C.S.C.2.   The CHI PACC® program does not require or advocate a "right way" for children/ adolescent and a family member to believe, cope, make decisions, grieve, or die but recognizes the deeply personal and individual nature of this experience. CHI PACC® team members provide counseling and supporting services which build upon each family member's own emotional and spiritual strengths, coping mechanisms, priorities, communication styles, belief and value systems, cultural and ethnic values, and social resources.

    C.S.C.3.   The CHI PACC® program facilitates the provision of adequate counseling and supportive services in all settings of care.

    C.S.C.4.   The CHI PACC® program has clinical expertise through competent counseling, social work and chaplain staff, as well as childlife and childcare specialists.

Volunteer Services

- **Principle:**

    Trained and screened volunteers provide an opportunity for members of the community, including children and adolescents, to become directly involved in the care of children/adolescents living with life-threatening conditions, their families and the bereaved, as well as to serve the CHI PACC® program in other supportive and organizational capacities.

- **Practice:**

    V.S.1.   The CHI PACC® program has a structured, organized and active volunteer program adequate to support the care needed by children/adolescents and their families, as well as to meet other needs within the CHI PACC® program for volunteer support.

    V.S.2.   The CHI PACC® volunteer program is managed by a designated, qualified supervisor/ coordinator that is a member of the CHI PACC® Interdisciplinary Team and meets regularly with them.

    V.S.3.   CHI PACC® program volunteers are considered non-salaried staff members and are managed and supervised accordingly.

    V.S.4.   All volunteers are appropriately recruited, screened, trained, assigned, supervised and evaluated on the basis of their roles and responsibilities.

    V.S.5.   Volunteers may include children and adolescents.

    V.S.6.   CHI PACC® volunteer services to children/adolescents and families are initiated according to the assessed need and consent of the child/adolescent and family.

    V.S.7.   CHI PACC® volunteers have access to an organized program of ongoing education and support.

    V.S.8.   CHI PACC® volunteer services are documented and reports provided on kinds of services provided, hours of services provided and other activities undertaken, as well as the financial value of these services to the program.

Bereavement Program

- **Principle:**

Family members of children/adolescents who die may continue to need supportive and/or professional services following the child's/adolescent's death for a period of time that varies among families and family members. The overall goal of bereavement care is to assist family members to reintegrate themselves into the communities of which they are a part and to find their long-term support in their communities.

- **Practice:**

  B.P.1. The CHI PACC® program has a structured, organized, adequate program of bereavement services for surviving family members and/or significant others, including linkage to support organizations and services in the community.

  B.P.2. The CHI PACC® bereavement program is managed by a designated, qualified supervisor/coordinator who is a functioning member of the CHI PACC® Interdisciplinary Team and meets regularly with them.

  B.P.3. The CHI PACC® bereavement program has professional and/or volunteer staff members adequate and competent to meet the range of services needed by family members, including siblings.

  B.P.4. The CHI PACC® Interdisciplinary Team members who were involved in the care of families before the child died provide an assessment of the level of risk and need for services of the bereavement program by family members.

  B.P.5. All CHI PACC® professional and volunteer staff members in other settings of care have access to bereavement services as needed.

  B.P.6. The CHI PACC® bereavement program establishes a written bereavement plan of care based on an assessment of needs for each family member receiving bereavement services until the person is discharged from the program.

  B.P.7. The CHI PACC® bereavement team members have access to an organized program of education, supervision, support and evaluation.

  B.P.8. CHI PACC® bereavement services are documented and reports provided on services and their utilization.

Research and Evaluation

- **Principle:**

The CHI PACC® care program acknowledges the importance of developing evidence to support the most effective care practices for children, families, providers, and health systems concerning comprehensive services for children diagnosed with life-threatening conditions and their families. CHI PACC® programs accept the responsibility to participate in a variety of research activities, including those that may have scientific value or others that may guide program improvements or meet reporting requirements. These diverse research activities will occur in community and clinical care settings, and shall extend to bereavement services as appropriate. While these research activities may vary in methodology and setting, they will all provide opportunities for patients, families and providers to assess the performance of programs and services in systematic, confidential, and valid ways. These research activities will share the general purposes of improving the quality of pediatric care and promoting optimum outcomes for patients, families, providers, and health systems. These research efforts will strive to be culturally competent and family-centered in their approach to conceptual and measurement issues. Because of the need to generate new knowledge in this area, CHI PACC® programs further accept the responsibility to protect the rights of patient privacy and to understand and guard against any potential harm, including psychological burden, to families and patients who participate in ongoing research and/or evaluation activities.

- **Practice:**

  R.E.1. The CHI PACC® program has a defined and timely research agenda, plan, and structure for implementation.

  R.E.2. The CHI PACC® program staff at all levels is educated to the importance and necessity of research, its different approaches and methods, and requirements for the protection of human subjects. CHI PACC® program staff also is encouraged to initiate and/or participate in research activities.

  R.E.3. The CHI PACC® program provides resources to support the research activities it undertakes.

  R.E.4. The CHI PACC® program encourages research collaborations locally and nationally to expedite the process of generating new knowledge and establishing clinical consensus.

  R.E.5. The CHI PACC® program has an organized and effective way to facilitate communication and sharing of tools and knowledge to others who are providing comprehensive pediatric care, including palliative and end-of-life care.

  R.E.6. The scope of outcomes that are relevant to the quality of care in pediatric services include outcomes across the care continuum and extend to bereavement care. The focus of outcomes are broad and span patient and family satisfaction, quality of life, provider satisfaction, cost-effectiveness, clinical performance, and health systems change.

  R.E.7. The CHI PACC® program participates in national cross-site type evaluation studies as needed and supports the collection of nationally-based data, criteria, and evaluation information over and above information needed for program specific goals.

  R.E.8. The CHI PACC® program has methods and procedures for monitoring, evaluating and improving its performance in meeting its most fundamental assumptions of access to a continuum of integrated disease management and palliative care from the time of diagnosis, with hope of cure, until the time of discharge from the program, as well as consistency of care across all settings of care and cost effectiveness.

  R.E.9. The CHI PACC® program has an organized, effective and consistent way in which professional and volunteer staff members evaluate the effectiveness and adequacy of its policies and procedures, outreach, services, programs, management, and governance.

  R.E.10. The CHI PACC® program has an organized, effective method by which primary care pediatricians, professionals in disease and treatment, and key staff members in other collaborative settings and/or programs of care evaluate the effectiveness of the CHI PACC® program, its operation and services.

  R.E.11. The CHI PACC® program provides all reports, data and documentation required by funders and constituents in a timely, accurate manner.

R.E.12.   The CHI PACC® program participates in all required activities which foster the development and expansion of the national CHI PACC® model.

R.E.13.   The CHI PACC® program has an up-to-date written program for program improvement and utilization review.

Governance and Administration

- **Principle:**

The governance and administration of, or for the CHI PACC® program, establishes, supports, and develops the program as a priority to meet the needs of children/adolescents and families in the community and/or region it serves. Governance may be achieved through an independent Board of Directors or an Advisory Board.

- **Practice:**

G.A.1.   The governance structure for the CHI PACC® program insures that its mission, vision, general policies, and range of services implement the national CHI PACC® program standards to meet the needs of children/adolescents with life-threatening conditions and the members of their families in the program's service area.

G.A.2.   The governance structure of the CHI PACC® program includes a broad representation of its service area, including diverse community representatives, professional and/or industry representatives, and children/adolescents and family members, while protecting against incurring conflicts of interest.

G.A.3.   The governance structure of the CHI PACC® program insures the integrity and functioning of the CHI PACC® program by providing the level of resources necessary to provide the level of care, mix of services, and range of collaboration needed to meet the needs of children/adolescents and families throughout its service area.

G.A.4.   The CHI PACC® program director is accountable to an appropriate institutional administrator or governance structure.

G.A.5.   The administration and organizational structure of the CHI PACC® program is adequate and appropriate for its mission, principal functions, goals and objectives, requirements for services, and size of program.

G.A.6.   The CHI PACC® program has suitable, adequate, appropriate space, work and service environments, equipment, supplies, security and safety systems, communication systems, and other essential resources.

G.A.7.   The governance and administration of the CHI PACC® program participates in the ongoing development, refinement, and positioning of the CHI PACC® model and vision of care for children/adolescents and their families.

From: Children's Hospice International. *Standards of Care and Practice Guidelines.* 2003. Available at http://www.chionline.org. Accessed May 24, 2005.

APPENDIX 4

STANDARDS OF HOSPICE AND PALLIATIVE NURSING PRACTICE[1]

Standards of Care

Standard I.   Assessment
The hospice and palliative nurse collects basic individual and family data.

Standard II.   Diagnosis
The hospice and palliative nurse analyzes the assessment data in determining diagnoses utilizing an accepted framework that supports hospice and palliative nursing knowledge.

Standard III.   Outcome Identification
The hospice and palliative nurse identifies expected outcomes relevant to the individual and family, in a partnership with the interdisciplinary/healthcare team.

Standard IV.   Planning
The hospice and palliative nurse develops a plan of care—a plan negotiated among the individual, family, and interdisciplinary/healthcare team—that includes interventions and treatments to attain expected outcomes.

Standard V.   Implementation
The hospice and palliative nurse implements the interventions identified in the plan of care.

Standard VI.   Evaluation
The hospice and palliative nurse evaluates the individuals' and families' progress in attaining expected outcomes.

Standards of Professional Performance

Standard I.   Quality of Care
The hospice and palliative nurse systematically evaluates the quality and effectiveness of hospice and palliative nursing practice.

Standard II.   Performance Appraisal
The hospice and palliative nurse evaluates one's own nursing practice in relation to professional practice standards and relevant standards and regulations.

---

[1] From: Hospice and Palliative Nurses Association, American Nurses Association. Scope and Standards of Hospice and Palliative Nursing Practice. Washington, DC: American Nurses Publishing; 2002.

Standard III.   Education
The hospice and palliative nurse acquires and maintains current knowledge and competence in hospice and palliative care nursing.

Standard IV.   Collegiality
The hospice and palliative nurse interacts with and contributes to the professional development of peers and other healthcare providers as colleagues.

Standard V.   Ethics
The hospice and palliative nurse demonstrates moral discernment, critical reasoning, and discriminating judgment in integrating ethics into hospice and palliative nursing during all interactions with the patient, family, organization, and community.

Standard VI.   Collaboration
The hospice and palliative nurse collaborates with patient and family, members of the interdisciplinary/healthcare team, and other healthcare providers in providing patient and family care.

Standard VII.   Research
The hospice and palliative nurse uses research findings in practice.

Standard VIII.   Resource Utilization
The hospice and palliative nurse considers factors related to safety, effectiveness, and cost in planning and delivering patient and family care.